ANTIBIOTICS IN
CLINICAL PRACTICE

ANTIBIOTICS IN CLINICAL PRACTICE

Hillas Smith, M.A., M.D., M.R.C.P.

Consultant Physician,
Royal Free Hospital,
Department of Infectious Diseases,
Coppetts Wood Hospital

Pitman Medical

First published 1969
Second Edition 1972

SIR ISAAC PITMAN AND SONS LTD
Pitman House, Parker Street, Kingsway, London, WC2B 5PB
P.O. Box 6038, Portal Street, Nairobi, Kenya

SIR ISAAC PITMAN (AUST.) PTY. LTD
Pitman House, 158 Bouverie Street, Carlton, Victoria 3053, Australia

PITMAN PUBLISHING COMPANY S.A. LTD
P.O. Box 11231, Johannesburg, South Africa

PITMAN PUBLISHING CORPORATION
6 East 43rd Street, New York, N.Y. 10017, U.S.A.

SIR ISAAC PITMAN (CANADA) LTD
495 Wellington Street West, Toronto 135, Canada

THE COPP CLARK PUBLISHING COMPANY
517 Wellington Street West, Toronto 135, Canada

Paperback: ISBN 0 272 76065 1
Library Edition: ISBN 0 272 76066 X

Printed by photo-lithography and made in Great Britain at
the Pitman Press, Bath
21 3452 11
21 3454 11

TO

D. H. R. S.

Preface

One has it seems to give a reason, or at least a pretext for writing a new book: not sufficient just to say that the subject seemed worth doing and leaving it at that. Certainly it could not be claimed that a new book on antibiotics fills a long-felt need; many books on the subject are available. The majority of these, however, deal with antibiotics from a strictly pharmacological or bacteriological viewpoint with little clinical emphasis. It has been my object to redress this balance. My approach, therefore, has been uncompromisingly clinical, especially in Part II which deals primarily with antibiotic management, while Part I provides a description of the major chemotherapeutic agents.

In clinical practice one has become accustomed to the manifestations of infection being obscured or altered by prior antibiotic therapy without cure of the patient. In many cases resolution of these difficulties is easily accomplished but sometimes the situation presents almost unmanageable perplexity so that any therapeutic approach is likely to be extremely hazardous. In this predicament the question is asked, "What should be done now?"; an attempt to provide an answer to this question is the real reason for writing this book.

I have tried to give, in more than customary detail, clinical aspects and antibiotic management of certain subjects which have appeared to me insufficiently well covered in available texts. These subjects include septicaemia and endocarditis, chemoprophylaxis and the difficulties encountered in antibiotic control of patients with liver and kidney disorders or in those with altered immunity states. Because of this there has been some repetition but this has been by design; also I have had to be selective—for instance, pulmonary infections and urinary tract infections are dealt with only indirectly.

The book has been written for doctors practising inside or outside hospital and for senior students. Many of the chapters form the basis for lectures given to students of the Royal Free Hospital during their training in infectious diseases at Coppetts Wood Hospital. The book is not primarily intended for microbiologists, nor for specialists in the antibiotic field.

Although the approach has been predominantly clinical parts of the subject have a marked biochemical or scientific bias and sections such as those dealing with the mode of action of drugs have been given in some detail. In these matters I have been fortunate in having assistance from Professor E. B. Chain and Dr G. N. Rolinson. I am most grateful to them for making time available to advise and assist me on many points especially those of historical biochemical and microbiological importance.

Many colleagues and friends have helped me with discussion, comments and advice. I am particularly grateful to Dr Sherwood Gorbach for reading many chapters and for his informed criticism. Dr Gordon Cook and Dr Peter Cavanagh read respectively the chapters relating to jaundice and to tuberculosis and I thank them for their comments. I am grateful also to Dr Clara Lowy who read several chapters and provided helpful suggestions. Drs A. M. Ramsay and R. T. D. Emond, my recent chiefs at Coppetts Wood Hospital, have helped with advice on specific points. I have been lucky in having as a colleague Dr Susan Young who has helped not only with criticism and discussion but in many other ways, particularly in compiling the index.

I express my gratitude to these colleagues, friends and associates but they cannot be held responsible for the opinions or any mistakes which may be found; these are mine.

H. S.

Preface to Second Edition

Not only the introduction of new drugs but alterations in the application of established drugs have been the main reasons for presenting a second edition of this book two and a half years after its first appearance.

These advances have resulted in changes in fifteen of the original twenty-one chapters; major changes have related to sections on trimethoprim/sulphamethoxazole, the rifamycins and other antituberculous agents, methicillin-resistant staphylococcal infections, and details of the more recently available tetracyclines. Opportunity has been taken to extend the scope of the book by introducing two new chapters, one on chemotherapy in pulmonary infections and another on urinary tract infections. Chapter 20 which deals with infections in special circumstances has been extended to include a detailed section on chemotherapy in the newborn infant. These various changes have involved a considerable amount of extra material but due to the new method of typography the total number of pages remains little changed.

My chief aim in this as in the first edition has been to provide a guide to clinicians dealing with bedside medicine; despite this clinical approach I have been pleased to note the interest in the book shown by microbiologists.

The new additions have been the result of discussions with colleagues both clinical and microbiological and I am most grateful to them for their criticism and help. Dr Susan Young has organised the redrafting and arranging the index; for this task and for her continued critical interest it is again a pleasure to express my thanks.

H. S.

Contents

Part One

1. Principles of Antibiotic Use

INTRODUCTION

In an age when the benefits of scientific endeavour make wider and more frequent impact than at any other time in history it is natural that antibiotic drugs, so clearly the product of scientific research, should be the subject of high public demand, much discussion, and some controversy. They have become part of the scientific miracle of our time; to some they are even status symbols of affluence.

The success of these drugs in many conditions, such as bacterial meningitis and tuberculosis, has lent them a certain aura so that their administration is often based on emotional rather than scientific assessment. Leaving aside the vexed question of whether it is possible or even desirable to practise medicine in a truly scientific manner, there would seem to be room for a large measure of improvement in the use of these much prescribed drugs.

Further, advances in science and medicine frequently result in complications and untoward responses when these advances are put into practical application. Antibiotics have not escaped this generalisation. Side effects and toxicity related to these drugs, alterations in bacterial flora, and the production of strains of bacteria resistant to antibiotic action are noted all too frequently. These two factors, a requirement for more objectivity in the administration of antibiotics, and a better understanding of untoward effects are the basic themes which recur throughout this book.

The modern era of chemotherapy began in 1935 with the discovery of prontosil by Domagk. The active principle proved to be para-aminobenze sulphonamide and in the following decade a number of sulphonamide compounds were synthesised and offered for clinical use. Thus, at that time, selection of an antibacterial agent involved choosing a drug from a number of compounds with similar antibacterial though somewhat different pharmacological activity. The introduction of penicillin to clinical use, delayed until eleven years after Fleming's original observations of 1929, greatly increased the therapeutic potential and widened the choice available to the clinician. He could now prescribe a sulphonamide or penicillin, or both. The importance of choice became clear when, in the late 1940's and 1950's many new antibiotics were introduced and today the doctor has to choose between innumerable compounds.

IS CHEMOTHERAPY REQUIRED?

This question should always be answered before prescribing an antibiotic. There are good reasons for withholding antibiotic drugs just as in some circumstances their use is imperative. There is no advantage in prescribing antibiotics when the patient's illness is not due to infection, or if infection, though present, results from agents such as viruses which are known to be unresponsive to antibiotic action. Another reason for not prescribing chemotherapeutic drugs is the presence of bacterial infection in an advanced stage of resolution.

It should be realised that it is not always simple to decide if infection is or is not present. Acute leukaemia, malignancy, collagen diseases and the like can mimic infection; fever does not necessarily indicate infection.

When the decision has been taken to use chemotherapy three other aspects of the situation should be considered in detail; these are: the patient, his disease, and the responsible pathogen.

THE PATIENT

Patients with apparently similar infections react differently. This results perhaps because of the patient's previous experience with the same organism or may reflect characteristics of an individual's host response. The vigour of this response may demand parenteral therapy in one while in another oral therapy may suffice.

The presence of underlying disease such as disorders of the liver or kidney demands modifications in dose or choice of drug. It is important to ascertain if there has been previous infection of a similar nature and how the patient responded to treatment. Were there any adverse reactions to drugs in the past? In this way an impression may be gained of the manner in which a particular patient is likely to respond to the drug selected and careful observation should be made of any deviation from the expected course.

THE DISEASE

A knowledge of the type of disease produced by the pathogenic micro-organism is vital for the clinician who is to get the best result from chemotherapy. This knowledge must extend not only to the clinical manifestations of infection but should include appreciation of the basic pathological and metabolic disorders accompanying infection and the changes which may occur during treatment. For instance, in some infections of the central nervous system a depressed serum sodium concentration can result from inappropriate secretion of antidiuretic hormone and lead to water intoxication if there is injudicious fluid administration, or, the apparent deterioration in the radiological appearances in patients with pulmonary tuberculosis may be due not to extension of the disease but to a pulmonary reaction to one of the drugs prescribed - most commonly aminosalicylate.

The response of typical infections to properly chosen therapy should be well known. For example, acute infections due to Group A streptococci or pneumococci respond rapidly to treatment with penicillin G usually within 48 hours, while in typhoid fever the temperature pattern may show no alteration for four or five days with chloramphenicol therapy, and with ampicillin the response is frequently more delayed.

THE MICRO-ORGANISM

Full bacteriological assessment is the basis for definitive chemotherapy. One would not treat infections due to *Treponema pallidum* with streptomycin nor use penicillin in tuberculosis. One might, however, use penicillin G to treat staphylococcal infection but not if there was evidence of penicillinase production.

Ideally, before starting treatment a full range of antibiotic sensitivity tests should be available. This, however, would make little difference to the treatment of proven pneumococcal or Group A streptococcal infections but would influence greatly the outcome of severe infections due to Gram-negative bacteria. This difference arises because many Gram-negative species have a much more varied antibiotic sensitivity than the two Gram-positive organisms mentioned above; further antibiotic sensitivity may change during treatment, thus demanding alternative therapy.

The clinician should be aware what bacteria are likely to be encountered in particular situations. For instance, in patients with extensive burns or skin lesions *Pseudomonas aeruginosa* can be cultured from the lesions sooner or later; blood stream invasion is common and often fatal. This same organism is frequently present in the sputum of children who have cystic fibrosis yet in the adult chronic bronchitic *Streptococcus pneumoniae* and *Haemophilus influenzae* are the usual pathogens. This type of information may be of use not only in planning chemotherapy but also in preventing superinfection or treating it at an early stage.

REASONS FOR FAILURE OF CHEMOTHERAPY

Five days' treatment will usually be sufficient to indicate if resolution is occurring. If, at the end of this period the patient's condition has not improved the following possibilities should be considered.

WRONG DIAGNOSIS

This is a common reason for failure of chemotherapy. For example, antibiotics do not influence the pyrexia in virus infections such as occurs in the prodromal stage of measles, nor does infectious mononucleosis respond to these drugs.

WRONG CHOICE OF DRUG

This occurs when the clinical diagnosis is correct, but the organism is not responsive to the drug selected. This is a problem with some severe complicated infections and correct management requires careful laboratory assessment. It is however often seen when simple infections like streptococcal pharyngitis or skin infections are treated with unsuitable drugs such as tetracyclines.

WRONG DOSE

Patients vary in their ability to absorb drugs and to some extent this is determined by the presence of food in the stomach or by gastro-intestinal upset. Even an appropriate antibiotic may fail if too little is administered. Some patients of course do not take their medicines and this will have similar results. Blood levels and in some cases urine tests for the drugs can settle this point.

In severe infections parenteral therapy is obligatory.

DEVELOPMENT OF RESISTANCE

Periodic determination of the antibiotic sensitivity of the pathogen should be carried out in patients with severe infections requiring prolonged treatment. Tuberculosis and infection with some Gram-negative bacilli often cause this type of problem.

INFECTION WITH MORE THAN ONE ORGANISM

If two or more organisms are responsible for infection antibiotics directed against one may not be curative. For example, mixed blood stream infection is not uncommon in septic abortion when coliform organisms may be present along with Clostridium welchii and staphylococci.

DRUG FEVER: SUPERINFECTION

These two complications of antibiotic therapy must be kept in mind when the response has been unsatisfactory. In both conditions all antibiotics should be stopped; fever will soon diminish if the drugs are responsible, if superinfection is suspected this is an opportune moment for obtaining fresh samples for culture and antibiotic sensitivity.

ASSOCIATED DISEASE

The presence of underlying disease may be the cause of apparent failure of antibiotic therapy. This often means that infection (which may have resolved) has complicated conditions such as lymphoma, malignant disease or leukaemia.

PRESENCE OF PUS

Collections of pus nearly always require surgical drainage. If present it is extremely unlikely that any antibiotic therapy can succeed.

COLLECTION OF SAMPLES

While it is often necessary to institute chemotherapy before there is bacteriological confirmation, treatment should never be started before appropriate samples have been obtained for examination and culture. This, of course, is a counsel of perfection and many infections are successfully treated without any laboratory aid. But this is a bad habit, for those infections seemingly trivial which do not respond may become insoluble chemotherapeutic problems because proper samples have not been examined initially. Patients with severe infections demand examination, not only of samples from the site of infection, but also culture of blood. Several samples should be obtained.

ANTIBIOTIC SENSITIVITY TESTS

Of the many methods available for estimating the sensitivity of micro-organisms to antibiotics the most commonly used are the tube dilution technique and especially the 'disc method'. This involves the application of discs impregnated with a known amount of drug to the surface of nutrient agar uniformly inoculated with a suspension of a culture of bacteria. The antibiotic diffuses into the agar and after incubation examination of the plates will show a clear area without growth surrounding those discs containing antibiotics to which the organism is sensitive. It must be remembered that while the width of the clear zone around the disc may be an indication of the sensitivity of the organism to a particular drug, the concentration of drug and the thickness and uniformity of the medium are also important variables. The 'disc' method will thus give an indication of sensitivity for a given antibiotic concentration; it is no guide to the inhibitory effects of the much greater antibiotic concentrations which are often easily achieved in clinical practice. Further, no distinction is possible between bactericidal and bacteriostatic effects; these may assume great importance in patients with serious systemic infections such as endocarditis but are not required in treatment of the majority of infections. This type of information can be obtained by using the tube dilution method. A practical technique in patients with severe systemic infections is to incubate the pathogen obtained from the patient in varying dilutions of the patient's own serum. In this way using the patient's antibiotic-serum complex an estimate can be made of the dilution at which a given antibiotic is bacteriostatic and bactericidal. A satisfactory dilution for a bactericidal effect is 1:4.

In some circumstances antibiotic sensitivity tests have little place in planning therapy. This is perhaps best exemplified by salmonella infections, especially those due to S. typhi. This bacillus often shows in vitro sensitivity to a large number of antibiotics, yet in the acute condition only chloramphenicol and to a lesser extent ampicillin produce consistent clinical response. Similarly one is sometimes faced with a seriously ill patient whose infection is resolving satisfactorily despite the apparent lack of sensitivity of the pathogen to the therapy selected. In this situation it is usually advisable to leave well alone. It should not be forgotten that the treatment of every patient with antibiotics is, finally, a separate biological experiment in which there are many variable factors, the majority of which are beyond the control of the physician.

2. Chemotherapeutic Mechanisms

MECHANISM OF CHEMOTHERAPEUTIC ACTION

The principle underlying chemotherapeutic action is selective toxicity, that is, the drugs should be toxic for pathogenic micro-organisms but non-toxic to the cells of the host. Ideally, these two effects would be independent, but in practice, chemotherapeutic substances exert a varying degree of toxicity on mammalian cells. The antibiotic which most frequently almost achieves this chemotherapeutic ideal is penicillin. Gale (1963) has classified antibiotics in current use on the basis of their mechanism of action. These include:

Group 1: those affecting the bacterial cell wall, such as penicillins and cephalosporins;

Group 2: agents affecting the cell membrane, such as polymyxins, colistin, and the antifungal agents nystatin and amphotericin B;

Group 3: includes antibiotics interfering with protein synthesis — chloramphenicol, tetracyclines, streptomycin;

Group 4: drugs which alter the biochemical environment, sulphonamides, isoniazid and para-aminosalicylic acid, and finally

Group 5: griseofulvin which affects nucleic acid metabolism.

INTERFERENCE WITH CELL WALL SYNTHESIS

It follows from what has been said that bacterial and mammalian cells must differ in some fundamental respect so that the principle of selective toxicity may function. One way in which these cells differ is an anatomical one — bacterial cells possessing a thick cell wall (10-25 mμ) while the mammalian cells of the host do not. It has been found that certain antibiotics – penicillins, cephalosporins, bacitracin, novobiocin, vancomycin, cycloserine, act by chemical interference with the bacterial cell wall (Gale, 1963). The action of penicillin has been most studied and the following comments refer to that antibiotic, although the other drugs listed above behave in a similar, though not identical, fashion.

Bacteria consist of an outer cell wall and internal to this a lipoprotein membrane which limits the interior of the cell. The 'outer' cell wall from Gram-positive cells contains a mixture of sugars, amino sugars, polyols and amino acids; it is thought that glucosamine, N-actylmuramic acid, D-glutamic acid and DL-alanine form a comon muco-peptide ground substance; this makes up about 65% of the wall in Staphylococcus aureus, but only 1% to 10% of the wall of Escherichia coli (Gale, 1963).

Penicillin acts by interfering with muco-peptide synthesis which results in the production of deficient cell walls. This exposes the cells to osmotic action — the cells swell, rupture and die. This bactericidal action occurs only when the cells are actively dividing. It is possible that differences in muco-peptide composition and its relation to the lipo-protein cell membrane are major factors in determining the response of Gram-negative and Gram-positive cells to the action of penicillin. Recent work suggests that an enzyme, named lysostaphin, produced by certain strains of staphylococci has a specific action on staphylococcal cell walls. This enzyme, which acts locally on susceptible organisms, is of considerable interest because it acts on the bacterial cell wall not only during the phase of synthesis, but also in the resting state.

INTERFERENCE WITH PROTEIN SYNTHESIS

Other antibiotics, such as chloramphenicol, streptomycin, the tetracyclines, kanamycin and neomycin, act not on the bacterial cell wall but inhibit protein synthesis within the cell. Ribosomal binding differs in both types of cell allowing selective activity. In both types of cell genetic instruction for protein synthesis is coded in the structure of the deoxyribonucleic acid (DNA) of the cell nucleus. DNA directs the production of template or messenger ribonucleic acid (RNA) containing the same information. This RNA becomes bound to ribosomes and forms a template for the assembly of amino acids in a determined sequence (Ochoa, 1962). The selective activity of antibiotics which inhibit protein synthesis in bacteria, can be reproduced as in vitro systems from both bacteria and higher organisms. This discrimination seems to arise as a result of differences in the ribosomes in the two systems; bacterial ribosomes differ from mammalian cell ribosomes in number and in other physical characteristics (Collins, 1965). Interference with protein synthesis results in failure of the organism to grow — this is a bacteriostatic effect and elimination of pathogenic organisms and resolution of infection depend on the host's defence system.

The difference between bacteriostatic and bactericidal effects is in practice not as great as might be supposed. If high concentrations of a bacteriostatic drug are used to treat an infection due to sensitive organisms the response is frequently as quick and satisfactory as when bactericidal drugs are used. Relapse is common after bacteriostatic drugs so that more prolonged therapy is desirable.

INTERFERENCE WITH CHEMICAL ENVIRONMENT

The sulphonamide drugs act by depriving susceptible bacteria of para-aminobenzoic acid (PABA) which is necessary for the formation of folic acid. Organisms which must synthesise folic acid are susceptible to sulphonamide action; organisms which use existing folic acid are not, and bacteriostasis resulting from sulphonamides can be reversed by providing PABA in the culture medium. Mammalian cells can use preformed folic acid — they are therefore in a similar position to insensitive micro-organisms which do not synthesise folic acid (Weinstein, 1965).

From these examples it will be appreciated that many of the chemotherapeutic substances in use can discriminate between mammalian and bacterial cells; penicillin attacks the cell wall of bacteria but not that of the host's cells; differences in the ribosomes of the two cells allow antibiotics, such as the tetracyclines, to form in some bacteria the 'wrong' protein; sulphonamides deprive organisms of PABA essential for their metabolism.

A list of the more commonly used bactericidal and bacteriostatic drugs is as follows:

Bactericidal	Bacteriostatic
The Penicillins	Sulphonamides
The Cephalosporins	Tetracyclines
Streptomycin	Chloramphenicol
Polymyxin	Erythromycin
Colistin	

COMBINED THERAPY

There are two chief reasons for using combined therapy: the prevention of antibiotic drug resistance, and to increase the intensity of chemotherapeutic action.

PREVENTION OF RESISTANCE

Bacteria being unicellular organisms are compelled to undertake a variety of metabolic processes; antibiotics act by interfering with some part of these processes. Within any population of bacteria mutations occur resulting in cells which are capable of producing metabolites by alternative pathways. If these pathways are not susceptible to antibiotic blockade, then mutation has produced resistance to the antibiotic used, and if this same drug is continued, susceptible bacteria will be removed and the infection dominated by the emergent resistant strains. It is plain that drugs which differ in their metabolic action are most likely, when used together, to prevent development of resistant organisms. However, even more important than the characteristics of the antibiotics are the nature and behaviour of the bacterial species.

Some organisms are not sufficiently versatile to alter their metabolism and avoid the metabolic block caused by antibiotics, while others have a high mutation rate, and resistance develops easily — notorious in this respect is Mycobacterium tuberculosis.

One reason for using drug combinations is the presence of infecting organisms known to have a high mutation rate. Alternatively, when the drugs to be prescribed are those to which resistance develops easily, then they should be used in combination. Before the introduction of the penicillinase-resistant penicillins, erythromycin and chloramphenicol were frequently recommended as a combination to treat staphylococcal infection, and Barber et al (1960) were able to show that this combination reduced the number of emergent resistant strains. Streptomycin and erythromycin are examples of drugs which can be used in combination with others; streptomycin and chloramphenicol is a useful combination in treating infections due to Klebsiella pneumoniae. In treating resistant pseudomonas infections there is some recent evidence (Shirley & Moore, 1965) that a combination of penicillin G and methicillin may be effective.

CROSS RESISTANCE

In choosing antibiotics to be used together it must be remembered that drugs showing cross-resistance should be avoided. Cross-resistance is the term applied to a phenomenon in which bacteria have become resistant to one drug, may be resistant to a second, although the organism has not been exposed to the second drug.

A list, quoted by Crofton (1965), showing the main drugs in which cross-resistance may occur is given below:

Cross-Resistance	
1. Between Tetracyclines	Complete
2. Tetracycline - Chloramphenicol	
Gram-negative:	Fairly often
Gram-positive:	None
3. Methicillin - Cloxacillin	Complete
4. Erythromycin - Oleandomycin - Carbomycin - Spiramycin	Very often (Barber & Garrod, 1963)
5. Erythromycin - Chloramphenicol (Staphylococci)	Sometimes (Barber et al, 1958)
6. Kanamycin - Neomycin - Framycetin - Paromomycin	Often

(If resistant K-N-F-P, resistant Streptomycin, not vice versa)

INCREASING CHEMOTHERAPEUTIC ACTION

At a time when penicillin and the sulphonamides were the only chemotherapeutic agents available it was natural that their combined action should be explored. There was some confusion in the results. For instance, Ungar (1943) reported that sulphapyridine increased the inhibitory action of penicillin against streptococci and staphylococci, whereas Garrod (1944) found that sulphathiazole reduced the bactericidal action of penicillin against staphylococci. Hobby and Dawson (1946) showed that the in vitro effect of a given combination depended on at least five variables which could be controlled only to a limited extent- less control could be exerted over the drugs when used in clinical practice, so that in effect combining penicillin with a sulphonamide was unlikely to increase the therapeutic usefulness of either drug. More recently Weinstein et al (1964) have shown that combining penicillin and sulphonamides leads to unpredictable chemotherapeutic action. These authors considered that some 'broad spectrum' effect was achieved, but that increased, indifferent or decreased antimicrobial action may be produced, and they recommend full doses of both drugs if this combination is used to avoid the risk of depression of antibacterial activity to a point where therapeutic efficiency may be lost.

In 1952 Jawetz and Gunnison proposed their laws of antibiotic action. They divided the drugs into bactericidal and bacteriostatic groups and on the behaviour of certain combinations in both clinical and laboratory evaluation concluded that:

1. A bacteriostatic antibiotic combined with another bacteriostatic antibiotic may bring about an additive effect.
2. A bactericidal antibiotic in combination with another bactericidal antibiotic may be synergistic.
3. A bacteriostatic antibiotic added to a bactericidal antibiotic may bring about antagonism.

   Synergism is the term used when the effect of two drugs exceeds the sum of the action of the individual components. The action of the whole, exceeds the action of the sum of the parts.

The application of these principles for a considerable period of time has had some use. For instance, the combination of penicillin and streptomycin in treating Str. faecalis infections, especially endocarditis has stood the test of time. A re-evaluation of penicillin-streptomycin treatment in enterococcal endocarditis by Jawetz and Sonne (1966) showed that in a series of nine patients bacteriological cure was effected in eight by penicillin in combination with another antibiotic. In vitro studies suggested that the addition of streptomycin to penicillin failed in three cases to produce a bactericidal effect, whereas the addition of erythromycin or bacitracin or both did achieve this result. The authors tested ten strains of enterococci and found that in 20: the bactericidal effect of penicillin alone was as good as that of penicillin and streptomycin in combination. For 40% of strains tested, however, the latter combination was essential for complete bactericidal action.

It is very doubtful if antagonism is an important clinical phenomenon although its existence cannot be doubted on the basis of careful laboratory observation.

Combined therapy has a place in severe acute infections or with infections due to mixed organisms. Patients whose lives are threatened by the severity of infection and in whom an accurate diagnosis cannot be made, indeed may never be made, are often best treated by a combination of antibiotics. In septicaemia, for instance, when a staphylococcal origin is suspected, a useful combination is penicillin G, and either methicillin or cloxacillin. In this way rapid response may be expected if the staphylococci are penicillin G sensitive, and the semi-synthetic drug can attack the penicillinase-producers. A purulent meningitis, when the organism is not known, may be treated with a combination of penicillin and chloramphenicol. The combination is used not so much to intensify antibiotic action, but to widen the cover to include most of the likely pathogenic organisms.

A recently reported in vitro effect of colistin sulphonamide synergism on Proteus vulgaris and P. mirabilis isolates, has an interesting therapeutic potential. Proteus isolates were shown to have a low order of sensitivity to sulphonamide and colistin when used separately; combining the two drugs led to much greater inhibition which could be overcome by PABA (Gale & Odell, 1966). Recently synergism resulting from the combination of sulphonamide and trimethoprim has led to the introduction of products containing both compounds. Trimethoprim blocks purine synthesis at a stage immediately after that of sulphonamide action.

Other reasons for using more than one antibiotic are to reduce side effects known to occur with full doses of a particular drug, and to reduce the cost of therapy.

A list of some useful combinations is given below:

Combination	Infection
Penicillin : Streptomycin	Str. faecalis (endocarditis)
Penicillin : Chloramphenicol	Purulent Meningitis (organism unknown)
Streptomycin : Chloramphenicol	Klebsiella pneumoniae
Penicillin G : Cloxacillin	Suspected Staphylococcal septicaemia
Penicillin G : Methicillin	Pseudomonas Urinary infections (Shirley & Moore, 1965)
Streptomycin : Tetracycline	Brucellosis
Streptomycin : PAS : INAH	Tuberculosis

DRUG RESISTANCE

Solutions of antiseptic like mercury or phenol kill bacteria if the concentration is high enough, and for antibiotics a similar principle holds, side effects and toxicity setting a limit to the concentrations permissible. The ability of these agents to kill micro-organisms is therefore relative; it appears that in any given population of bacteria some will be killed more easily than others, that is the sensitivity of any population is made up by considerable variation in the sensitivity of individual cells. Resistance to antibiotic drugs is a result of genetic inheritance so that in any population of cells a proportion of them may be genetically constituted so that they are not susceptible to antibiotic action. Alteration in this state of affairs can only occur by modification in the genetic information within the cell and this may be brought about in two ways, mutation, or by acquisition by the cell of certain particles of nuclear material containing genetic information relating to drug resistance. The second of these processes has received a good deal of emphasis recently and occurs chiefly in Gram-negative bacilli present predominantly though not exclusively in the bowel.

Mutation in cells is random and its frequency may be influenced by such factors as ionising radiation but not by any known antibacterial drugs. These drugs can influence bacterial populations only by inhibiting the growth of cells sensitive to their action while permitting the insensitive cells to flourish. In this way the proportion of sensitive to insensitive cells is altered and in time resistant organisms dominate the cell population. The rapidity of this change depends on such factors as the number of resistant mutants in the original population and the degree of resistance exhibited by individual cells.

The biochemical alterations in the cell result from a number of different reactions and some of the mechanisms involved are explained below.

THE MECHANISM OF BIOCHEMICAL RESISTANCE

ALTERED METABOLISM

If bacteria can alter their metabolism so that the process which the antibiotic interferes with is no longer essential, then bacteria will be able to survive and multiply in the presence of the antibiotic. This is what very frequently happens with streptomycin.

It is thought that streptomycin becomes bound to ribosomes in the sensitive bacterial cell producing specific misreadings in the genetic code. The ribosome-streptomycin complex in sensitive cells cannot react normally with messenger RNA, thus protein synthesis is blocked, or perhaps unacceptable proteins are formed. Streptomycin insensitive cells are unable to bind streptomycin, and protein synthesis continues normally (Spots & Stanier, 1961).

PRODUCTION OF ESSENTIAL GROWTH FACTOR BY ORGANISMS

The inhibition of utilisation of PABA essential for the growth of certain organisms, which is the basis of sulphonamide action, may be overcome if the organisms produce PABA in sufficient quantity. This appears to be the mechanism of resistance of some strains of staphylococci.

Chloramphenicol resistance of some bacteria appears to result from failure of the antibiotic to penetrate the cell; ribosomes from resistant strains bind the antibiotic to the same extent as those from sensitive ones (Vasquez, 1964).

DESTRUCTION OF THE DRUG

The ability of organisms to produce enzymes capable of destroying antibiotics is the best studied mechanism of drug resistance. The β-lactamases which have penicillin and cephalosporin as substrate, produced by resistant staphylococci provide the model for this form of drug insensitivity. Some Gram-negative organisms such as Bact. aerogenes, Pseudomonas aeruginosa also produce penicillinase; E. coli forms penicillinase, and also rarely, penicillin amidase. Some strains of this organism may also produce chloramphenicol reductasse, an enzyme which results in inactivation of the drug. Doubts have been expressed as to whether this is the only mechanism responsible for the marked variation in resistance in strains of E. coli to chloramphenicol (Pollock, 1960).

THE β-LACTAMASES

The penicillin nucleus comprises a 5-membered thiazolidine ring fused to a 4-membered β-lactam ring and a side chain (Figure 1).

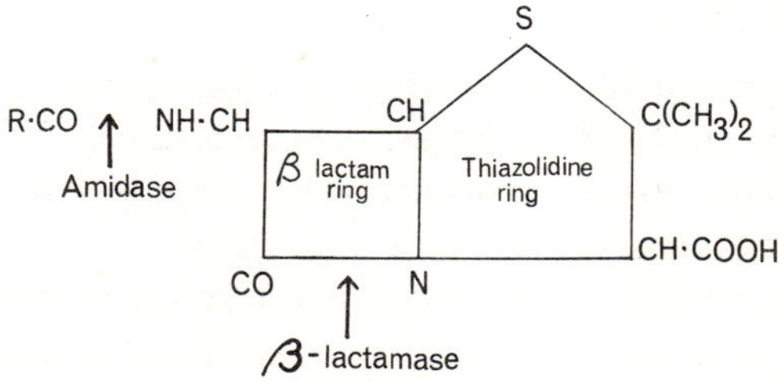

Figure 1. Penicillin Molecular Structure and site of action of enzymes.

The property which confers on this simple compound the ability to attack the bacterial cell wall in dividing cells, resulting in the organisms' death, rests in the β-lactam ring. This particular configuration is susceptible to attack by β-lactamase (penicillinase) which splits the β-lactam ring hydrolytically, converting active benzyl penicillin to the corresponding inactive penicilloic acid.

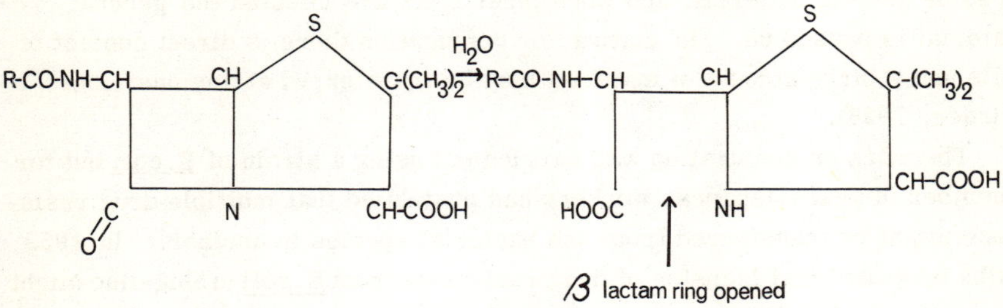

Figure 2. Hydrolysis of penicillin to produce open chain inactive penicilloic acid.

The importance of this reaction is that the compounds formed – the penicilloic acids – are chemotherapeutically inactive resulting in a loss of all antibacterial action. Penicillinase-producing organisms not only survive the action of penicillin but also protect susceptible, non-penicillinase-producing strains from the action of penicillin.

AMIDASE

Various micro-organisms and moulds are capable of forming amidase; this removes the side chain from penicillin producing 6-aminopenicillanic acid (6 APA) which, unlike penicilloic acid, retains some antibacterial action. Amidase obtained from such organisms as E. coli has now an important commercial use in producing 6 APA — the 'penicillin nucleus' being the starting point for many semi-synthetic derivatives.

β-lactamase is in some bacteria produced inducibly, that is the presence of substrate induces enzyme formation; amidase is a constitutive enzyme and its production is independent of the presence of substrate. Amidase production is uncommon for the majority of bacteria and the end product (6 APA) has some antibacterial activity.

TRANSMISSION OF DRUG RESISTANCE

Genetic information in the DNA or RNA of bacterial cells can be transferred from one cell to another. The agents involved in transmission of drug resistance known as resistance or R factors are extrachromosomal genetic elements similar to other plasmids or episomes of bacteria (Jacob & Wollman, 1961; Datta, 1965). R factors consist of two parts, resistance transfer factors (RTF) responsible for the transfer of DNA between conjugating cells, and a variable number of drug resistant markers or resistance determinants.

There are three ways in which genetic material may be passed from one cell to another. In **transformation**, the cell disrupts and the material lies free of the cell and a piece may enter another cell. In **transduction** (Lederberg & Tatum, 1946) viruses infecting a bacterial cell are capable of taking up some genetic material, and when other cells are infected the genetic material is passed on. In **mating**, or conjugation there is direct contact of cells and a large amount of material may be transferred at any one time (Zinder, 1958).

The work on conjugation was carried out using a strain of E.coli but for a number of years Japanese workers had postulated that multiple drug resistance might be transferred from one bacterial species to another. In 1959 Akiba proposed that transfer of drug resistance from E.coli to Shigellae might occur, and in fact this was demonstrated (Ochiai et al, 1959; Akiba et al, 1960). So far this form of infectious drug resistance seems to be confined to Gram-negative bacteria whose normal habitat is the bowel and has been demonstrated in strains of Salmonella typhi-murium isolated in London (Datta, 1962), Munich (Lebek, 1963), and Holland (Manten et al, 1962, 1964). There are reports of transferable R factors in enteric bacteria causing infection of the genito-urinary tract (Smith & Armour, 1966). Datta (1965) reviewing the subject commented on the increasing number of strains of Salmonella typhi-murium which showed multiple drug resistance. Table I is taken from her review.

Table I. Salmonella typhi murium isolated in Britain, 1961-1964

Year	Number examined	Number resistant*	Number where transfer to E.coli K-12 was demonstrated
1961	916	35 (2.7%)	17
1962	645	18 (2.8%)	13
Nov. 1963 Feb. 1964	712	133 (18.7%)	97

*Resistant to one or more of the following drugs:
streptomycin, tetracycline, chloramphenicol, sulphonamides, kanamycin, neomycin and ampicillin
(Reproduced by kind permission of the author and editor Brit. Med. Bull.)

Transmission of drug resistance appears to be increasing in frequency in particular pathogenic bowel organisms. Is this reflected in an increasing number of clinical treatment failures? It is very difficult to obtain accurate data but recently difficulty in treating Shigella sonnei infections was commented on (Smith & Young, 1966), no therapy producing results comparable to that of using a variety of antibiotics, although Moorehead and Parry (1966) claim very high clearance rates using a number of drugs — most notably streptomycin.

PRACTICAL IMPLICATIONS OF DRUG RESISTANCE

PREVENTION OF MULTIPLICATION OF RESISTANT MUTANTS

Every physician who uses antibiotics has a duty not only towards his patient whom he should cure as quickly and efficiently as possible, but also a duty towards the community, potential future patients, in prevention of multiplication and dissemination of resistant bacterial mutants. Antibiotics should be given when their therapeutic potential outweighs their disadvantages; they should not be used in self-limiting infection where the only effects may be side effects. In my view this refers, for instance, to the vast majority of infections due to Shigella sonnei and Salmonella infections other than those due to Salmonella typhi and paratyphi (see Chapter 15).

If laboratory experience is to be relied on the use of low doses of antibiotics will increase the proportion of resistant mutants and would appear to be a clear indication for not using the drugs in this way. This raises the vexed question of prophylactic antibiotic therapy about which more will be said later (Chapter 21). Judicious use of drug combinations (page 12) prevents the emergence of resistant strains.

PREVENTION OF INACTIVATION OF DRUG BY ENZYMES

There are as yet no known substances which prevent bacteria from producing drug destroying enzymes but the introduction of the sterically hindered penicillin derivatives has opened a new chapter in the fight against penicillinase-producing organisms. These compounds have less antibacterial action than has penicillin G on sensitive organisms, but their molecular structure is such that the β-lactam ring is not hydrolysed, and so antibiotic action is maintained (see Chapter 3).

It seems that by combining a hindered penicillinase-resistant compound with a hydrolysable penicillin, the anti-bacterial effect on certain organisms may be enhanced. Sutherland and Batchelor (1964) showed a synergistic effect when ampicillin or benzyl penicillin was used against several strains of Gram-negative bacteria in the presence of methicillin or cloxacillin. This in vitro demonstration was, however, shown in only a small proportion of 350 freshly isolated strains of Gram-negative bacteria, and because of this the authors doubted the usefulness of this synergism in routine clinical application.

It has also been shown that penicillinase obtained from Pseudomonas aeruginosa could be inhibited by a β-lactamase inhibitor (methicillin or cloxacillin) with a number of derivatives of 6 APA which are susceptible to enzymatic hydrolysis (Sabath & Abraham, 1964). These authors doubted if this synergism would be effective in man unless unusually large doses were given, but suggested that useful concentrations could be obtained in the urine. Of some interest therefore is the report by Shirley and Moore (1956) of the successful treatment of a 55-year old patient with Pseudomonas aeruginosa urinary tract infection using a combination of large doses of penicillin G and methicillin over a fourteen day period. Many other antibiotics had failed but the urine was sterile three months after combined penicillin therapy. Although of potential importance this particular combined therapy of pseudomonas infection has been overshadowed by the introduction of carbenicillin active in high concentrations against many strains of pseudomonas and which may be used synergistically with gentamicin.

The penicillinase-producing staphylococci would appear in this context to involve different problems. Sabath et al could not demonstrate synergism using a combination of either methicillin or oxacillin with penicillin G, against penicillinase-producing staphylococci (Sabath et al, 1963); Citri and Garber (1962) showed that penicillinase-resistant penicillins are capable of inactivating penicillinase as well as resisting its action. Gourevitch et al (1963) extended this work showing that penicillinase-resistant penicillins act as enzyme activators, but only if introduced prior to the hydrolysable penicillin.

If this work is confirmed and other penicillinase destroying penicillins are found, it could open the way for another therapeutically significant advance against penicillinase-producing staphylococci.

REFERENCES

Akiba, T. (1959) in 'Proceedings of the 15th General Meeting of the Japan Med. Ass.', Vol. 5, page 299

Akiba, T., Koyama, K., Ishiki, Y., Kimura, S. and Fukushima, T. (1960) Jap. J. Microbiol., **4**, 219

Barber, Mary, Csillag, Anna and Medway, A. J. (1958) Staphylococcal Infection Resistant to Chloramphenicol, Erythromycin and Novobiocin. Brit. med. J., **2**, 1377

Barber, Mary, Dutton, A. A. C., Beard, M. A., Elmes, P. C. and Williams, R. (1960) Reversal of Antibiotic Resistance in Hospital Staphylococcal Infection. Brit. med. J., **1**, 11

Barber, Mary and Garrod, L. P. (1963) In 'Antibiotic and Chemotherapy'. 1st Edition. E. & S. Livingstone, Edinburgh

Citri, N. and Garber, N. (1962) The interaction of penicillinase with penicillins. I. Effects of substrates and of a competitive inhibitor on native and urea-treated enzyme. Biochim. biophys. Acta., **62**, 385

Collins, J. F. (1965) Antibiotics, Proteins and Nucleic Acids. Brit. med. Bull., **21**, 223

Crofton, J. W. (1965) The Choice of Antibiotics for the Clinician. in 'Symposium on Advanced Medicine'. Page 114. Pitman Medical, London

Datta, N. (1962) Transmissible drug resistance in an epidemic strain of Salmonella typhi-murium. J. Hyg. (Camb), **60**, 301

Datta, N. (1965) Infectious Drug Resistance. Brit. med. Bull., **21**, 254

Gale, E. F. (1963) Mechanisms of Antibiotic Action. Pharmacol. Rev., **15**, 481

Gale, G. R. and Odell, C. A. (1966) Antagonism of Colistin-sulphonamide Synergism by para-Aminobenzoic Acid. Nature (Lond.), **209**, 1357

Garrod, L. P. (1944) Action of Penicillin. Lancet, **ii**, 673

Gourevitch, A., Hunt, G. A., Parsitano, T. A. and Lein, J. (1963) Combined action of penicillinase-sensitive and penicillinase-resistant penicillins against Staph. aureus. Proceedings of the Third Interscience Conference on Antimicrobial Agents and Chemotherapy. Page 485

Hobby, G. L. and Dawson, M. H. (1946) The Effect of Sulphonamides on the action of penicillin. J. Bact., **51**, 447

Jacob, F. and Wollman, E. L. (1961) Viruses and Genes. Sci. Amer., **204**, 93

Jawetz, E. and Gunnison, J. B. (1952) Studies on Antibiotic synergism and antagonism: a scheme of combined antibiotic action. Antibiot. Chemother. (N.Y.), **2**, 243

Jawetz, E. and Sonne, M. (1966) Penicillin - Streptomycin Treatment of Enterococcal Endocarditis. New Engl. J. Med., **274**, 710

Lebek, G. (1963) Zbl. Bakt. Abt. 1. Orig. **188**, 494

Lederberg, J. and Tatum, E. L. (1946) Novel genotypes in mixed cultures of biochemical mutants of bacteria. Cold Spring Harbor Symp. Quant. Biol., **11**, 113

Manten, A., Kampelmacher, E. H. and Guinee, P. A. M. (1962) Antonie van Leeuwenhoek, **28**, 428

Manten, A., Kampelmacher, E. H. and Guinee, P. A. M. (1964) Antonie van Leeuwenhoek, **30**, 10

Moorehead, P. J. and Parry, H. E. (1965) Treatment of Sonne Dysentery. Brit. med. J., **1**, 913

Ochiai, K., Yamanaka, T., Kimura, K. and Sawada, O. (1959) Nippon lji, **1861**, 34 (in Japanese)

Ochoa, S. (1962) in 'Basic Problems in Neoplastic Disease'. Columbia University Press

Pollock, M. R. (1960) Mechanisms of Drug Resistance. Brit. med. Bull., **16**, 17

Sabath, L. D. and Abraham, E. P. (1964) Synergistic Action of Penicillins and Cephalosporins against Pseudomonas pyocyanea. Nature (Lond.), **204**, 1066

Sabath, L. D., Steinhauer, B. W. and Finland, M. (1963) Combined Action of Penicillin G with Methicillin or Oxacillin against Staph. aureus. New Eng. J. Med., **268**, 284

Shirley, R. L. and Moore, J. W. (1965) Pseudomonas aeruginosa urinary tract infection. New Engl. J. Med., **273**, 283

Smith, D. H. and Armour, S . E. (1966) Transferable R factors in Enteric bacteria causing infection of the genito-urinary tract. Lancet, **ii**, 15

Smith, Hillas and Young, S. E. J. (1966) Treatment of Sonne Dysentery (C). Brit. med. J., **1**, 481

Spotts, G. R. and Stanier, R. Y. (1961) Mechanisms of Streptomycin action on bacteria, unitary hypothesis. Nature (Lond.), **192**, 633

Sutherland, R. and Batchelor, F. R. (1964) Synergistic activity of Penicillins against penicillinase-producing Gram-negative bacilli. Nature (Lond.), **201**, 868

Ungar, J. (1963) Synergistic Effect of Para-Aminobenzoic Acid and Sulphapyridine on Penicillin. Nature (Lond.), **152**, 245

Vasquez, D. (1964) Uptake and binding of Chloramphenicol by sensitive and resistant organism. Nature (Lond.), **203**, 257

Weinstein, L. (1965) The Pharmacological Basis of Therapeutics. 3rd Edn. (Ed) L. S. Goodman and A. Gilman. Page 1148. Collier-Macmillan Ltd., London

Weinstein, L., Samet, C. A. and Chew, W. H. (1964) Studies of the Effects of penicillin-sulphonamide combinations in man. Amer. J. med. Sci., **248**, 408

Zinder, N. D. (1958) Transduction in Bacteria. Sci. Amer., 199, 38

3. Penicillins and Cephalosporins

PENICILLIN

HISTORY

The story of penicillin has been told many times; because it is an interesting, and indeed a romantic story, it will be repeated here, if only in outline.

In 1928 Alexander Fleming, working in Almroth Wright's department in St Mary's Hospital, Paddington, noted that some colonies of staphylococci were lysed when the medium was contaminated by a mould – later classified as Penicillium notatum. Fleming's cultures, exposed probably for several weeks, demonstrated a lytic phenomenon, an effect which attracted Fleming's interest, his mind having been conditioned by his earlier work on the bacteriolytic enzyme lysozyme. He isolated the mould, showed that the culture fluid beneath it had antibacterial properties and that it was non-toxic to mice when injected even in the undiluted state. He did not however demonstrate that this material protected infected mice; it may be that the orientation in Almoth Wright's department, predominately involved with vaccines, was not conducive to the investigation of potential antibacterial agents.

Others, notably Pasteur and Joubert (1877) and Lister (1871) had already described the phenomenon of antibiosis – using the products of one living organism to kill another living organism – and the mould itself Penicillium had been used by Gossio (1896) in an unsuccessful attempt to produce an antibacterial substance. Fleming must have been aware of the single-dose antibacterial treatment envisaged by the great German pathologist Paul Ehrlich. Whatever may have been the reasons for the particular note that Fleming took of his contaminated staphylococcal cultures, it is lucky for us that he was aware of the possibilities and was able to pursue the subject in his own diligent and painstaking way. Professor Gordon T Stewart in a recent publication (Stewart, 1965) describes delightfully Fleming's accomplishment, and I cannot do better than quote the piece verbatim: 'the importance lay less in Fleming's observation than in his action. Being at heart a good Presbyterian, he felt in an entirely unpretentious way that Destiny entered his laboratory that day; not least among his endearing qualities was his candid admission, years later, that, "the fates were wonderfully kind to me"'.

In 1929 Fleming published an account of his work; he described the antibacterial action of the substance which he named penicillin, mentioned its lack of toxicity for human leucocytes and wounds, and was impressed by the possibility that it could be used to suppress bacterial growth in cultures, but allowed the influenza bacillus to flourish. During the years up to 1937 Fleming continued work on penicillin; attempts to purify the mould extracts were not successful, but he did have some success in treating wounds with a topical application, and publications continued to appear in 1930, 1932 and 1937.

The observations of Fleming appear to have been virtually unnoticed by the majority of the medical profession; there was a noticeable absence of demand for increased research — the subject was too new for an impact of this nature. However, the early experiments had been noted in Oxford, and a team of research workers at the Sir William Dunn School of Pathology, including Florey, Chain and Heatley, became engaged in extracting and purifying penicillin from cultures of the mould. Because of the impurity of the product large quantities of material were required for fermentation — 100 litres being used to produce enough penicillin for one day's treatment. Bedpans and such utensils were pressed into service. By February 1941 enough penicillin was available to treat an Oxford policeman dying of staphylococcal pyaemia; the infection was arrested, the patient rallied, but when supplies of penicillin failed the infection advanced and the patient died.

The result of treating this patient and some others convinced the Oxford workers of the effectiveness and lack of toxicity of penicillin; because the large scale fermentation required for increased production could not be carried out in England at that time, Florey and Heatley went to America in 1941 and obtained the cooperation of government and university departments as well as several pharmaceutical firms. Not only was the production on a large scale carried out, but the conditions of fermentation altered, especially the deep fermentation process developed at the Research Laboratories of the Department of Agriculture, Peoria, Illinois, which resulted in a vastly improved yield of penicillin. Clinical trials in America confirmed the previous studies at Oxford. The main problem was to obtain sufficient quantity, and because of this supplies were limited to British and American armed forces until about 1946. By that time, supplies became sufficient for civilian use; the indications for treatment and the military experience in treating a large number of infections led to fairly well defined methods of clinical use of the drug.

NOMENCLATURE

Units

The Oxford workers devised a system of unitage – still referred to as Oxford or Florey Units. This was very similar to the standard adopted by the International Conference on the Standardisation of Penicillin in 1944. The international unit of penicillin is the specific penicillin activity contained in 0.6 μg of the crystalline sodium salt of penicillin G.

Because of impurities in early samples of penicillin some form of unitage was desirable; today when the substance can be obtained in pure form it is probably more convenient to express amounts of penicillin in milligrams: this is sometimes done today for penicillin G and has been adopted for routine use with the later penicillins. One milligram of pure sodium penicillin G is equivalent to 1667 units. One million units of penicillin is frequently referred to as one mega unit.

Terms

The fused β-lactam and thiazolidine rings are common to all compounds termed penicillins. Different side chains result in altered antibacterial properties. Used alone the term penicillin usually refers to penicillin G. It had been found in 1944 that the penicillins produced in Britain and America differed and these differences led to the discovery of several natural penicillins. The American workers used capital letters to designate their different penicillins, thus penicillin G, F, K, X, were compared. Penicillin X, for instance, had the lowest activity; penicillin K the highest, but was so closely bound to protein that its therapeutic efficiency was reduced. Penicillin G, which possessed a benzyl side chain, had consistently high antibacterial activity, and seemed the obvious choice for routine therapeutic purposes. Penicillin G as the free acid is unstable but converting it to the sodium or potassium salt makes it quite stable. When we refer to penicillin G, we are therefore referring to the sodium or potassium salt of benzyl penicillin.

6 APA

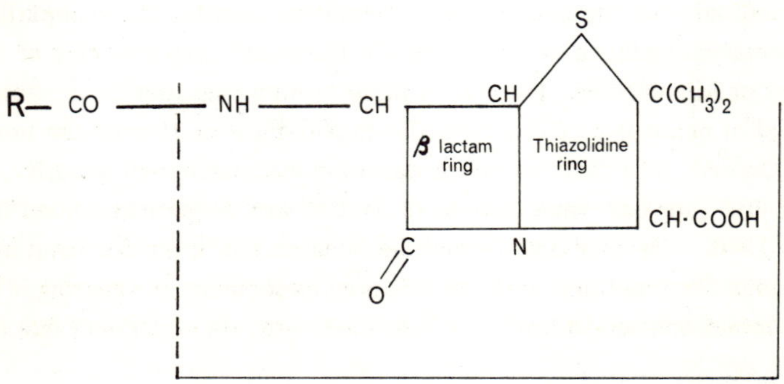

The key to understanding the chemistry of the penicillins lies in 6-amino-penicillanic acid (6 APA) for to this compound, the so-called penicillin nucleus, may be added various side chains to produce the other active compounds in use today. The isolation of this compound has led to the introduction of the newer penicillins (Batchelor et al, 1959).

The first compound in general use was penicillin G which was found to have a benzyl side chain:

Benzyl Penicillin

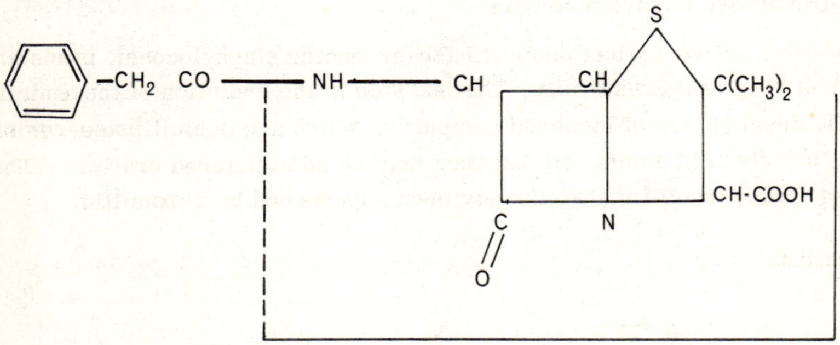

The enzyme β-lactamase splits the β-lactam ring producing inactive penicilloic acid, and amidase removes the side chain to produce 6 APA (Chapter 2, page 15).

Certain alterations in the side chain were found to increase acid stability – thus the first 'oral' penicillin came into use when phenoxy-methyl or phenoxy-ethyl groups were substituted in the side chain:

Penicillin V

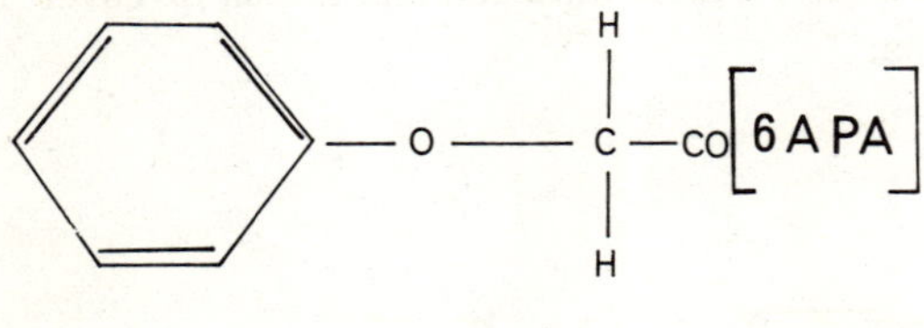

a-Phenoxy-methyl

The labile C-N bond gives penicillin its intrinsic activity and its dissolution by penicillinase results in complete loss of antibacterial activity. The C-N bond can be protected, to a large extent, by bulky side chains, a process known as steric hindrance. This process gave the first penicillinase resistant penicillin:

Methicillin

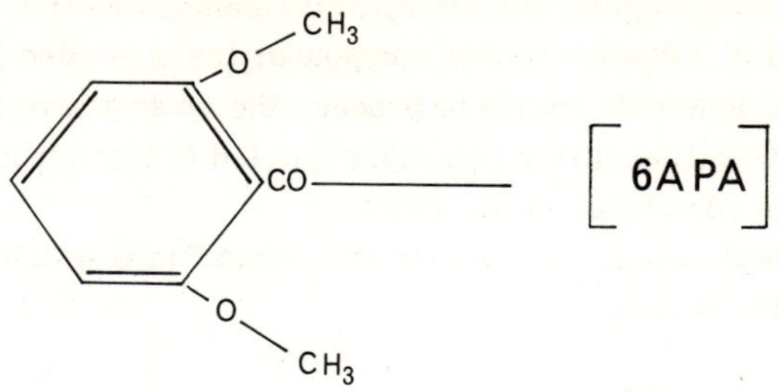

2,6 - Dimethoxy Phenyl penicillin

Methicillin, active against penicillinase-producing staphylococci, is unstable and must be given parenterally. The next step in the evolution of the penicillins was the development of hindered compounds which are penicillinase-resistant and relatively acid stable, so that they may be administered orally. The first of these, oxacillin, has largely been superseded by cloxacillin:

Cloxacillin

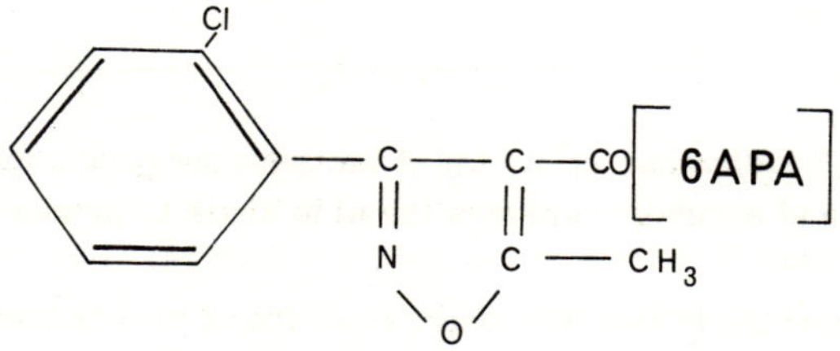

3 - Chlorophenyl - 5 methyl 4 isoxazolyl penicillin

The addition of an alpha NH_3 group has led to what no doubt will turn out to be only the first of penicillins with 'wide spectrum' activity. This compound, ampicillin, extends the range of antibacterial action to cover many Gram-negative organisms:

Ampicillin

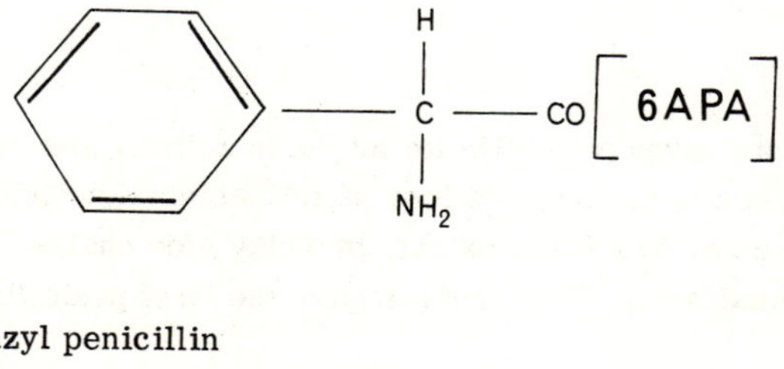

a - Amino benzyl penicillin

Carbenicillin (disodium α-carboxybenzyl penicillin) introduced in 1967 is a semi-synthetic penicillin with a wider range of activity than ampicillin and is particularly active against Pseudomonas aeruginosa. It is administered by injection and there are a number of papers describing its clinical use:

Carbenicillin

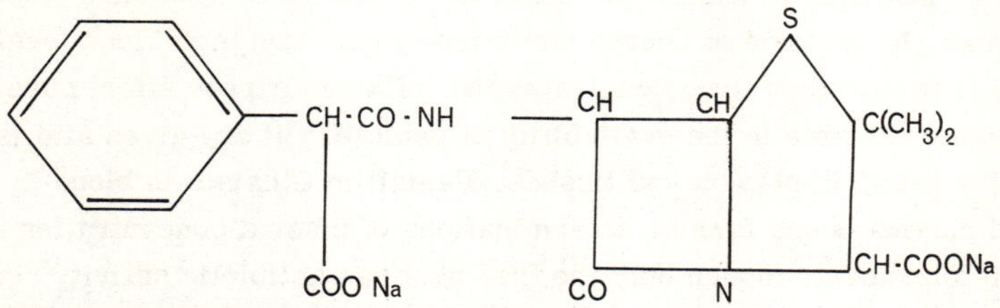

Disodium α-carboxybenzyl penicillin

It could be argued that we have enough penicillins, but will no doubt get more; patients continue to die, as Petersdorf and Turk (1966) comment 'not for lack of effective antimicrobials but for deficiency in knowledge of the pathophysiology of the diseased host'.

PENICILLIN G

Pharmacology

The crystalline, soluble salts of benzyl penicillin are, when injected, rapidly absorbed, diffuse easily into body cavities and joint spaces and are very quickly excreted by the renal tubules. Very little penicillin crosses from the blood into the cerebrospinal fluid (CSF) when the meninges are intact. Raising the serum concentration to 122 units/ml by intravenous infusion led to simultaneous cerebrospinal fluid concentration of less than one unit per ml in two normal subjects. When meningitis is present appreciable quantities are detectable in the cerebrospinal fluid (Chapter 17) but the values are unpredictable; in young children higher CSF concentrations seem to be reached for a given serum level.

The level of penicillin in bile is usually several times that of the plasma; if there is obstruction to the bile ducts no penicillin may reach the bile.

Because of very rapid renal excretion, high blood levels of penicillin G can only be maintained by injecting large doses at frequent intervals or by reducing the rapidity of renal excretion. A planned pharmacological approach by Beyer led to the discovery of carinamide and later the more effective probenecid (Beyer et al, 1951) which depresses renal tubular excretion, but does not eliminate glomerular filtration of penicillin. Excretion of antibiotics other than penicillins, cephalothin and aminosalicylic acid is not affected. The effective adult dose of probenecid is usually 2 g per day, orally in divided doses.

Tissue Availability

Although the blood level and the level in various body fluids may be estimated, it is not at all clear what happens in an area of inflammation. Penicillin may be found in inflammatory exudate (Florey et al, 1946), but the vascularity of the part, modified by local toxins or by pressure from tissue oedema must reduce any attempts to assess the penicillin concentration inside a lesion to guess work. In practice of course one tries to maintain high blood levels in the hope that sufficient drug penetrates the inflamed part to effect cure.

Another variable in the availability of penicillin at any given site is the proportion bound in plasma and tissues. Penicillin G exists in blood in both free and plasma bound forms; determinations of plasma concentration estimate the total level, though only the free part has antibiotic activity, but in some situations the total concentration in the plasma may be of interest (Lithander, 1963). The bond between penicillin and serum is reversible so that an equilibrium is established between the protein and free antibiotic on one hand, and the protein-bound drug on the other. The proportion of unbound drug at a particular time will depend on the concentration of the drug present and on the concentration and to a lesser extent the nature of the protein. Binding occurs not only to proteins in the serum but also to other proteins in tissues and fluids in a similar manner.

Long-Acting Preparations of Penicillin G

Instead of giving large doses frequently, or reducing renal excretion by using probenecid, longer lasting plasma penicillin levels may be obtained by using a relatively insoluble salt which allows slow release from the site of injection. Early attempts to produce this type of effect involved mixtures of penicillin G and beeswax; better results have been obtained with procaine penicillin. Procaine combines mole for mole with penicillin resulting in a compound which is very poorly soluble in water, and the quantity of procaine used is not usually a cause of toxicity. Procaine penicillin, in conventional doses of 300,000 units, reaches its highest plasma concentration in about four hours and declines slowly over a period of twenty-four hours. The addition of aluminium monostearate to procaine penicillin further slows absorption and detectable plasma penicillin levels may be recorded a month or more after a single injection. A similar long-lasting effect may be obtained by using benzathine penicillin G suspension. Various combinations of penicillin salts with different solubilities are available to give both rapid as well as prolonged plasma levels.

Range of Activity of Penicillin G

It is an extraordinary fact that the first antibiotic discovered should be not only one of the most useful and least toxic, but also that it should remain so after very many other antibiotics have come into use. In general terms penicillin sensitive organisms are Gram-positive, penicillin insensitive organisms are Gram-negative, notable exceptions being meningococci and gonococci.

Streptococci

The incidence of haemolytic streptococcal infection had been on the decline before the introduction of penicillin, but the treatment of established infection was still a major problem despite the use of sulphonamides. The introduction of penicillin altered this situation in a way that can only be described as dramatic. This position is maintained today with regard to group A haemolytic streptococci which probably accounts for more than 90% of human streptococcal infections, many such infections when treated by penicillin disappearing as if by 'magic'.

Infections due to alpha-haemolytic streptococci (Str. viridans) such as subacute bacterial endocarditis will usually, but not always, respond to penicillin therapy. Organisms isolated from blood culture must be submitted for antibiotic sensitivity as occasionally group D streptococci, non-haemolytic streptococci or anaerobic streptococci may be isolated, all of which show very variable patterns of penicillin sensitivity.

Pneumococci

Penicillin G is the antibiotic of choice in treating infections due to Str. pneumoniae. Resistant strains have not been encountered.

Meningococci

Meningococci are sensitive to penicillin G; the fact that small though useful quantities are demonstrated in cerebrospinal fluid samples taken from patients with meningitis (see page 208) means that when this drug alone is used to treat meningococcal meningitis, large doses are given frequently, sometimes by the intravenous route. Other clinicians prefer more conventional penicillin doses combined with a sulphonamide which diffuses easily into the cerebrospinal fluid.

Gonococci

The vast majority of strains of gonococci are sensitive to penicillin, indeed a single injection will often cure gonococcal urethritis in both male and female patients. In recent years, however, there have been reports from many countries of in vitro resistance of gonococci to penicillin G, and the number of treatment failures seems to be increasing. It is not unusual to find minimum inhibitory concentrations of 0.5 u/ml - 0.8 u/ml.

Staphylococci

When penicillin was first introduced the majority of infections due to Staphylococcus aureus responded to penicillin G. Resistant strains were soon encountered and today it has been estimated that some 90% of staphylococcal infections acquired inside hospital are resistant to penicillin G; 20% of infections due to staphylococci encountered outside hospital are thought to result from resistant strains.

This presents a considerable problem for penicillin G is the drug of choice for treating infections due to **sensitive** staphylococci but has little or no effect against penicillinase-producing organisms. The drugs of choice in this context are the newer sterically hindered compounds such as methicillin or cloxacillin; these drugs have considerable antibacterial effect, though less than that of penicillin G against non-penicillinase-producing staphylococci.

In recent years Staphylococcus albus, an organism often considered non-pathogenic, has been isolated from culture in patients with blood stream infection due to contaminated prostheses inserted by cardiac or neurosurgical procedures (Quinn et al, 1965). These infections are difficult to treat, and cure is not usually effected until the prosthesis is replaced; a proportion of these organisms are sensitive to penicillin G, and this may in the first instance be the drug of choice; sensitivity tests are essential.

Less Common Organisms

Penicillin G is also effective in treating clostridial infections, fusio-spirochaetosis, diphtheria (in conjunction with diphtheria antitoxin), anthrax, actinomycosis and infection due to Listeria monocytogenes, and Treponema pallidum.

Gram-Negative Infections

Infections due to organisms such as Escherichia coli, Alkaligenes aerogenes, Alk. faecalis, Salmonella, Shigella, Proteus and Pseudomonas are not usually treatable by penicillin G used in conventional doses. However, Weinstein et al (1964) by using intravenous doses of twenty to sixty mega units per day and obtaining plasma concentrations ranging from 30 to 500 units per ml were able to show that severe infections with some of these organisms could be cured. Pseudomonas and indole-positive proteus infections were resistant to doses even in this range.

MODE OF ACTION OF PENICILLIN

The mode of action of penicillin has already been touched upon in Chapter 2 (page 7), but will be dealt with in greater detail here.

Morphological Changes

Fleming discovered not only penicillin but also the enzyme lysozyme. It was recognised that lysis resulting in bacteria from the action of lysozyme was caused by the disruption of the bacterial cell wall (Salton, 1952). When the cell wall is impaired or destroyed, the organism is unable to withstand osmotic action if the surrounding medium is hypotonic in relation to the interior of the cell. It assumes a spherical shape, enlarges and finally ruptures. Similar morphological changes had been observed by early workers in penicillin treated organisms, that is the formation of spheroplasts, and in 1946 Duguid speculated that the action of penicillin might result in failure to form rigid outer cell walls. These changes occurred in both Gram-positive and in Gram-negative bacteria, indeed were most marked in Gram-negative organisms which showed most resistance to lysis by penicillin (Stewart, 1947). Eriksen (1946) demonstrated that destruction of staphylococci was dependent on bacterial growth and that the degree of lysis depended on the concentration of penicillin. These observations on the morphological changes in bacteria subjected to the action of penicillin focused attention on the cell wall and interest was then centred on the biochemical and metabolic behaviour of this structure.

Biochemical Changes

Gale and Taylor (1947) showed that penicillin prevented the uptake of glutamic acid in staphylococci but not in Gram-negative coliform bacilli, and in 1949 Park and Johnson found that phosphates accumulated in staphylococci grown in low concentrations of penicillin. Further work showed that these phosphates had the same basic structure, namely uridine 5 phosphate attached to an unusual acetamido sugar in combination with a nucleotide (Park, 1952). These 'Park nucleotides' were found in trace quantities in the cell wall of staphylococci and in increased quantities in the wall of penicillin-treated staphylococci. It was therefore proposed that uridine diphospho-acetylmuramyl-pentapeptide, the major accumulated peptide, was a cell wall precursor, and its accumulation resulted from inhibition of cell wall synthesis by penicillin (Park & Strominger, 1957; Strominger et al, 1959). This hypothesis has been confirmed by isotopic measurements of cell wall synthesis in Gram-positive and in Gram-negative bacteria (Strominger & Tipper, 1965).

Recent studies suggest that the rigidity of the cell wall is at least in part accounted for by cross linking between the various mucopeptide structures, and it seems probable from recent work that a transpeptidation is inhibited by the action of penicillin (Salton, 1961; Work, 1961).

Other components of the bacterial cell wall are teichoic acids and in Gram-positive cocci treated with penicillin there is an accumulation of cytidine nucleotides which may be precursors of teichoic acids.

In conclusion the action of penicillin G may be summarised by the observed physical changes: swelling of the cell, inhibition of cell divisions and production of spheroplasts. The biochemical factors include the accumulation of nucleotide precursors of both mucopeptide and teichoic acids, and in the breaking of the transpeptide bridge between two glycopeptide chains.

The possession of mucopeptide by bacterial cells appears to be a unique factor distinguishing it from human cells. It is this difference which confers on penicillin its ability to be selectively toxic for bacterial cells.

This account, a simplified version of present thought, leaves a good deal unexplained. Nearly all the work on which the account is based has been done with penicillin G and staphylococci; it is usually accepted that the newer penicillins have similar action to penicillin G but how then does one reconcile this with the effect of ampicillin on Gram-negative bacteria? How does the addition of an NH_2 group confer on ampicillin its wider spectrum and in what way does this differ from the definite, though clinically less useful, effect of penicillin G on Gram-negative bacteria? Can spheroplasts or L forms produced by the action of penicillin survive, return to a state of multiplication and result in recrudescence of clinical infection? These are examples of some unanswered, and as yet unanswerable questions, regarding the action of penicillin.

ACID STABLE PENICILLINS

Penicillin G when given orally is absorbed in small and unpredictable quantities; it is largely destroyed by the acid in the stomach. A search for acid stable compounds has produced several useful drugs relatively well absorbed when given by mouth, but with an altered or restricted antibacterial spectrum in comparison with penicillin G.

Phenoxymethyl Penicillin. Penicillin V

Introduced in 1953 it produces two to five times the blood levels of similar oral doses of penicillin G; it is most active when the potassium salt is used. Peak levels occur one hour after oral administration and vary somewhat according to the state of stomach. Sixty mg of penicillin V is approximately equal to 100,000 units of penicillin G.

Its antibacterial range is similar to that of penicillin G, but it is less active against the gonococcus, the meningococcus and *Haemophilus influenzae*. Penicillin V is supplied for usal use as tablets of 125 mg or 250 mg; it may also be obtained as a suspension or in granule form.

Phenoxyethyl Penicillin. Phenethicillin

This phenoxyethyl analogue of penicillin G introduced in 1959 was the first clinically useful modification derived biosynthetically from 6 APA. It is relatively well absorbed, better than penicillin V and has a similar antibacterial range to penicillin G and V. It is more active than penicillin G against penicillinase-producing organisms. In practice these differences offer little advantage. Potassium phenethicillin is available as tablets of 125 mg or 250 mg, or as a powder for paediatric use.

Phenoxypropyl Penicillin. Propicillin

Propicillin has a similar antibacterial spectrum of phenethicillin. It is well absorbed — peak blood levels are found at about one hour. It has a similar effect to phenethicillin against penicillinase-producing staphylococci. It is available as tablets of 125 mg or 250 mg, or as a syrup.

Phenbenicillin

Very similar to phenethicillin in antibacterial spectrum phenbenicillin is very well absorbed and maintains a high plasma concentration after oral administration; 125 mg are claimed to give higher peak levels than double the dose of penicillin V.

Ampicillin

The introduction of the reactive NH_2 group into the penicillin molecule leads to widening of the antibacterial spectrum and the most useful compound to emerge so far is -amino phenylacetamido-penicillanic acid (Ampicillin).

This compound, so far unique among the penicillins for the range of its antibacterial action, is in this respect comparable to the tetraycyclines and chloramphenicol.

It is active against non-penicillinase-producing staphylococci, and most streptococci, group A strains being universally inhibited. Pneumococci, meningococci and gonococci are also sensitive, but ampicillin is less active against these cocci than penicillin G.

It is highly active against H. influenzae and many strains of E. coli. It is inactive against pseudomonas and some strains of proteus.

It shows in vitro activity against shigella and salmonella, but its clinical usefulness in infections due to these organisms has been disappointing.

Ampicillin is well absorbed when given by mouth, peak blood levels appear in 1-3 hours and detectable amounts persist for about 6 hours. It is excreted for the most part unchanged in the urine and reaches quite high levels (up to ten times the plasma level) in bile. Little ampicillin crosses the intact blood-brain barrier. Probenecid reduces urinary excretion.

Ampicillin has several disadvantages:

1. It is destroyed by some penicillinases.
2. Resistance to coliform bacteria develops rapidly.
3. While the drug is relatively non-toxic, hypersensitivity reactions when they occur may be severe and there is cross allergenicity with other penicillins.
   The author has treated 15 patients from a mental hospital, suffering from acute typhoid fever, with intramuscular ampicillin in daily doses ranging from 4 to 6 g. Of the 15 patients, 6 developed

eruptions, one of them sufficiently severe for the drug to be withdrawn. This high incidence of rashes may have resulted not only from the effect of ampicillin therapy, but may also reflect that these patients were a 'hospital population', being patients for long periods of time with exposure to many drugs.

It is available for oral use as capsules containing 250 mg; daily oral doses for an adult range from 2-6 g. The drug can also be given intramuscularly and intravenously.

Cloxacillin. Orbenin

Modification of the penicillin molecule by substituting various groups so arranged as to protect the labile C-N bond, that is steric hindrance, has produced a number of new penicillins. The first of these was methicillin, which is not acid stable, and will be described later.

Table II. Oral Penicillins

Official Name (Trade Names)	Usual dose	Antibacterial Activity	Comments
Penicillin V (Crystapen V; Distaquaine V)	250 mg 6 hourly	Similar to Penicillin G Not active against penicillinase producers	Variable absorption. Not suitable serious infection. Use in prophylaxis.
Phenethicillin (Broxil)	250 mg 4-6 hourly	Less active than Pen. G and V against cocci	Variable absorption
Propicillin (Ultrapen)	250 mg 4-6 hourly	Range as for phenethicillin. Some increase in activity against penicillinase producers	Variable absorption
Oxacillin (Prostaphlin; Resistopen)	250-500 mg 6 hourly	High activity against penicillinase-producing Staphs. Narrow spectrum	Variable absorption 60-70% protein bound
Cloxacillin (Orbenin)	250-500 mg 6 hourly	High activity against penicillinase-producing Staphs.	Narrow spectrum
Nafcillin (Unipen)	250-500 mg 6 hourly	High activity against penicillinase-producing Staphs.	More variable absorption than other penicillinase resistant drugs
Ampicillin (Penbritin; Polycillin)	250-500 mg 6 hourly	'Wide' spectrum. Not penicillinase resistant	Gram-negative, organism may develop resistance

Oxacillin was the first isoxazole derivative, but this has been superseded by cloxacillin. The great advantage of these 'hindered' products is that they resist cleavage of the C-N bond by penicillinase, making them eminently suitable for treating infections due to penicillinase-producing staphylococci. Cloxacillin is well absorbed when administered orally, peak levels being higher than with oxacillin. Intramuscular injection provides double the plasma level of a comparable oral dose.

In antibacterial spectrum cloxacillin resembles penicillin G but is less active against those organisms for which penicillin might be considered specific, such as pneumococci and haemolytic group A streptococci. In chronic pulmonary infections cloxacillin may not always remove all staphylococci and the drug has little effect on nasal carriers of staphylococci. The usual dose is 500 mg every 6 hours when given by the oral route. The drug may be given intrathecally and into infected cavities.

Other semisynthetic derivatives such as nafcillin and quinacillin which have similar antistaphylococcal properties are less useful because of differences which primarily relate to inadequate absorption by the oral route. They offer no advantages over cloxacillin and will not be described in detail.

Flucloxacillin

This isoxazole penicillin was introduced late in 1970 (Sutherland et al, 1970) and is similar in antibacterial range to cloxacillin. Its use is primarily in the treatment of penicillin-resistant staphylococcal infections. After oral or intramuscular administration of flucloxacillin high plasma levels of free antibiotic occur. The available data suggest that flucloxacillin may well be effective at lower dosage than any of the isoxazole penicillin in current use. There are as yet no publications describing its clinical use.

Methicillin

Methicillin was the first penicillin, produced by steric hindrance, which was not destroyed by penicillinase. It is water soluble, unstable in acid conditions and is not absorbed when given by mouth.

It is a narrow spectrum drug, active against penicillinase-producing staphylococci and on a weight basis less active than other penicillins against the usual penicillin-sensitive organisms. Staphylococci may exhibit in vitro resistance which is not related to penicillinase production; methicillin induces the production of this enzyme. In practice cloxacillin has largely replaced methicillin.

Carbenicillin

Since its introduction in 1967 this semi-synthetic penicillin has been widely used to treat infections due to a number of Gram-negative species particularly those due to <u>Pseudomonas aeruginosa</u>.

Carbenicillin is not absorbed after oral administration and is given parenterally, usually by the intravenous route. The minimum inhibitory concentration for many strains of Ps. aeruginosa is 50 μg/ml or more and this requires that large doses of carbenicillin be given in the treatment of systemic infections. Daily doses of the order of 24 to 30 g may be given by the intravenous route in the treatment of septicaemia; plasma levels are enhanced by simultaneous administration of probenecid.

In pulmonary Pseudomonas infections Pines and colleagues (1970) reported on the treatment of 81 patients and claimed that carbenicillin in daily doses up to 8 g intramuscularly plus 4 g by inhalation, and blood levels enhanced by probenecid was more successful than colistin and gentamicin in clearing Pseudomonas from the sputum. In pulmonary nosocomial infections associated with ventilatory equipment Duma and colleagues (1970) reported on 16 respiratory infections due to Ps. aeruginosa treated by intravenous injections of carbenicillin up to 1 g per hour. This regime was effective clinically in 75% and bacteriologically in 50% of infections.

In reviewing urinary tract infections treated by carbenicillin Demos and Bryan (1970) assessed 73 courses of treatment, Pseudomonas was present in 35, Proteus in eight and mixed Proteus and Pseudomonas in eight. There were also 22 other mixed infections including those due to E. coli, Pseudomonas or mixed Proteus/Pseudomonas infections cleared in approximately 86% of cases. The highest relapse rate was in the Pseudomonas/Proteus group. Of five patients with pure Pseudomonas infections who were not cured the dose in every case was less than 100 mg/kg administered by intramuscular injection.

Carbenicillin has been used to treat Pseudomonas meningitis (Richardson et al, 1968). The drug was given in high doses intravenously and intrathecal or intraventricular injections (50 mg 8 hourly) were combined with oral probenecid. Ross and associates (1970) treated four infants with Proteus meningitis with intravenous carbenicillin. Intrathecal therapy was used in only one case and all four recovered.

Infection with Pseudomonas aeruginosa in other sites, such as bones (Grump & Christmas, 1970), burns (Copeland, 1970) have also been treated with carbenicillin.

There is no doubt this antibiotic has improved the outlook in many patients with acute Pseudomonas infections. However the very nature of Pseudomonas infections which usually occur in ill patients with gross underlying disease, together with the problems associated with the drug itself ensure that the treatment of these infections is a formidable task. There is a tendency for resistance to carbenicillin to occur during prolonged therapy and sometimes bacteriological and clinical improvement do not coincide. Combined therapy with gentamicin my be required in some cases.

Side effects have been few and include transient rashes and increased serum transaminase levels without other evidence of hepatic dysfunction. Spontaneous bleeding has been reported after high doses (McClure et al, 1970). The drug is painful when injected intramuscularly, particularly in doses greater than 1 g. In patients with reduced renal function high doses can produce encephalopathy with fits (Hoffman et al, 1970); doses in these circumstances must be appropriately reduced.

Carbenicillin is available as the disodium salt in vials of either 1 g or 5 g.

Daily doses by the intravenous route (with normal renal function) range from 20 g to 30 g. In children the daily intravenous dose is calculated on the basis of 250 mg to 400 mg per kg body weight in divided doses.

Intrathecal doses are given in single daily doses as follows:

Adult:	40 mg
Age 2-10 years:	20 mg
Up to 2 years:	10 mg

CLINICAL USE OF PENICILLINS

For infections proven bacteriologically or suspected on clinical grounds to result from Group A haemolytic streptococci, pneumococci, gonococci, Vincent's organisms, Treponema pallidum, the anthrax bacillus, or Coryn. diphtheriae penicillin G is the first drug of choice and should be given parenterally. Some infections may respond to oral penicillin, but the failure rate suggests that virtually all infections should be treated at least initially by the intramuscular route; oral penicillins may be used to continue treatment and they have considerable place in chemoprophylaxis.

In infections due to clostridia or meningococci penicillin G is a logical first choice, the drug should be included in any therapeutic regime, but there are good alternatives.

Ampicillin has its chief use in 'blind' therapy of patients with exacerbation of chronic pulmonary disease and urinary tract infections; it may have a place in the prevention of exacerbations of chronic bronchitis (see Chapter 21) and it deserves trial in typhoid carriers.

For treating staphylococcal infections which are not severe and not acquired inside hospital, penicillin G should be tried. For severely ill patients one of the hindered compounds is advised: cloxacillin either orally or intramuscularly is the drug of choice. Petersdorf and Turck (1966) recommend that one of these compounds should be considered in all Gram-positive infections before the precise bacteriology is known, and go so far as to suggest using one of these drugs in every case of staphylococcal infection until the sensitivity to penicillin G of the infecting strain is determined.

SPECIAL USES

1. Intrathecal penicillin

Penicillin G may be given intrathecally in single daily doses of up to 20,000u dissolved in a few ml of sterile water. For children the dose should be proportionately lower.

Cloxacillin and ampicillin can be given by the same route in doses of 10 mg.

There is very little indication to use any of these drugs intrathecally; penicillin G crosses into the cerebrospinal fluid in useful amounts if the dose is high and when the meninges are inflamed. Ampicillin is sometimes used in the treatment of *Haemophilus influenzae* meningitis and intrathecal injections will be required; it is not recommended. Chloramphenicol is a superior alternative and need not be given intrathecally.

Cloxacillin may be used intrathecally when resistant staphylococci are the cause of meningitis.

These drugs may also be injected into body cavities, joints or abscess cavities.

2. Intravenous Use of Penicillin

Penicillin G may be given intravenously in high doses in the treatment of meningitis, septicaemia, endocarditis or some Gram-negative infections. In some patients, critically ill, this may well be the treatment of choice. In using this form of therapy there are two methods commonly employed for administering the drug — either intermittent injection of the desired dose of penicillin dissolved in physiological saline or 5% dextrose, and given in a volume of 50 to 100 ml intravenously in 20 to 30 minutes, or alternatively continuous intravenous infusion (Weinstein et al, 1964; Smith, 1967; Smith et al, 1967).

In using penicillin this way, especially for prolonged periods, certain simple facts should be remembered. The patient will be receiving an additional fluid and electrolyte load, and the osmolality of the infusion should be close to that of plasma. In treating a patient for bacterial endocarditis the author has given penicillin G in doses of 100 mega units intravenously for a period of approximately three months without ill effect. The daily dose of penicillin was divided into three and dissolved in three half litre bottles of 0.18% of saline. In this way during each 24-hour period the patient received 1.5 litres of water, 154 mEq of sodium and 84 mEq of potassium when the total penicillin ration was divided equally between the potassium and sodium salts. This infusion gives an osmolality of 283 mOs/litre. Using this treatment there was no hyponatraemia or other electrolyte disturbance, no neurotoxicity and no observed haemolytic effect (Smith, 1967).

The chief danger of using high doses of intravenous penicillin are neurotoxic effects such as fits, which usually occur when penicillin doses are very high especially if there is impaired renal excretion of the drug when hyponatraemia develops or in those with pre-existing neurological disorders.

TOXICITY : SIDE EFFECTS : HYPERSENSITIVITY

The penicillins are among the least toxic of antibiotics; untoward effects are chiefly of two kinds — allergic — hypersensitivity phenomena which are common, and direct toxicity which is rare.

HYPERSENSITIVITY REACTIONS

Hypersensitivity reactions are usually of the urticarial-oedema type resembling serum reactions. In mild reactions the only manifestation may be an erythematous or urticarial eruption; the skin lesions are frequently seen on the face and facial swelling and oedema are common. Severe reactions may be accompanied by joint swelling. In one patient seen by the author there was a very intense skin reaction with petechial elements, oedema and joint pain. This patient had been given both penicillin G and ampicillin and had a previous history of topical penicillin therapy. Lupus erythematosus cells were found in the blood during the height of the reaction, but not when it had subsided.

In highly sensitised people anaphalyxis may occur and may cause death. Contact dermatitis may result in those in close frequent contact with penicillin — especially nurses.

Any of these reactions may occur in patients from whom no history of previous penicillin therapy is obtained, but this almost certainly means that they become sensitised by previous contact with the drug, and it is usually assumed that the consumption of milk containing penicillin is the common method. Penicillin given by any route may cause any of these reactions, intravenous administration being associated with the severest reactions. Aqueous penicillin G has been estimated to cause reaction in 2 to 2.5% of patients while the procaine salt may cause reaction in twice that proportion.

The skin manifestations of hypersensitivity of ampicillin would appear to differ somewhat from those resulting from other penicillins. Ampicillin may cause mild eruptions which do not necessarily require treatment to be stopped; on the other hand, very intense and prolonged rashes may appear and may require treatment with corticosteroid drugs. The relative frequency of these reactions has not been established.

In some cases hypersensitivity is for the most part confined to a particular organ such as the lung or the brain; tachypnoea while commoner in asthmatics is not confined to them; confusion, toxic psychosis and coma are usually attributed to cerebral oedema. Much more difficult to classify is the nephropathy which has been described in association with penicillin therapy.

Hewitt and his associates reported oliguria in three patients receiving methicillin, only one of the patients being hypersensitive to penicillin. The urine contained fresh blood and casts — all cleared when the drug was withdrawn (Hewitt et al, 1961). In a review of the literature Schrier (Schrier et al, 1966) was able to find twenty-three cases with renal disorders which were thought to relate to penicillin therapy. There was a previous history of penicillin therapy in only twelve of the twenty-three patients. Haematuria, albuminiuria, pyuria, oliguria, were the common clinical manifestations; there were two cases of the nephrotic syndrome. These authors described four cases of nephropathy, one due to methicillin and three due to benzyl penicillin; they stress that absolute causal relation was not established.

DIRECT TOXICITY

Direct toxicity due to penicillin G is very rare and probably only occurs after prolonged therapy with high doses administered intravenously.

Neurotoxicity is important because if its relationship to therapy is not recognised it can prove fatal. In a review of this subject it was pointed out that cerebrospinal fluid penicillin concentrations above 10 u/ml should be avoided (Smith et al, 1967).

There have been several reports of haematological effects. Penicillin G may interfere with blood coagulation (Fleming & Fish, 1947); Coombs-positive haemolytic anaemia due to the development of λ G (7S) penicillin antibodies has been described in two patients receiving large doses of penicillin intravenously (Petz & Fedenberg, 1966; Swanson et al, 1966). Methicillin and oxacillin have been associated with granulocytopenia (McElfresh & Huang, 1962; see Medical Letter, 1962). Agranulocytosis has been recorded during allergic reactions (Sigal, 1963).

Abnormalities of hepatic function tests, such as raised transaminase levels have been recorded with oxacillin (Ten Pas & Quinn, 1965).

Any antibiotic when taken by mouth may alter the intestinal bacterial flora; this is most important when wide spectrum drugs are used and may result in superinfection with resistant bacteria; fungal infections and enterocolitis may occur.

PREVENTION OF PENICILLIN REACTIONS

Although it has been accepted that hypersensitivity is commonly produced by topical penicillin application, it is now thought that penicillin metabolites such as penicillanic acid, rather than penicillin itself, are more likely to be involved in the antigenic complex (Parker et al, 1962). This theory is at the moment the most acceptable one, explaining hypersensitivity to degradation products of 6 APA, and also the cross allergenicity that exists between the various penicillins. Penicillin intradermal and skin tests are of doubtful value in predicting hypersensitivity reactions; if positive they are helpful, in some individuals they provoke severe reactions, and if negative they are useless. Using penicillanic acid as the antigen may cause similar reactions, but a penicilloyl-polypeptide compound — penicilloyl-polylysine — may prove more reliable in detecting penicillin hypersensitivity (Parker, 1963).

In a study of eighty patients with past history of penicillin allergy and who required penicillin therapy, Voss et al (1966) used several objective tests to predict those who would have an allergic response. Using both penicilloyl-polylysines and a mixture containing benzyl penicillin and some of its degradation products, these authors showed that sixty-eight patients with negative skin tests tolerated penicillin without immediate or accelerated reactions. Patients with positive skin tests had a high incidence of allergic reactions. There are, however, at least two reports in the literature of adverse reactions to penicilloyl-polylysine. Ettinger and Kayer (1964) reported a generalized urticarial reaction and Resnik and Shelley (1966) described an anaphylactic response to the antigen while the patient was not clinically sensitive to penicillin G, either by laboratory tests, skin test or oral challenge.

An in vitro test for penicillin hypersensitivity has been developed by Shelley (1963). This indirect basophil test requires one drop each of the patient's serum, of the penicillin solutions and of rabbit leucocytes. A positive reaction is shown by progressive degranulation in the basophil cells. This test which can be applied to any of the penicillins is doubtful in its reliability and specificity, but has not been widely enough evaluated to form a clear view of its usefulness. The work of Batchelor and associates (1967) and Stewart (1967) has shed new light on the problem of penicillin hypersensitivity. These workers were able to isolate two high molecular-weight residues from 6-aminopenicillanic acid and penicillin G. Neither of these residues had antibacterial activity and one provoked reactions in subjects known to be hypersensitive to penicillins. Allergic individuals gave a significantly reduced weal-and-erythema skin reaction to the purified penicillin (Purapen-G'). However, the purified preparation is still capable of provoking some hypersensitivity reaction.

The importance of this work lies in that when purified penicillin is widely adopted there should be a reduced incidence of hypersensitivity and that some subjects known to be allergic may be given the new preparation with impunity. This latter course cannot at the moment be recommended. The following measures may be of practical help:

1. Avoid topical application of penicillin; lozenges should not be used.
2. Before prescribing penicillin enquire if previous penicillin therapy has caused upset. If there has been a reaction do not use penicillin; we have now sufficient alternative drugs.

3. Desensitisation may be undertaken, using minute doses together with an antihistamine (O'Driscoll, 1955) in those working in close continued contact with penicillin.

THE CEPHALOSPORINS

DISCOVERY

A sewage effluent in Sardinia was found by Brotzu to have antibacterial activity which was due to a cephalosporium species. A culture of this mould was sent to Oxford, and Florey was able to report on the identification of three antibiotics (Florey, 1955). One of these was cephalosporin P, a steroid-like molecular structure similar to fucidic acid; cephalosporin N, really a penicillin, was found to be identical to an antibiotic isolated by Gottshall and colleagues and named synnematin B (Gottshall et al, 1951).

Cephalosporin C was found to have a similar structure to the penicillins — having instead of the five membered thiazolidine ring a six membered dihydrothiazine ring fused to a β-lactam ring. The interest in this structure lay in its ability to resist hydrolysis by β-lactamase. This compound was not very active against bacteria, large doses being required for a useful effect. The isolation of the active nucleus of cephalosporin C, 7 aminocephalosporanic acid (7 ACA) led to the production and testing of semisynthetic compounds. Three of these have been introduced to clinical practice: cephaloridine, cephalothin and cephalexin.

CEPHALORIDINE (Ceporin)

PHARMACOLOGY

This derivative of 7 ACA was introduced in 1964. It is soluble in water, slightly acid but stable at pH 4.5-5.0. It is inactivated in the gut and has to be given parenterally; intramuscular injection is remarkably well tolerated.

Peak serum levels are reached in about an hour after intramuscular injection, useful concentrations being maintained for six hours or more after a 500 mg injection. Approximately 80% of the antibiotic is excreted unchanged by the kidneys, resulting in high urine concentrations. Excretion is by glomerular filtration and is not affected by probenecid; lower doses may be adequate in renal insufficiency. Cephaloridine does not cross the intact blood-brain barrier in appreciable amounts: levels of 0.03 to 0.25 μg/ml occur one to two hours after an intramuscular dose of 500 mg. To date, cerebrospinal fluid levels do not seem to be available in patients with meningitis. Twenty-four hours after intrathecal injection of 50 mg Murdoch (1964) found a mean cerebrospinal fluid concentration of 5.7 μg/ml; after 100 mg the mean concentration was 20.3 μg/ml. Following the higher dose two patients developed hallucinations and nystagmus which cleared spontaneously when the drug was withdrawn.

The drug does not show a significant degree of protein binding; it is widely distributed in the tissues and experimentally inflamed muscle was found to contain more antibiotic than non-inflamed tissue. Bile concentrations are very low; satisfactory pleural penetration was found in two patients with pleural effusions (Murdoch et al, 1964).

IN VITRO SENSITIVITY

Cephaloridine is bactericidal in action causing a rapid kill of bacteria at or near the minimum inhibitory concentration. In vitro concentrations of 1 μg/ml cephaloridine inhibit most strains of the following organisms, Staph. aureus, Str. pneumoniae, Str. viridans, Coryn. diphtheriae, Cl. welchii. Concentrations of 8 μg/ml or less inhibit most strains of E. coli, Proteus mirabilis, Haemophilus influenzae, N. gonorrhoeae and N. meningitidis. It is usually inactive against most strains of Proteus vulgaris and Pseudomonas aeruginosa. Strains of Str. faecalis and Aerobacter aerogenes vary in sensitivity; there is little activity against Mycobacterium tuberculosis. In vitro activity can also be demonstrated against Salmonella typhi and paratyphi, Salmonella typhimurium and some strains of Shigella.

CLINICAL USE

This wide-spectrum bactericidal antibiotic, active against penicillinase-producing staphylococci, with low toxicity is a welcome newcomer to our range of antibacterial drugs.

There are three situations when cephaloridine is likely to prove its worth, in respiratory infections, in renal tract infections and in patients with septicaemia and endocarditis.

Respiratory Infections

Cephaloridine may be expected to produce good results with infections due to the usual Gram-positive cocci, but if the causative organism is one of the cocci (other than staphylococci) penicillin G is a more logical first choice than cephaloridine. It is when staphylococci of unknown sensitivity, Klebsiella pneumoniae, or coliform organisms are present or when blind therapy has to be instituted in severely ill patients, especially in those who have had previous antibiotic therapy that cephaloridine is most useful. It is a good alternative for treating patients who are allergic to penicillin.

Urinary Tract Infections

The control or eradication of urinary tract infections due to Gram-negative organisms is extremely difficult, but cephaloridine has a definite place in treating such infections. Infections due to Aerobacter aerogenes may be treated with kanamycin, but a better choice is the less toxic cephaloridine.

In a series of 62 patients with urinary tract infections treated by various authors, 39 had satisfactory results; of 22 patients with unsatisfactory response to cephaloridine 11 had anatomical abnormalities. Most of these infections had failed to respond to other antibiotics. It should be pointed out, however, that cephaloridine, like cephalothin, may be inactivated by β-lactamase produced by Gram-negative bacteria, and the precise nature of this inactivation in a number of Gram-negative organisms is still being investigated (Hamilton-Miller et al, 1965).

Endocarditis and Septicaemia

In treating these severe infections the attractiveness of cephaloridine is obvious; not only the wide spectrum of antibacterial activity including penicillinase-producing staphylococci but also the strong bactericidal action especially against Gram-negative organisms is most useful. In these situations the dose for an adult should be not less than two grams per day and much more may be required: Seftel (1965) gave up to 15 grams per day intravenously. In treating a child successfully with a Staph. aureus infection of a Spitz-Holter valve Stewart and Holt used doses of 10 to 30 mg/kg given intramuscularly and intravenously. The author has also seen a similar infection eradicated, without removal of the valve, with intramuscular doses alone.

Endocarditis

The experience of Apicella and colleagues (1966) suggests that cephalosporin derivatives may have considerable importance in treating endocarditis in patients allergic to penicillin. They report four cases, one treated with cephalothin and three with cephaloridine, suffering from endocarditis due to Gram-positive cocci. All four patients were allergic to penicillin. They comment that the minimum effective dose of these antibiotics in treating endocarditis is unknown, but in their experience it should be 120 to 300 mg of cephalothin, or 90 to 100 mg cephaloridine per kilogram of body weight per day.

Miscellaneous Infections

Seftel and Sieff (1966) report on the use of cephaloridine in early syphilis and acute gonorrhoea. In 21 patients with syphilis, mucocutaneous lesions healed rapidly and motile spirochaetes usually disappeared with twenty-four hours. In 29 patients with gonorrhoea treated with cephaloridine in whom the effect of the drug could be assessed, 25 were clinically cured, and the remaining four were markedly improved before they defaulted. There was recurrence in three patients, probably due to reinfection rather than treatment failures.

In treating fifty consecutive cases of whooping cough with cephaloridine,

Miller (1966) reported a mortality rate of 6%, compared with an overall mortality of 17% in 398 cases treated during a four-and-a-half year period, with various other antibiotics including tetracycline, chloramphenicol, penicillin, streptomycin and erythromycin. The severity of the cases in both groups was thought to be similar.

In treating meningitis, cephaloridine may have a place, but we do not have sufficient experience to be emphatic. Meningitis due to pneumococci or meningococci can be treated by well established alternative regimes; in neonatal meningitis cephaloridine may well prove very useful especially in Gram-negative infections. Intrathecal therapy will be necessary.

DOSE/24 HOURS

		Route
Adults	1 - 2 grams	I.M.
	2 - 4 grams (severe infection)	I.M. or I.V.
	25 - 50 mg	Intrathecal
Children	10 - 30 mg/kg	I.M.
	0.5 mg/kg	Intrathecal

The above dose schedule is only a guide — larger doses may be used (with the exception of intrathecal injections) without ill effect.

Cephaloridine is available in vials of 250 mg, 500 mg and 1 gram.

SIDE EFFECTS: TOXICITY

Although cephaloridine is a relatively safe antibiotic it may be responsible for a number of minor reversible side effects and is capable of causing serious renal disturbance.

Erythematous rashes, abnormalities in liver function tests and in blood coagulation and transient leucopoenia may occur. Positive Coombe tests have been described usually in elderly patients receiving large doses or in those with impaired renal function. This phenomenon has been associated with haemolytic anaemia in at least one case, and can interfere with cross-matching of blood.

Intrathecal injection of 100 mg may give rise to drowsiness and mental confusion.

In one azotaemic patient (serum creatinine 6.4 mg/100 ml) treated with 8 grams intravenously daily encephalopathy developed on the thirteenth day. Improvement occurred with peritoneal dialysis and the patient survived (Gabriel et al, 1970).

Although cephaloridine may cause hypersensitivity responses clinical usage indicates that it is a safe drug to administer to patients who are hypersensitive to the penicillins.

RENAL EFFECTS

Cephaloridine is capable of causing renal tubular abnormalities in man and animal – the rabbit seems particularly susceptible. In a detailed study in rabbits Silverblatt Turk and Bulger (1970) concluded that in high doses cephaloridine causes a dose dependent lesion of the second segment of the proximal tubule.

In man the available evidence suggests that renal tubule damage is also dose dependent – Kaplan, Reisberg and Weinstein (1968) reported that microscopic haematuria, proteinuria, or cylindruria cleared when the drug was stopped. They also give an example of progressive renal failure with shutdown in a patient who received 226 grams of cephaloridine in 23 days.

The situation may be summarised as follows: prolonged administration of very high doses (in excess of 12 grams daily) may be capable of causing tubule damage even in patients with normal renal function.

When renal insufficiency is present evidence of further renal damage occurs at much lower doses. The presence of casts and proteinuria related to cephaloridine therapy indicates that dosage is too high. The dose schedule in patients with impaired renal function recommended by the manufacturers is given in the table.

Table III. Dose of Cephaloridine in Renal Failure

Serum Creatinine in mg%	Creatinine clearance in mls/min	Blood Urea in mg%	Cephaloridine Serum half life in hours	Cephaloridine maximum daily dosage in gms
1.1 to 3	75 to 40	42 to 75	2 to 5	2 to 3
3.1 to 6	40 to 20	75 to 110	4 to 6	1 to 2
6.1 to 9	20 to 10	110 to 160	5 to 10	1
> 9	< 10	> 160	8 to 20	0.5

Cephaloridine present in the urine may give rise to a brown-black colour when testing for glucose with Benedict's solution and with 'clinitest'. This does not occur when 'clinistix' is used.

CEPHALOTHIN (Keflin)

This semi-synthetic derivative of 7 ACA – (7-(thiophene-2-acetamido) cephalosporanic acid was the first clinically useful compound derived from the cephalosporins and was introduced in 1962.

It has many similarities to cephaloridine – rapid bactericidal action against many Gram-positive and Gram-negative bacteria, including penicillinase-producing staphylococci and no antibacterial action against Pseudomonas aeruginosa. There are many reports in the literature describing useful clinical application.

Cephalothin is rather more closely bound to protein and is rather less active in antibacterial action than cephaloridine. It is rapidly excreted by the renal tubules and excretion may be blocked by probenecid. It is now clear that cephaloridine is considerably more toxic to renal tubules than cephalothin though the latter may occasionally produce renal damage. There is little information regarding the penetration of the drug into the cerebrospinal fluid but thereapeutic levels in the fluid have been commented upon after parenteral doses (Weinstein, 1965).

Cephalothin, like cephaloridine, may cause a number of reversible side effects, though none of the effects noted were serious. Eosinophilia, fever, urticarial rashes and serum sickness have been reported; Davis et al (1963) reported neutropoenia which returned to normal in three cases when the drug was withdrawn.

It was first suggested by Abraham and Newton (1956) that some organisms produced an enzyme which specifically destroyed the antibacterial action of cephalosporin C. This work was further extended by Chang and Weinstein (1963) who reported on the isolation of cephalosporinase - a specific enzyme twelve times more active against cephalothin than against benzyl penicillin. Purified penicillinase had little effect on cephalothin. Cephalosporinase appears to be a β-lactamase acting on the β-lactam ring of cephalothin, and produced by organisms including Staph. aureus, Enterococcus, Herellea, Shigella, Aerobacter aerogenes, Klebsiella group, and Salmonella. Cultures of Pseudomonas do not contain cephalosporinase.

CEPHALEXIN

Cephalexin is an analogue of Cephalosporin C, a white crystalline solid with antibacterial action against a wide range of Gram-positive and Gram-negative bacteria. It may in some instances be more stable to staphylococcal penicillinase than cephaloridine. It has a relatively low in vitro activity against many pathogens but because it is extremely well absorbed after oral administration, with a small degree of protein binding and high urine concentrations its major use is in treating urinary tract infections. Probenecid delays excretion and enhances plasma concentrations of cephalexin.

Cephalexin is available as capsules containing 250 mg or 500 mg; it is also issued as granules so that when reconstituted each 5 ml contains 250 mg cephalexin. The usual adult daily dose ranges from one to four grams in divided doses.

Side effects include intestinal upset, rashes, and reversible neutropoenia.

When renal function is markedly impaired cephalexin may accumulate in the serum and tissues. Cephalexin may give rise to a false positive reaction for glucose in the urine with Benedict's and Fehling's solution and with 'clinitest' tablets but not with 'clinistix'.

REFERENCES

PENICILLINS

Batchelor, E. P., Doyle, E. P., Naylor, J. H. and Robinson, G. N. (1959) Synthesis of penicillin: 6-amino-penicillanic acid in penicillin fermentations. Nature (Lond.), **183**, 257

Beyer, K. H., Russo, H. F., Tillson, Elizabeth K., Miller, A. Katherine, Verwey, W. F. and Gass, S. R. (1951) 'Benemid' p-(di-n-propylsulfamyl)-benzoic acid: its renal affinity and elimination. Amer. J. Physiol., **166**, 625

Copeland, C. E. (1970) Carbenicillin therapy in burn patients. Excerpta Medica Foundation (Symposium). Page 116

Demos, C. H. and Bryan, J. E. (1970) Survey of urinary tract infection treated with Pyopen. Excerpta Medica Foundation (Symposium). Page 56

Duguid, J. P. (1946) The Sensitivity of Bacteria to the action of penicillin. Edinburgh med. J., **53**, 401

Duma, R. J., Warner, J. F. and Utz, J. P. (1970) Carbenicillin (Pyopen) in Pseudomonas aeruginosa respiratory infections. Advances in the management of pseudomonas and proteus infections. Excerpta Medica Foundation (Symposium). Page 16

Eriksen, K. R. (1947) Proceedings 4th International Congress Microbiol. Rosenkilde and Bagger, Copenhagen (1949). Page 100

Ettinger, E. and Kaye, D. (1964) Systemic manifestations after a skin test with Penicilloyl-Polylysine. New Engl. J. Med., **271**, 1105

Fleming, A. (1929) On antibacterial action of cultures of penicillium, with special reference to their use in isolation of B. influenzae. Brit. J. exp. Path., **10**, 226

Fleming, A. (1932) On the specific antibacterial properties of penicillin and potassium tellurite. J. Path. Bact., **35**, 831

Fleming, A. (1937) Proceedings of the 2nd International Congress Microbiol. Page 33

Fleming, A. and Fish, E. W. (1947) Influence of Penicillin on the coagulation of the blood with special reference to certain dental operations. Brit. med. J., **2**, 242

Fleming, A. and Maclean, I. H. (1930) On the occurrence of influenza bacilli in the mouths of normal people. Brit. J. exp. Path., **2**, 127

Florey, M. E., Turton, E. C. and Duthie, E. S. (1946) Penicillin in Wound Exudates. Lancet, **ii**, 405

Gale, E. T. and Taylor, E. S. (1947) The Assimilation of Amino-Acids by Bacteria 5. The action of penicillin in preventing the assimilation of gentamic acid by Staphylococcus aureus. J. gen. Microbio., **1**, 314

Gossio, B. (1896) Riv. Iq. San. pub. 7., **825**, 961

Grump, D. W. and Christmas, W. A. (1970) Treatment of osteomyelitis with carbenicillin. Excerpta Medica Foundation (Symposium). Page 101

Hewitt, W. L., Finegold, S. M. and Mouzou, O. T. (1961) Untoward side effects associated with Methicillin therapy. Antimicrobiol agents and Chemotherapy. Page 765

Hoffman, T. A. and Bullock, W. E. (1970) Carbenicillin Therapy of Pseudomonas and other Gram-negative bacillary infections. Ann. intern. Med., **73**, 165

Lister, J. (1950) Commonplace Book 1871. November 25th: In Ann. roy. Coll. Surg. England 6

Lithander, Arne (1963) Determination of the concentration of penicillin in blood-plasma, cerebrospinal fluid and brain substance in the rabbit. Acta path. microbiol. scand., **59**, 229

McClure, P. D., Casserly, J. G., Monsier, C. and Crozier, D. (1970) Carbenicillin-induced bleeding disorder. Lancet, **ii**, 1307

McElfresh, A. E. and Huang, N. (1962) Bone marrow depression resulting from the administration of Methicillin. New Engl. J. Med., **266**, 246

Medical Letter (1962) **4**, 29

O'Driscoll, B. J. (1955) Desensitization of nurses allergic to penicillin: a report of a case. Brit. med. J., **2**, 473

Park, J. P. and Strominger, J. W. (1957) Mode of action of penicillin: a biochemical basis for the mechanism of action of penicillin and for its selective toxicity. Science, **125**, 99
Park, J. T. (1952) Uridine-5' pyrophosphate Derivatives. I. isolation from staph. aureus. II. amino-acid containing derivatives. J. biol. Chem., **194**, 885
Park, J. T. and Johnson, M. J. (1949) Accumulation of labile phosphate in Staph. aureus grown in the presence of penicillin. J. bio. Chem., **179**, 585
Parker, C. W . (1963) Penicillin allergy. Amer. J. Med., **34**, 747
Parker, C. W., DeWeck, A. L., Kern, M. and Eisen, H. N. (1962) The preparation and some properties of penicillanic acid derivatives relevant to penicillin hypersensitivity. J. exp. Med., **115**, 803
Pasteur, L. and Joubert, J. E. (1877) C.R.Acad. Sci. (Paris), **85**, 101
Petersdorf, R. G. and Turck, M. (1966) The new penicillins and their proper use. Ann. int. Med., **64**, 207
Petz, L. D. and Fudenberg, H. H. (1966) Coombs positive haemolytic anaemia caused by penicillin administration. New Engl. J. Med., **274**, 171
Pines, A., Raafat, H., Siddiqui, G. M. and Greenfield, J. B. S. (1970) Treatment of severe pseudomonas infections of the bronchi. Brit. med. J., **1**, 663
Quinn, E. L., Cox, F. and Fisher, M. (1965) The problem of associating Staph. albus with disease. Ann. NY Acad. Sci., **128**, 428
Resnik, S. S. and Shelley, W. B. (1966) Penicilloyl-Polylysine skin test: anaphylaxis in the absence of penicillin sensitivity. J. Amer. med. Ass., **196**, 740
Richardson, A. E., Spittle, C. R., James, K. W. and Robinson, O. P. W. (1968) Experiences with carbenicillin in the treatment of septicaemia and meningitis. Postgrad. med. J., **44**, 844
Ross, S., Kraybill, E. N. and Khan, W. (1970) Treatment of proteus meningitis with carbenicillin: a report of four cases. J. infect. Dis., **22**, suppl. Page 62
Salton, M. R. J. (1952) Cell wall of M. lysodeikticus as the substrate of lysozyme. Nature (Lond.), **170**, 746
Salton, M. R. J. (1961) Studies of the bacterial cell wall VIII reaction of the walls with hydrazine and fluorodinitrobenzine. Biochim. biophys. Acta, **52**, 329
Schrier, R. W., Bulger, R. J. and Van Arsdel, P. P. Jr. (1966) Nephropathy associated with penicillin and homologues. Ann. intern. Med., **64**, 116
Shelley, W. B. (1963) Indirect basophil degranulation test for allergy to penicillin and other drugs. J. Amer. med. Ass., **184**, 171
Sigal, E. S. (1963) Chronic recurrent agranulocytosis as a manifestation of increased sensitivity to penicillin in a nursing sister. Kszan med. Zh., **1**, 59
Smith, Hillas (1967) Intravenous penicillin: the use of large doses in the treatment of endocarditis. Postgrad. med. J., **43**, 785
Smith, Hillas, Lerner, P. I. and Weinstein, L. (1967) Neurotoxicity and 'massive' intravenous therapy with penicillin. A study of possible predisposing factors. Arch. intern. Med., **120**, 47
Stewart, G. T. (1947) Studies on effect of penicillin upon Gram-negative bacteria; penicillin-sulphonamide synergy. J. Hyg. (Cambs.), **45**, 282
Stewart, G. T. (1965) The penicillin group of drugs. Elsevier Publishing Co., London
Strominger, J. L., Park, J. T. and Thompson, R. E. (1959) Composition of the cell wall of Staphylococcus aureus: its relation to the mechanism of action of penicillin. J. biol. Chem., **234**, 3263
Strominger, J. L. and Tipper, D. J. (1965) Bacterial cell wall synthesis and structure in relation to the mechanism of action of penicillins and other antibacterial agents. Amer. J. Med., **39**, 708
Sutherland, R., Croydon, E. A. P. and Rolinson, G. N. (1970) Flucloxacillin, a new isoxazole penicillin, compared with Oxacillin, Cloxacillin, Dicloxacillin. Brit. med. J., **4**, 455

Swanson, M. A., Chanmougan, D. and Schwartz, R. S. (1966) Immunohaemolytic anaemia due to antipenicillin antibodies. Report of a case. New Engl. J. Med., **274**, 178
Ten Pas A. and Quinn, E. L. (1965) Cholestatic hepatitis following the administration of Sodium Oxacillin. J. Amer. med. Ass., **191**, 674
Voss, H., Redmond, A. P. and Levine, B. B. (1966) Detection of potential penicillin allergy. J. Amer. med. Ass., **196**, 679
Weinstein, L., Lerner, P. I. and Chew, H. W. (1964) Clinical and bacteriological studies of the effect of 'massive' doses of Penicillin G on infections caused by Gram-negative bacilli. New Engl. J. Med., **271**, 525
Work, E. (1961) The mucopeptides of bacterial cell walls: a review. J. gen. Microbiol., **25**, 167

CEPHALOSPORINS

Abraham, E. P. and Newton, G. G. F. (1956) A comparison of the action of penicillinase on benzyl penicillin and cephalosporin N and competitive inhibition of penicillinase by cephalosporin C. Biochem. J., **63**, 628
Chang, T. W. and Weinstein, L. (1963) Isolation characterisation and distribution of cephalosporinase. In 'Antimicrobial Agents and Chemotherapy'. Page 278
Davis, A., Seligman, S. J., Hewitt, W. L. and Finegold, S. M. (1963) Neutropoenic reaction to Cephalothin therapy. In 'Antimicrobial Agents and Chemotherapy'. Page 272
Florey, Sir H. W. (1955) Antibiotic products of a versatile fungus. Ann. intern. Med., **43**, 480
Gabriel, R., Foord, R. D. and Joekes, A. M. (1970) Reversible encephalopathy and acute renal failure after Cephaloridine. Brit. med. J., **4**, 283
Gottshall, R. Y., Roberts, J. M., Portwood, L. M. and Jennings, J. C. (1951) Synnematin: an antibiotic produced by Tilachlidium. Proc. Soc. exp. Biol. (NY), **76**, 307
Hamilton-Miller, Smith, J. T. and Knox, R. (1965) Interaction of cephaloridine with penicillinase-producing Gram-negative bacteria. Nature (Lond.), **208**, 235
Kabins, S. A. and Cohen, S. (1964) Cephalothin serum levels in the azotemic patient. Antimicrob. Agents Chemother., 207
Kaplan, K., Reisberg, B. and Weinstein, L. (1968) Cephaloridine. Studies of therapeutic activity and untoward effects. Arch. intern. Med., **121**, 17
Kunin, C. M. and Atuk, N. (1966) Excretion of cephaloridine and cephalothin in patients with impaired renal function. New Engl. J. Med., **274**, 654
Merrill, S. L., Davis, A., Smolens, B. and Finegold, S. M. (1966) Cephalothin in serious bacterial infection. Ann. intern. Med., **64**, 1
Miller, G. B. (1966) Severe whooping cough with complications. Cephaloridine in treatment. Med. Proc. (S.Africa), **12**, 36
Murdock, J. McC., Spiers, C. F., Geddes, A. M. and Wallace, E. T. (1964) Clinical trial of a cephaloridine (Ceporin) a new broad-spectrum antibiotic derived from Cephalosporin C. Brit. med. J., **2**, 1238
Perkins, R. L. and Saslaw, S. (1966) Experience with Cephalothin. Ann. intern. Med., **64**, 13
Perkins, R. L., Smith, E. J. and Saslaw, S. (1969) Cephalothin and Cephaloridine: comparative pharmocodynamics in chronic uremia. Amer. J. med. Sci., **257**, 116
Seftel, H. C. (1965) A clinical trial of Cephaloridine, a new broad-spectrum antibiotic. Med. Proc. (S.Africa), **11**, 41
Seftel, H. C. and Sieff, B. (1966) Treatment of early syphilis and acute gonorrhoea with Cephaloridine. Med. Proc. (S.Africa), **12**, 29
Silverblatt, F., Turck, M. and Bulger, R. (1970) Nephrotoxicity due to Cephaloridine: a light and electron-microscopic study in rabbits. J. infect. Dis., **122**, 33
Stewart, G. T. and Holt, R. J. (1964) Laboratory and clinical results with Cephaloridine. Lancet, ii, 1305

Tuano, B. S., Brodie, J. L. and Kirby, W. M. M. (1966) Cephaloridine versus cephalothin: relation of kidney to blood level differences after parenteral administration. Antimicrob. Agents Chemother., 101

Walters, E. D., Romonsky, M. J. and Johnson, A. C. (1963) Cephalothin - Laboratory and Clinical Studies in 109 patients. In 'Antimicrobial Agents and Chemotherapy'. Page 247

Weinstein, L. (1965) In 'Pharmacological Basis of Therapeutics'. (Ed) L. Goodman and A. Gillman. Third Edition. Collier-Macmillan Limited, London. Page 1271

4. Streptomycin

INTRODUCTION

The failure of penicillin to control infections due to a large number of Gram-negative organisms led to a search for an antibiotic effective in this range. The discovery of streptomycin was therefore not an accident but the result of a carefully planned search in the laboratory of S. A. Waksman, a soil microbiologist, working at Rutgers University, New Brunswick. His work on the production of soil humus led his interest to the group of streptomycetes which are predominantly concerned in this process. Many of the strains in this group had antibiotic properties and between 1939 and 1943 a number of antibiotics were isolated, but were too toxic for clinical use. In 1943 a strain of Streptomyces griseus was isolated which produced an antibacterial substance, and the following year the first announcement of the discovery of the new antibiotic — streptomycin — was made by Schatz, Bugie and Waksman.

During the next three years, the effect of streptomycin not only on Gram-negative and Gram-positive organisms, but also on the tubercule bacillus was confirmed. Centres were established for testing the sensitivity of freshly isolated strains of M. tuberculosis to streptomycin, and in 1946 came the report on the first hundred cases of tuberculosis treated with the new antibiotic (Hinshaw et al, 1946). The evaluation of this antibiotic was carried out by a coordinated programme with the cooperation of the US Government, and a number of private pharmaceutical firms supervised by the National Research Council, an essay in collaboration that appears to be unique.

Dihydrostreptomycin, introduced in 1947, has similar antibacterial properties to streptomycin. Although less likely than streptomycin to damage the vestibular branch of the auditory nerve, permanent deafness may result from damage to the cochlear branch. Dihydrostreptomycin, or combinations of dihydrostreptomycin and streptomycin have therefore no place in clinical practice.

PHARMACOLOGY

Streptomycin is a basic substance composed of three compounds, streptidine, streptose and N-methyl glucosamine.

In the dry state it remains stable at room temperature for at least one year; in solution at or below 28° C at pH 3 to 7 activity is retained for several months.

Streptomycin is very poorly absorbed from the intestinal tract, but is well absorbed after intramuscular, subcutaneous, or intrapleural injection. In adults with normal renal function an intramuscular injection of 1 g gives peak concentrations of 25 to 30 μg/ml one or two hours after injection.

Streptomycin is distributed into the plasma and extra-cellular fluids; even when meningitis is present virtually no streptomycin reaches the cerebrospinal fluid after intramuscular injection.

Approximately half the parenteral dose is excreted within 24 hours; streptomycin clearance is about 30% lower than the glomerular filtration; tubular reabsorption does not occur. About one third of the amount absorbed becomes protein bound and is not filtered by the glomerulus. When renal insufficiency is present the blood level of streptomycin remains high and little is excreted in the urine; use of the drug in these conditions is hazardous, and if undertaken should be controlled by estimation of the plasma concentration after the initial dose.

PREPARATIONS

Streptomycin sulphate is available either as a sterile powder or in sterile solution. The powder is put up in quantities of either 1 or 5 g; the solution contains the equivalent of 0.5 g streptomycin per ml.

ROUTES OF ADMINISTRATION

Streptomycin is usually administered by intramuscular injection; it may be given subcutaneously or intravenously. Intrathecal injection can be used in the treatment of meningitis. For intrapleural injection 1 g of streptomycin is dissolved in a few ml of sterile physiological saline and injected after aspiration of the pleural sac.

As very little streptomycin is absorbed from the bowel after oral administration the drug has been used for prophylaxis of infection in abdominal surgery and in the treatment of intestinal infections such as those due to <u>Shigella sonnei</u>; it is not recommended for either.

MODE OF ACTION

The mode of action of streptomycin has been the subject of dispute. The theory probably most widely accepted at the time of writing is that streptomycin is an inhibitor of protein synthesis (Spotts & Stanier, 1961). It is thought that as a result of binding of streptomycin, probably to ribosomal subunit 30s, the coding for protein synthesis is altered in such a way that unacceptable proteins are formed (Chapter 2, page 8). This is what happens in sensitive organisms, whereas in streptomycin-dependent organisms the antibiotic is required for the interaction between ribosomes and RNA. Organisms resistant to streptomycin have ribosomes that are unable to bind the drug.

In its antibacterial action streptomycin may be bacteriostatic or bactericidal — the precise effect depending on such factors as the length of time of contact between organism and antibiotic, the organisms involved, and the concentration of streptomycin. In low concentration streptomycin may stimulate bacterial growth; some strains require streptomycin for multiplication — the so-called streptomycin-dependent organisms.

RESISTANCE TO STREPTOMYCIN

The development of bacterial resistance to streptomycin causing therapeutic failure was first demonstrated in the treatment of urinary tract infections. Finland and colleagues found that resistance to streptomycin developed rapidly in eight of twelve patients with such infections (Finland et al, 1946). This finding has been confirmed many times and unless urinary tract infections can be cured within two or three days of starting treatment with streptomycin, bacterial resistance is likely to make treatment ineffective.

A high degree of bacterial resistance, occurring early in many other infections has also been recorded (Paine et al, 1947; Buggs et al, 1946). Weinstein (1946) reported that highly sensitive strains of H. influenzae responsible for meningitis became resistant to concentrations of greater than 1000 μg/ml within 48 to 72 hours of starting streptomycin therapy.

In vitro studies have shown that bacteria cultured serially in media containing increasing quantities of streptomycin may develop insensitivity very quickly, but in some cases resistance may occur relatively slowly and is to some extent dependent on inoculum size. Small inocula may produce stepwise resistance, but when the inoculum size is increased, sudden, early, 'one-step' resistance is almost invariable.

Most organisms developing resistance to streptomycin retain it even though the antibiotic is withdrawn, unlike organisms which become resistant to penicillin and revert to sensitivity when the antibiotic is not present.

M. tuberculosis frequently develops resistance to streptomycin during treatment; to reduce the frequency of this occurrence streptomycin should be used in combination with other antituberculous drugs. Using streptomycin alone, drug resistant bacilli have been cultured as early as the 29th day of treatment (Waksman, 1949). When maximum doses of 3.0 g per day for 120 days were used, more than 80% of patients excreting tubercule bacilli gave drug-resistant cultures (Muschenheim et al, 1947).

The sensitivity of tubercule bacilli obtained from different sites in the same patient may show different degrees of streptomycin sensitivity; cultures from different sites taken at autopsy usually show the same sensitivity, but occasionally marked differences are noted. Patients who have definite pulmonary cavities are more likely to produce resistant cultures than those without cavities, and drug resistance is more frequent in those who start treatment with large numbers of bacilli in the sputum. Tubercule bacilli lodged in the central nervous system become resistant less readily than those in the lungs (Waksman, 1949). To explain these anomalies it is usual to mention such variables as the size of the lesion and the number of tubercule bacilli present, the local concentration of the drug, the length of time of contact between the organism and antibiotic, and the proliferation of naturally resistant bacilli. It is unlikely that these factors are the complete explanation.

IN VITRO RANGE

Organisms, all strains of which are sensitive to concentration of streptomycin obtainable in man include: Brucella, Erysipelothrix, _Haemophilus ducreyi_, _Listeria monocytogenes_, _Actinobacillus mallei_, Nocardia, _Pasteurella pestis_ and _tularensis_, _Mycobacterium tuberculosis_ and Shigellae. Concentrations of up to 15 μg/ml will inhibit these organisms, but even in this range there is considerable variation, _Pasteurella pestis_ for instance usually being inhibited by concentrations in the range 0.5 to 1.5 μg/ml whereas Nocardia may require concentrations ranging from 4 to 12.5 μg/ml.

Even greater variation in in vitro sensitivity may be seen in strains of such organisms as _Str. pneumoniae_, _H. influenzae_, _E. coli_, _Proteus vulgaris_, _Staph. aureus_ and _albus_, and various streptococci including _Str. pyogenes_, _Str. faecalis_ and _Str. viridans_. The wide range of variation is exemplified by _Staph. aureus_, the sensitivity for which is given as between 0.5 to 128 μg/ml (Murray et al, 1947). Organisms insensitive to the action of streptomycin include Clostridia, Rickettsiae, Candida, Torula, _Entamoeba histolytica_ and all viruses.

CLINICAL APPLICATION

The clinical uses of streptomycin have become less as more suitable drugs have become available; nonetheless it has several important and useful applications. These are limited by the ease and rapidity with which bacterial resistance develops; for this reason streptomycin will seldom be used alone.

TUBERCULOSIS

Its most important use is in the treatment of tuberculosis; it was the first drug to have activity against _M. tuberculosis_ and it remains one of the principal antituberculous agents. Both human and bovine strains are usually sensitive to a concentration of 10 μg/ml of streptomycin; atypical mycobacteria are not sensitive.

Whatever drug regime is decided upon, one principle is clear in treating tuberculosis: streptomycin should never be used alone. Used in combination with other antituberculous drugs such as isonicotinic acid hydrazide (INAH) or sodium aminosalicylate (PAS), resistance to streptomycin is delayed but is not prevented.

GENERAL PRINCIPLES IN TREATING TUBERCULOSIS

In treating this disease it must be remembered that while chemotherapy may be the most important single factor, the principles evolved before the introduction of antituberculous agents should not be entirely neglected; nor should the natural history of the disease be forgotten, the chronicity of which will often lead those in charge of patients who get well to comment 'apparently' cured. Thus the majority of patients with tuberculosis should be in hospital or a sanitorium at least in the initial stages of their treatment. This ensures adequate diet and rest, that the drugs prescribed are taken by the patient, that frequent assessment of both clinical progress and special investigations can be carried out and that surgical measures, if required, may be performed.

If possible the sensitivity of the organism to streptomycin should be tested. This is most important in those who have had previous therapy with antituberculous drugs. If insensitivity is demonstrated there is little use in prescribing streptomycin; but in new cases, before this information is available, therapy should be started with one of the drug combinations, which may include streptomycin.

The usual daily intramuscular dose of streptomycin is 1 g for an adult; after a period of one month, this is reduced to 1 g two or three times weekly. During this initial period 70 to 80 g of streptomycin will be given over a period of 4 to 5 months.

Concurrently with streptomycin, at least one other 'first line' drug will be given. Thus, isoniazid 250-350 mg per day in divided doses may be given, or alternatively PAS in daily doses of 10 to 16 g. PAS may cause gastric irritation and a low starting dose, 6 to 8 g, may be necessary to avoid this upset. Therapy should usually be continued for periods of 1 to 2 years.

Some authorities treat pulmonary tuberculosis with PAS and isoniazid alone; for discussion of these various programmes and details of the chemotherapy of tuberculosis the reader is referred to Chapter 18.

MENINGITIS

Streptomycin may be used in the treatment of tuberculous meningitis, or in meningitis due to a number of Gram-negative organisms, particularly H. influenzae, Kl. pneumoniae, E. Coli, Proteus and Ps. aeruginosa. Intrathecal therapy in tuberculour meningitis has been discarded by most authorities, but some advise an intrathecal dose of 50 mg each day for the first two weeks of therapy.

Alternative drugs are available for treating Gram-negative meningitis and in the case of H. influenzae the author considers chloramphenicol the drug of choice. This drug is effective and intrathecal therapy is unnecessary. There is no doubt, however, that a combination of streptomycin parenterally and intrathecally, used with a sulphonamide can produce excellent results. Used in this way Weinstein recommended an initial intrathecal dose of streptomycin, freshly prepared in a volume of no less than 10 ml, to be injected over a period of 10 minutes, an equal volume of cerebrospinal fluid having previously been withdrawn. The intrathecal dose is as follows: infants less than 1 year of age 10 to 15 mg; children 1 to 3 years 15 to 25 mg; children 4 to 10 years up to 50 mg; adults 75 to 100 mg. A single intrathecal injection is usually sufficient, but if repeated, the interval between injections should be no less than 12 hours (Weinstein, 1965). In children 30 mg of streptomycin per kg of body weight and 1 to 2 g in adults are given intramuscularly daily. Sulphadiazine (0.1 g/pound body weight per day in 6 divided doses) is also given. Treatment with both drugs continues for two weeks.

In treating meningitis due to other Gram-negative organisms such as E. coli, Proteus and Ps. aeruginosa, streptomycin may well have a useful role when it is administered in a similar manner to that described for H. influenzae meningitis. It must be emphasised that these infections are usually very difficult to treat, that several courses of drugs may be required, and that in vitro sensitivity tests offer the best guide to successful therapy. The position is discussed in further detail in the section on meningitis (Chapter 17).

URINARY TRACT INFECTIONS

Acute urinary tract infections may respond to treatment with streptomycin, but it can seldom be the drug of first choice. Because of the prevalence of resistant strains of the common organisms causing urinary tract infections, sensitivity tests should be carried out. It must be remembered that resistance to streptomycin frequently develops within forty-eight hours of exposure to the drug, and that organisms which have developed resistance usually retain it. The pH of the urine is important; in one series (Hewitt, 1949) treated without alkalinisation of the urine sterilisation occurred in 20%; when alkali was given simultaneously with streptomycin bacilluria disappeared in 73%. An attempt to achieve a urinary pH of 7.5 or more should be made using sodium bicarbonate or potassium citrate.

If streptomycin is going to be effective, this will usually be obvious within 48 hours of starting treatment. The usual dose for an adult, with normal renal function is 2 g daily in 4, 0.5g intramuscular doses; for children the total daily dose is 30 mg/kg. The maximum period of treatment is ten days.

BACTERIAL ENDOCARDITIS: SEPTICAEMIA

Endocarditis due to group D streptococci is best treated by a combination of drugs, streptomycin and penicillin are probably the most useful in this context. Str.faecalis may be sensitive to one or other of these drugs, but a combination of the two is more usually effective. The position has been reviewed by Jawetz and Sonne who conclude that for 20% of enterococcal strains selected at random, the bactericidal effect of penicillin alone was as good as that of penicillin and streptomycin. For 40% of strains, however, the latter combination was essential for complete bactericidal action (Jawetz & Sonne, 1966). In treating this type of infection which is notoriously intractable, the best guide to effective antibiotic management is the estimation of the effect of the patient's serum on the infecting organism, both bacteriostatic and bactericidal dilutions should be recorded. The dose of streptomycin for an adult is 1 to 2 g/day in divided doses combined with high doses of penicillin. The author has treated a patient with Str.faecalis endocarditis with 80g of streptomycin combined with very high doses of penicillin G intravenously for a period of three months (see Chapter 16).

MISCELLANEOUS INFECTIONS

Surgical infections such as peritonitis, diverticulitis, or subphrenic abscess, may respond to streptomycin and penicillin combined. This is usually an adjunct to surgical measures; of course many other antibiotics may be used in this situation, especially the tetracyclines, ampicillin or chloramphenicol.

Pulmonary infection with Kl.pneumoniae is best treated with streptomycin and chloramphenicol combined.

Brucellosis is very difficult to treat if the chronic stage of the illness has been reached; streptomycin, 2 g/day, combined with tetracycline, 2-3 g/day, is sometimes effective when given for 2-3 weeks.

Infections due to Pasteurella pestis (plague) and tularensis (tularaemia) respond to streptomycin.

It will be observed that excepting for tuberculosis, Str.faecalis endocarditis, Kl.pneumoniae infections, brucellosis and a limited number of other infections, streptomycin is seldom a first choice. In the author's view a case can be made for restricting its use, for very wide-spread prescribing of streptomycin increases the risk of patients who develop tuberculosis starting their treatment with streptomycin-resistant mycobacteria.

TOXICITY: SIDE EFFECTS

ACUTE TOXICITY

The acute toxicity resulting from streptomycin administration to animals has some similarity to the acute disasters reported after large doses in humans (McDermott, 1947; Farrington et al, 1947). The critical toxicity seems to occur in the range of 150-200 mg/kg, resulting from daily intramuscular doses of 6-8 g, more than double the maximum dose advised.

The manifestations of acute streptomycin toxicity are those of reduction in renal function. Various other symptoms, presumably from depression of medullary function have been described: listlessness, tachycardia, slowed respiration, stupor and coma (Bunn & Westlake, 1949).

CHRONIC TOXICITY

The most frequent serious toxic effect of streptomycin sulphate is on the eighth cranial nerve. Both vestibular and auditory functions may be upset, the former being more vulnerable.

VESTIBULAR UPSET

The earliest **symptoms** of vestibular disorder are usually giddiness in the upright position; because of the absence of sensation of rotation there is misrepresentation of movement — the patient fails to appreciate the end of movement — the so-called 'mental past pointing'. Headache, nausea and vomiting precipitated by movement occur in the acute stage. This stage usually lasts about ten days, and is followed by a chronic phase characterised by symptoms after sudden movements, ataxia being common. This stage usually becomes less troublesome as the patient compensates for his deficiency; it lasts about two months.

The first **sign** is usually evidence of 'mental past pointing' when the patient's eyes drift before focusing. Romberg's sign may be positive, nystagmus is rare.

The labyrinthine disturbance of streptomycin toxicity is a bilateral symmetrical depression of function; caloric, rotation and electrical stimulation confirm the abnormality.

There is wide variation in these toxic manifestations; reactions have been reported as early as the seventh day and as late as six months. There is, however, an impressive relation to total dosage. Most patients can tolerate a daily dose of 1 g for four to six weeks without clinical evidence of toxicity; if the dose is increased to 2 g per day depression of vestibular function may occur after four weeks, and if the period of administration is extended to between 60 and 120 days 75% of patients may be expected to show clinical manifestations of toxicity.

Reduced renal excretion of the drug and repeated intrathecal injection lead to earlier and more severe vestibular upset. Therapy should be stopped at the first complaint of headache and dizziness. The practical limitations imposed on the clinical use of streptomycin by these toxic manifestations are obvious.

DEAFNESS

Deafness is less common than vestibular upset as a manifestation of streptomycin toxicity; however, careful audiometric examination will reveal a reduced auditory acuity in a number of patients given the drug for more than seven days. Tinnitus is usually the first sign of toxicity, and is an indication for stopping therapy.

Deafness from dihydrostreptomycin is commoner than from streptomycin; it is not preceded by a 'warning' tinnitus, and may even occur when the drug has been stopped. There have been no reports of recovery from deafness following dihydrostreptomycin, but auditory defect resulting from streptomycin sulphate may lessen, and hearing eventually return to normal (Brown et al, 1946).

OTHER NERVOUS SYSTEM EFFECTS

Optic nerve dysfunction causing blurred vision due to enlargement of the blind spot has been recorded; peripheral neuritis and paraesthesia sometimes results. The latter sensation is commonly noted on the face, often on the lips and occurs within an hour of intramuscular injection.

Blockade of the neuromuscular junction has resulted in patients in whom as little as 2 g of streptomycin have been instilled into the peritoneal cavity post-operatively. This most commonly occurs in patients given skeletal muscle relaxants, and is similar to the block caused by the magnesium ion, being a combination of a competitive block with a reduction in release of acetylcholine. It is antagonised by calcium (Vital Brazil & Corrado, 1957).

An acute encephalopathy, with headache, fits and coma may result when too large doses of streptomycin are instilled into the cerebrospinal fluid. More than 50 mg should not be used in an adult, proportionately less in children, in any single injection. Even injections in this range cause some irritation and a pleocytosis of up to 400 cells per c.mm may be found after a single intrathecal injection.

HYPERSENSITIVITY REACTIONS

A large variety of rashes, eosinophilia, fever and even anaphylactic shock may occur during streptomycin therapy, often in patients giving a history of allergy.

Morbilliform, erythematous and other rashes develop in about 5% of

Table IV. Streptomycin (Sulphate)

Usual dose		Route	Frequency	Precautions	Side effects
Adult	Child				
1 - 2 g	30 mg/kg	I. M.	Daily reduce to 2-3 g/week after one month Total 70-80 g (adults) (tuberculosis)		Vestibular upset
1 - 2 g in 1 litre		I. V.	Daily		Deafness
25 - 50 mg	10 - 50 mg	Intrathecal	Not more than 12 hourly	Dissolve in 10 ml Prepare fresh. Inject slowly (10 min)	Rashes
0.5 - 1 g	0.25 - 0.5 g	Intrapleural			

patients and usually occur within two weeks of the first course of drug. Exfoliative dermatitis occasionally occurs and has caused death.

Contact dermatitis may be troublesome in those handling the drug; the use of rubber gloves is helpful; desensitisation is possible though tedious.

Blood dyscrasias such as aplastic anaemia and thrombocytopoenia occasionally occur.

Albuminuria, oliguria, cylindruria may be seen, usually as a result of large doses.

SUPERINFECTION

Superinfection is a relatively common result of streptomycin therapy. This may be related to the fact that irrespective of the route of administration there is a significant change in the bacterial flora of the gastrointestinal and respiratory tracts.

REFERENCES

Brown, H. A. and Hinshaw, H. C. (1946) Toxic reaction of streptomycin on the eighth nerve apparatus. Mayo Clin. Proc., **21**, 347

Buggs, C.W., Bronstein, B., Hirshfeld, H.W. and Pilling, M.A. (1946) The in vitro action of Streptomycin on bacteria. J. Amer. med. Ass., **130**, 64

Bunn, P. A. and Westlake, R. E. (1949) in 'Streptomycin'. (Ed) S.A. Waksman. Bailliere, Tindal & Cox, London. Page 526

Farrington, R. F., Hull-Smith, H., Bunn, P. A. and McDermott, W. (1947) Streptomycin Toxicity. J. Amer. med. Ass., **134**, 679

Finland, M., Murray, R., Harris, H. W., Kilham, L. and Meads, M. (1946) Development of streptomycin resistance during treatment. J. Amer. med. Ass., **132**, 778

Hewitt, W. L. (1949) in 'Streptomycin'. (Ed) S. A. Waksman. Bailliere, Tindal & Cox, London. Page 451

Hinshaw, H. C., Feldman, W. H. and Pfuetze, K. H. (1946) Treatment of tuberculosis with streptomycin. A summary of observations in 100 cases. J. Amer. med. Ass., **132**, 778

Jawetz, E. and Sonne, M. (1966) Penicillin-streptomycin treatment of enterococcal endocarditis: a re-evaluation. New Engl. J. Med., **274**, 710

McDermott, W. (1947) Toxicity of streptomycin. Amer. J. Med., **2**, 491

Murray, R., Paine, T. F . Jr. and Finland, M. (1947) Streptomycin, I: Bacteriologic and pharmacologic aspects. New Engl. J. Med., **236**, 701

Muschenheim, C., McDermott, W., Hadley, S. J., Hull-Smith, H. and Tracy, A. (1947) Streptomycin in the treatment of tuberculosis in humans. Ann. intern. Med., **27**, 989

Paine, T. F., Murray, R., Seeler, A. O. and Finland, M. (1947) Streptomycin in the treatment of meningitis: Report of 27 cases treated at the Boston City Hospital. Ann. intern. Med., **27**, 494

Schatz, A., Bugie, E. and Waksman, S. A. (1944) Streptomycin, a substance exhibiting antibiotic activity against Gram-positive and Gram-negative bacteria. Proc. Soc. exp. Biol. (NY), **55**, 66

Spotts, C. R. and Stanier, R. Y. (1961) Mechanism of streptomycin action on bacteria: a unitary hypothesis. Nature (Lond.), **192**, 633

Vital Brazil, O. and Pinto Corrado, A. (1957) The curariform action of streptomycin. J. Pharmacol. exp. Ther., **120**, 452

Waksman, S. A. (1949) 'Streptomycin. Nature and Practical Applications'. Bailliere, Tindall & Cox, London

Weinstein, L. (1946) The treatment of meningitis due to Haemophilus influenzae with streptomycin. New Engl. J. Med., **235**, 101

Weinstein, L. (1965) in 'The Pharmacological Basis of Therapeutics'. 3rd Edition. Collier-Macmillan, London

5. Tetracyclines

INTRODUCTION

The tetracyclines are a group of drugs with similar antibiotic action, though differing somewhat in pharmacology. The first member of this family was chlortetracycline (aureomycin), derived from the soil organism Streptomyces aureofaciens and introduced in 1948. This was followed by oxytetracycline (terramycin) produced from Streptomyces rimosus. The elucidation of the chemical structure of chlortetracycline led to molecular modification by removing the chlorine atom from the parent substance to produce tetracycline (achromycin) which was introduced in 1953.

Investigation of mutant strains of Streptomyces aureofaciens led to the discovery in 1957 of a new group of antibiotics, the demethyltetracyclines, one member of which, demethylchlortetracycline (ledermycin) became available for general use in 1959.

More recently two other tetracycline compounds have become available, methycycline (rondomycin) and lymecycline (tetralysal).

PHARMACOLOGY

The crystalline bases of the tetracyclines are yellow, bitter compounds, slightly water soluble at pH 7, and form soluble sodium salts and hydrochlorides. There is considerable variation in loss of activity of these compounds with altering conditions of temperature and pH. Demethylchlortetracycline, for instance, is stable over a wide range of pH, whereas at 37°C and pH 2.5 the half life of oxytetracycline hydrochloride is 12 days and this is reduced to 33 hours at pH 8.5. In the dry state, the bases and hydrochlorides are stable under normal storage conditions for several years.

Oral administration of tetracyclines results in incomplete absorption which takes place for the most part in the stomach and small intestine; absorption is reduced by aluminium hydroxide and milk, and increased, at least for oxytetracycline and tetracycline, by glucosamine 2-amino-d-glucose. Simultaneous administration of ferrous sulphate reduces the absorption of tetracycline, oxytetracycline, methacycline, and doxycycline (Neuvonen et al, 1970). There is considerable variation in plasma levels after similar oral doses of the tetracyclines. Expressing the antibiotic activity of a given plasma sample in terms of the activity of a solution of tetracyclines of known concentration Figure 3 gives the levels obtained for four different tetracyclines.

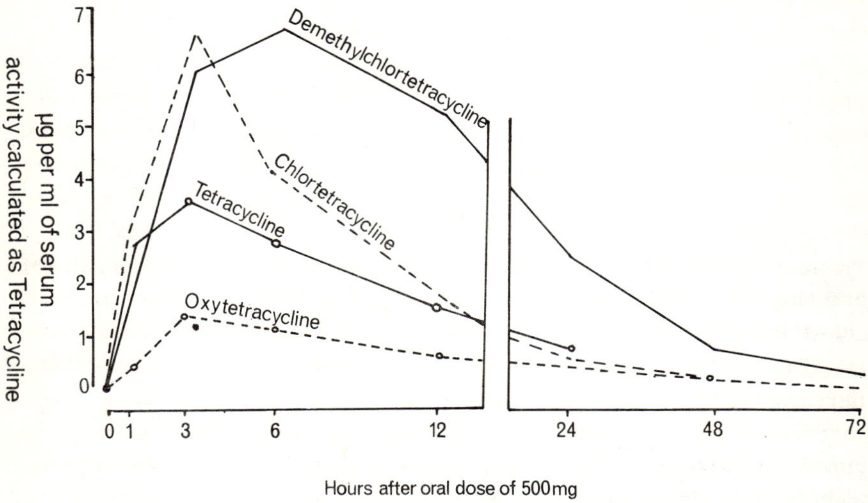

Figure 3. Average levels of antibacterial activity, calculated as tetracycline, in blood of same subjects after single oral doses of 500 mg of four tetracycline analogues. (Reproduced by kind permission of the authors Finland et al, Antibiotics Annual 1959-60)

Methacycline appears to behave similarly to demethychlortetracycline, but there is some conflicting evidence here, at least two studies favouring methacycline in obtaining higher concentrations, while two others favour demethylchlortetracycline.

Lymecycline which is a compound of tetracycline and the amino acid lysine has a higher solubility than any of the other tetracyclines, in solution has a pH of 7.8. This facilitates parenteral absorption, but absorption from the intestinal tract is probably of the same order as tetracycline when equivalent doses are used.

Clomocycline, similar to lymecycline, is highly water soluble and unstable in solution. It is claimed that because of its instability the amount of deposition in bones is reduced. More information is required for full assessment of this analogue. Clomocycline is supplied as capsules containing 170 mg, the usual adult daily dose is one capsule four times a day.

Doxycycline is a tetracycline compound which is well absorbed from the intestine and slowly excreted. A half life of 15 hours after a single dose has been claimed. Doxycycline is available as capsules containing 100 mg; the usual adult dose is two capsules on the first day of treatment and one capsule on subsequent days.

Minocycline is an analogue not yet commercially available. It is exceptionally well absorbed after oral administration and interestingly has antibacterial activity against many species which are tetracycline-resistant, most notably staphylococci and some streptococci.

Pyrrolidinomethyl tetracycline is a compound which has been used for a number of years on the continent particularly in Germany. It is highly water soluble, giving a neutral solution and is suitable for direct intravenous injection. High blood and tissue levels are obtained and a single intravenous injection may suffice for one day's treatment. Weizel and Dana (1961) reported blood levels averaging more than 4 μg/ml two hours after a single 275 mg intravenous injection of pyrrolidinomethyl tetracycline and detectable levels persisted for 24 hours.

This compound is most suitable for intravenous injection, does not commonly cause thrombosis or irritation of the tissues, but may be administered intramuscularly, even in children.

Toxic effects, including enterocolitis, occur; liver damage does not seem to have been reported, but must be expected if large doses are used.

Separate preparations of pyrrolidinomethyl tetracycline nitrate, each containing 350 mg, are issued for either intramuscular or intravenous use. The usual adult daily dose is one injection of 350 mg by either route; in severe infections two intravenous injections may be administered at 12 hourly intervals.

An intravenous dose of 500 mg of any of the four earlier analogues may be expected to produce plasma concentrations of 15-30 μg/ml, and detectable levels persist for periods of up to twelve hours. Chlortetracycline is irregularly absorbed after intramuscular injection; lymecycline is probably the most suitable tetracycline for intramuscular use.

The tetracycline analogues show varying degrees of protein binding with low values for oxytetracycline high for methacycline, are distributed in body fluids and are, to some extent, stored in tissues. Appreciable quantities of these drugs appear in the cerebrospinal fluid even when meningitis is not present. In patients with meningitis 1 g of oxytetracycline given intravenously every 12 hours produced a cerebrospinal concentration of up to 3.8 μg/ml; demethylchlortetracycline appears in the cerebrospinal fluid in small quantities only.

There is good penetration of the brain, saliva, pleural fluid and prostatic fluid by these drugs; concentrations in breast milk of lactating mothers is approximately half the simultaneous plasma level. They diffuse across the placental barrier and appear in foetal blood. Oxytetracycline has been found in high concentrations in human skin, but penetration into the ocular fluids is poor.

The tetracyclines are stored in reticulo-endotholial cells, in bone, in dentine and enamel of unerupted teeth.

These drugs are excreted in the urine and faeces; as renal excretion is by glomerular filtration renal insufficiency sets limitations to dosage. Chlortetracycline, which is least dependent on renal excretion is the safest in these circumstances; demethylchlortetracycline is more slowly excreted than either tetracycline or chlortetracycline. Tetracycline, but not chlortetracycline, can be removed by haemodialysis.

Excretion in the faeces occurs even when the drugs are given parenterally as they are secreted into bile.

MODE OF ACTION

The mode of action of the tetracyclines is not fully understood; it is usually said that they inhibit protein synthesis without interfering with nucleic acid synthesis (Liberman & Ove, 1959). The basic disturbance seems to be the prevention of synthesis of ribosomal protein from aminoacyl to RNA, an effect which occurs not only in bacterial, but also to some extent in mammalian cell-free systems (Rendi & Ochoa, 1962; Franklin, 1963).

These antibiotics are known to bind magnesium, manganese and calcium, and it has been suggested that their antibacterial activity is related to their ability to combine with divalent metallic cations, removing them from sites where they are required for the activation of enzymes (Weinberg, 1954).

The tetracyclines in concentrations in which they are commonly used are bacteriostatic; higher concentration obtained by parenteral injection may achieve a bactericidal effect.

RESISTANCE TO THE TETRACYCLINES

In vitro resistance to the tetracyclines develops slowly in step-wise manner, similar to the way resistance develops to the penicillins. Bacteria resistant to one tetracycline usually show resistance to others in the group; there is some cross resistance between the tetracyclines and chloramphenicol for Gram-negative organisms, none for Gram-positive ones (Chapter 2, page 10).

Tetracycline-resistant organisms are most likely to be acquired from other individuals in a population where tetracycline has been widely used. Some bacteria, rarely according to Lepper (1956), become insensitive in vivo as a result of exposure to the tetracyclines.

ADMINISTRATION: DOSE

The tetracyclines are usually given orally; they may be given parenterally, intramuscularly or intravenously; they should not be used intrathecally.

The usual dose of chlortetracycline, tetracycline and oxytetracycline is 250 mg/6 hourly; in severe infections double this dose may be used. The comparable doses for demethylchlortetracycline, methacycline and lymecycline are 150 to 300 mg/6 hourly, but the interval between doses can be increased to eight or even twelve hours. The larger doses may induce considerable gastro-intestinal upset, and in many cases a compromise will have to be reached in which some useful antibacterial effect is achieved, but at the expense of some side effects. Tolerance varies.

When given intravenously the maximum adult dose is 2 g/14 hours; for children 10 to 20 mg/kg per day may be given. Intravenous administration of the tetracyclines often causes thrombophlebitis, and intramuscular injection is painful; there are few indications for subjecting patients to these discomforts today, when alternative drugs are available.

In treating patients with renal insufficiency chlortetracycline, because it is least dependent on the kidney for its excretion, is most suitable. It is not suitable for intravenous therapy, being relatively unstable in solution.

Topical application of the tetracyclines is not generally recommended but they may be useful for local application in ophthalmic conditions.

Some of the preparations available for clinical use are given at the end of this chapter.

IN VITRO RANGE

The tetracyclines are among the antibiotics with the widest antibacterial spectrum, being active against many Gram-positive and Gram-negative bacteria, Rickettsiae, Mycoplasmas and the agents of the psittacosis-lymphogranuloma venereum group of conditions. In general all the members of the tetracycline group have a similar antibacterial range; demethylchlortetracycline and methacycline appear to have about twice the antibacterial activity of tetracycline (Finland & Garrod, 1960; Chang & Weinstein, 1962; Limson & Guevara, 1963); lymecycline has activity similar to that of tetracycline (Cassano et al, 1961).

Many strains of Proteus vulgaris, Pseudomonas aeruginosa, staphylococci and enterococci are for the most part resistant to the action of the tetracyclines. There has been some increase in the number of resistant strains of E. coli, Kl. pneumoniae, pneumococci, and especially group A streptococci.

CLINICAL APPLICATION

The clinical usefulness of the tetracyclines is almost entirely due to their wide range of activity; there are some infections, such as those due to Mycoplasmas, Rickettsiae, and the larger viruses of the psittacosis group, for which the tetracyclines might be considered 'specific', but even in these infections a tetracycline may be chosen only because the alternative chloramphenicol is even more undesirable.

The chief use of the tetracyclines can therefore be summarised in the following groups: acute and chronic infections, especially mixed infections, when the bacteriology is uncertain; infection due to Rickettsiae, Mycoplasmas, the larger viruses, and when combined with other drugs, Brucella, and E. histolytica; the tetracyclines have a 'second line' use in a number of infections when patients are hypersensitive to the more active penicillin, in such conditions as syphilis, gonorrhoea, anthrax and actinomycosis; they have little place in the treatment of infections due to Group A streptococci, pneumococci and in the treatment of bacterial endocarditis. In compiling a list of drugs with antituberculous action the tetracyclines might be included, but they have no place in therapy.

INFECTIONS OF UNCERTAIN BACTERIAL CAUSE

PULMONARY INFECTIONS

For acute chest infections when the pathogenic organisms are unknown and the patient's clinical condition demands treatment, a wide spectrum antibiotic is indicated. The tetracyclines are certainly useful here, and are widely prescribed. To some extent they have been replaced by ampicillin, which has a similar antibacterial range, bactericidal action, and greater efficacy against the pneumococcus, a common pathogen in this type of infection. When the tetracyclines are used in this context, they should be given in full doses, at least for the first forty-eight hours.

Acute exacerbation of chronic bronchitis must be treated along the same lines. Many of these patients may be already taking a tetracycline prophylactically, and a decision will have to be made as to whether the tetracycline be continued, albeit in increased doses, or an alternative drug prescribed. If the patient is very ill, it is probably wiser to assume that bacteria, resistant to the tetracyclines are responsible and use an alternative such as cephaloridine.

PERITONITIS

When perforation of the bowel occurs as a result of injury or surgery, or in the course of some infection such as diverticulitis or appendicitis, the tetracyclines have a definite place in therapy. In these circumstances a large number of bacteria are spilled into the peritoneal cavity, and the tetracyclines given by the intravenous route are indicated.

URINARY TRACT INFECTIONS

In acute urinary tract infections the tetracyclines offer a fair chance of performing a 'holding operation' until the pathogenic organisms and their antibiotic sensitivities have been established. They are becoming less useful in this context due to the prevalence of resistant pathogens.

RICKETTSIAE: MYCOPLASMAS: PSITTACOSIS GROUP

The various forms of typhus fever, rickettsial pox, and Q fever respond satisfactorily to the tetracyclines.

Mycoplasma pneumoniae, a pleuropneumonia-like organism (PPLO), is the commonest cause of primary atypical pneumonia and infections with these agents respond to treatment with tetracyclines.

The tetracyclines are the treatment of choice in lymphogranuloma venereum; acute cases respond quickly, but chronic cases may require treatment for several months, the dose being 2 g/day.

Psittacosis may be effectively treated by the tetracyclines: 2 g/day for two weeks is the commonly used dose.

Trachoma, which probably responds best to the sulphonamides may be treated satisfactorily with the tetracyclines. The ophthalmic ointment (0.5%) is applied to the conjunctiva several times per day for one month. Treatment with tetracycline or sulphonamide by mouth is usually added to the regime.

Inclusion conjunctivitis, produced by an agent similar to that responsible for trachoma, responds to topical administration of tetracycline.

Brucellosis may respond to the tetracyclines alone. In the acute stage of the illness a good response may be expected, but in the later stages it is doubtful if any treatment can eradicate the organism, but a tetracycline (2-3 g/day) combined with streptomycin (1-2 g/day) given for up to three weeks may sometimes be effective.

The tetracyclines have a place in the drug regime used in treating intestinal amoebiasis. They are usually given in conjunction with emetine or chloroquine; some suggest that tetracyclines improve the efficiency of amoebicidal drugs. Infections due to Shigella flexneri may respond to treatment with tetracycline.

TETRACYCLINES NOT INDICATED

The tetracyclines are not indicated in the treatment of infections proved to be due to streptococci, or pneumococci; the staphylococcus, being virtually a law unto itself, is also best treated with alternative drugs. Conditions such as tonsillitis, erysipelas and cellulitis, all caused by haemolytic streptococci, respond in an indolent, unsatisfactory manner if tetracyclines are used. When these drugs are stopped relapse is common; the antibiotic of choice in these infections is penicillin G.

Although some of the bacteria responsible for bacterial endocarditis may be shown to have in vitro sensitivity to the tetracyclines, it is preferable to avoid these drugs in treating this condition. Some patients have been cured of endocarditis with these compounds, but their bacteriostatic action frequently allows relapse to occur. An exception to this is Rickettsial endocarditis when the tetracyclines are indicated.

PROPHYLACTIC USE OF TETRACYCLINES

The tetracyclines have been used prophylactically, before bowel surgery, in preventing secondary bacterial infection in patients with mucoviscidosis, and most widely in prevention of exacerbation of infections in patients with bronchitis and chronic pulmonary disease.

In these conditions, prophylactic antibiotic therapy has to be considered in terms of its efficiency and its ill effects. In preparation of the bowel for surgery the evidence for a good effect is far from conclusive, whereas the side effects and dangers of tetracycline therapy are fairly clear cut. These drugs are not recommended in pre-operative bowel preparation.

In mucoviscidosis the tetracyclines may well have some place in prophylaxis. Given intermittently and alternated with other antibiotics, which will be indicated by in vitro sensitivity tests, a useful result may sometimes be obtained.

Patients with bronchitis and other chronic pulmonary infections are often treated with the tetracyclines to prevent exacerbation of infection. There are a number of studies showing that this can be effective. The drugs are sometimes given continuously, others prefer to prescribe them only in the winter months. Instead of offering indiscriminate long-term prophylaxis, patients should be selected and trained in the intermittent use of antibiotics. Thus, at the very onset of recurrence or reinfection, when symptoms first appear — sputum increasing in volume or becoming frankly purulent — the selected drug should be started. Similarly any upper respiratory tract infection, or influenza would be an indication for starting antibiotic therapy. These patients should try to avoid crowds when respiratory virus infections are common.

This plan of therapy may seem to be not so much true prophylaxis as early frequent treatment of infection. It seems to the author a rational approach to a very difficult subject. (For further discussion of chemoprophylaxis see Chapter 23.)

CHOICE OF TETRACYCLINE

There is little difference between the various tetracyclines with regard to antibacterial spectrum and their ability to produce side effects. Selection therefore will be dependent on such factors as convenience of dosage, cost, and the physician's previous experience with the drugs.

Demethylchlortetracycline and methacycline are similar drugs and because of their relatively good absorption can be effectively used in doses of 150 mg four times, or 300 mg twice daily. In prophylaxis 150 mg twice daily may suffice. These factors make these two analogues most suitable for the majority of infections where a tetracycline is indicated.

For the intravenous route the tetracyclines of choice are tetracycline and oxytetracycline; for intramuscular injection lymecycline is probably the drug of choice, but at the time of writing there is not sufficient data generally available to be emphatic on this point.

TOXICITY: SIDE EFFECTS

Side effects and superinfections, related to size of dose and length of treatment are common when the tetracycline drugs are used; serious toxic effects are relatively rare despite the metabolic effects produced by these drugs.

GASTRO-INTESTINAL UPSET

The commonest side effects are those related to the gastro-intestinal tract. Nausea, abdominal distention, diarrhoea and occasionally vomiting may result when full oral doses are given 6-hourly for as short a period as 48 hours. Sometimes these symptoms become less as treatment continues, more often the dose must be reduced, and in some cases the drug withdrawn. Irritation of the perianal region and sore mouth may occur, and these symptoms do not always seem to be related to candida infection. Administering the drugs with milk may alleviate some of these irritative effects, but this also leads to reduced absorption of the antibiotics. Tetracyclines given parenterally may cause intestinal upsets as these compounds are excreted into the bowel through bile.

Diarrhoea occurring in any patient who is having a wide spectrum antibiotic must be regarded with respect, for in a minority of patients this may be due to staphylococcal enterocolitis. This dangerous complication usually occurs in severely ill patients given these drugs for prolonged periods; the patient's condition deteriorates markedly, and profuse watery diarrhoea leading to rapid water and electrolyte loss becomes apparent. The diagnosis may be confirmed by examination of a Gram stain of a stool smear when many leucocytes and Gram-positive cocci can be identified. In mild cases withdrawal of the antibiotic may be sufficient to allow the patient to recover; other cases require energetic intravenous replacement of electrolytes and water and the use of an antibiotic effective against penicillinase-producing staphylococci; cloxacillin both orally and parenterally is suitable, vancomycin has also been used successfully.

SUPERINFECTIONS

Superinfection is commoner when the tetracyclines are used than when penicillin or streptomycin is given; a better comparison would be between the tetracyclines and ampicillin, but data for this comparison are not available.

Moniliasis, most commonly affecting the mouth, ano-rectal region, and the vagina frequently occurs. This may be troublesome, but is not usually dangerous. A few cases of intestinal moniliasis may occur, most often in patients with severe illness; diabetes mellitus, leukaemia, or the simultaneous use of immunosuppressive drugs are commonly the setting for this type of superinfection. Long continued intravenous infusions may be associated with generalised systemic candidiasis. Pulmonary candidiasis is often seen in those patients with chronic broncho-pulmonary disease. There is considerable difficulty in deciding when monilia isolated from sputum is pathogenic; small numbers of these yeasts do not appear to be harmful, and are frequently found in patients with chronic bronchitis.

Bacterial superinfection of the bowel is usually due to staphylococci. A condition independent of staphylococcal infection, pseudomembraneous enterocolitis may sometimes occur, but its relation to antibiotics is not clear, for it may be seen post-operatively when no antibiotics have been given (Editorial New Engl. J. Med., 1953).

HEPATIC AND RENAL UPSET

Tetracyclines given to rats have been shown to produce accumulation of fat in the liver (Seto & Lepper, 1954); Lepper (1951) showed that large intravenous or oral doses of tetracycline resulted in clinical manifestations of liver upset. Pregnant women appear to be particularly susceptible. Microscopic changes include vacuolation and increase in liver fat. Azotaemia, jaundice and shock have also been described in patients receiving large doses of tetracycline intravenously, and fatty changes in the liver lobules were the chief microscopical findings (Schultz et al, 1963).

Tetracyclines act by inhibiting protein synthesis and there is now considerable evidence that this inhibition is not confined to bacterial cells. Shils (1963) considered that in patients with renal disease tetracycline causes decreased utilisation of amino acids and that this results in an increased load of products of amino acid metabolism being presented to the kidney. Manifestations of this upset include increasing azotaemia, phosphataemia, acidosis, anorexia, nausea and vomiting, weight loss, and increased urinary losses of nitrogen and sodium. These changes are often delayed, and in patients with advanced renal disease may not cause maximum disturbance until up to six days after termination of tetracycline therapy. Anabolic steroids may prevent or delay some of the symptomatic and clinical manifestations.

In six subjects with normal renal function given demethylchlortetracycline Roth and associates (1967) observed renal abnormalities in two who received the drug for 28 days. These changes included impairment of urinary concentrating ability and in one case this was accompanied by a decrease in creatinine clearance and a rise in blood urea nitrogen level. These effects in normal subjects were reversible and produced no signs or symptoms.

The degradation products anhydrotetracycline and epianhydrotetracycline from the use of outdated tetracyclines have caused renal tubular damage with clinical manifestations of polyuria and vomiting. Proteinuria, glycosuria

Table V. Tetracyclines

DRUG	PREPARATION (ORAL)	PREPARATION (PARENTERAL)	OPHTHALMIC
1. Chlortetracycline (Aureomycin)	Caps: 50 mg, 250 mg Syrup: 125 mg/5ml		
2. Oxytetracycline (Terramycin) also Imperacin	Caps: 250 mg Syrup: 125 mg/5 ml Tabs: 50, 100 & 250 mg Paediatric Drops: 1g/10 ml Suspension: 250 mg/5 ml	Vials (I.M.) 100 mg Vials (I.V.) 250 mg	Vials (Soln) 250 mg/5 ml Ointment: Oxytetracycline 30 mg Polymyxin B. sulph. 10,000 U
3. Tetracycline (Achromycin) also Ambramycin Steclin, Tetracyn, Tetrex, Totomycin	Caps: 50 mg, 250 mg Soluble Tabs: 50 mg Syrup: 125 mg/5 ml Paediatric Drops: 100 mg/ml Tabs: 50 mg, 250 mg Troches: 15 mg	Vials (I.M.) 100 mg Vials (I.V.) 250 mg	i. Powder for soln. 0.5% dissolve in 5 ml sterile water ii. Oil suspension 1% iii. Ointment 1%
4. Demethylchlor-tetracycline (Ledermycin)	Tabs/Caps: 150 mg Tabs: 300 mg Syrup: 75 mg/5 ml Drops: 0.6 g/10 ml		
5. Methacycline hydrochloride (Rondomycin)	Caps: 150 mg Syrup: 75 mg/5 ml		
6. Lymecycline (Tetralysal) also Mucomycin	Caps: 204 mg = 150 mg tetracycline base	Ampoules (I.M.) 100 mg	
7. Clomocycline (Megaclor)	Caps: 170 mg		
8. Pyrrolidinomethyl-tetracycline (Tetrex)		Vials (I.M.) 350 mg Vials (I.V.) 350 mg	

DOSES

	Adults	Children
Chlortetracycline Oxytetracycline Tetracycline	250-500 mg 6 hrly	12.5-20 mg/kg/24 hr
Demethylchlortetracycline Methacycline Lymecycline	150-300 mg 6-8 hrly	6-12 mg/kg/24 hr
Clomocycline	170 mg 6 hrly	
	Intramuscular	
Oxytetracycline Lymecycline Tetracycline	400 mg/24 hr in divided doses	
	Intravenous	
Oxytetracycline Tetracycline	0.5-1 g/24 hr	
Pyrrolidinomethyltetracycline	350 mg-700 mg/24 hr	

and amino-aciduria are present and the condition has been likened to the Fanconi syndrome. When the drug is stopped the condition clears in about a month (Frimper et al, 1963). Change in colour of these antibiotics from light yellow to dark brown suggests the presence of these toxic degradation products.

HYPERSENSITIVITY

Hypersensitivity may be manifest as various forms of skin eruption, including exfoliative dermatitis. Phototoxic reactions may occur on exposure to sunlight in patients taking these drugs, especially demethylchlortetracycline.

DEPOSITION IN TISSUES

Brown discolouration of the teeth may occur in children taking tetracyclines; this is most likely to occur when large doses are given before the appearance of the first teeth. Pigmentation may result in the permanent teeth if these drugs are taken between the ages of two months and two years. Pregnant women treated with tetracyclines may give birth to infants with pigmented teeth. If treatment is prolonged some deposition of metabolites occurs in nails which very occasionally may show staining; deposition in growing bones also occurs.

MISCELLANEOUS EFFECTS

Large doses of tetracyclines may occasionally produce leucocytosis, thrombocytopoenia, eosinophilia; drug fever may occur.

Increase in intracranial pressure has been described in young children receiving conventional doses (Fields, 1961). Teratogenic effects cannot be accepted as proved on the basis of one case report (Wilson, 1962).

REFERENCES

Cassano, A., Filice, A., Costa, C. and Trimarco, C. (1961) Attivita antibatterica in vitro; assorbimento, diffusione ed eliminazione nell'uomo. Rif. med., **75**, 1383

Chang, T. W. and Weinstein, L. (1962) A comparison of the in vitro and in vivo activity of Methacycline and other tetracycline compounds. Antibiotic and Chemother., **12**, 676

Editorial (1953) Antibiotics, staphylococcal enteritis, and pseudomembraneous enterocolitis. New Engl. J. Med., **249**, 37

Fields, J. P. (1961) Bulging Fontanelle, a complication of tetracycline therapy in infants. J. Pediat., **58**, 74

Finland, M. and Garrod, L. P. (1960) Demethylchlortetracycline. Brit. med. J., **2**, 959

Franklyn, T. J. (1963) The inhibition of the incorporation of leucine into protein of cell-free systems from rat liver with Escherichia coli by chlortetracycline. Biochem. J., **87**, 449

Frimper, G. W., Timpanelli, A. E., Eisenmenger, W. H., Stein, H. S. and Erhlich, L. I. (1963) Reversible 'Fanconi Syndrome' caused by degraded tetracycline. J. Amer. med. Ass., **184**, 111

Lepper, M. H. (1951) Effect of large doses of aureomycin on human liver. Arch. intern. Med., **88**, 271

Lepper, M. H. (1956) Aureomycin (chlortetracycline). Med. Encyclopaedia Inc., New York

Liberman, I. and Ove, P. (1959) Isolation and study of mutants from mammalian cells in culture. Proc. nat. Acad. Sci. (Wash.), **45**, 867

Limson, B. M. and Guevara, R. Jr. (1963) Evaluation of Methacycline, a new analogue of oxytetracycline. Curr. ther. Res., **5**, 249

Neuvonen, P. J., Gothoni, G., Hackman, R. and Bjorksten, K.af (1970) Interference of Iron with the absorption of Tetracyclines in man. Brit. med. J., **4**, 532

Rendi, R. and Ochoa, S. (1962) Effect of chloramphenicol on protein synthesis in cell-free preparations of Escherichia coli. J. biol. Chem., **237**, 3711

Roth, H., Becker, K. L., Shalhoub, R. J. and Katz, S. (1967) Nephrotoxicity of Demethylchlortetracycline Hydrochloride. Arch. intern. Med., **120**, 433

Schultz, J. C., Adamson, J. S., Workman, W. W. and Norman, T. W. (1963) Fatal liver disease after intravenous administration of tetracycline in high dosage. New Engl. J. Med., **269**, 999

Seto, J. T. and Lepper, M. H. (1954) The effect of Chlortetracycline, Oxytetracycline and Tetracycline administered intravenously on hepatic fat content. Antibiotics and Chemotherapy, **4**, 666

Shils, M. E. (1963) Renal disease and the metabolic effects of Tetracycline. Ann. intern. Med., **58**, 389

*Weinberg, E. D. (1954) The influence of inorganic salts on the activity in vitro of oxytetracycline. Antibiot. and Chem., **4**, 35

Weizel, H. A. E. and Dana, D. (1961) Clinical and laboratory experience with a new intravenous tetracycline derivative. Canad. med. Ass. J., **85**, 1091

Wilson, F. (1962) Congenital defects in the newborn. Brit. med. J., **2**, 255

6. Chloramphenicol

INTRODUCTION

Soil collected from a field near Caracas, Venezuela, was found to contain a new actinomycete which Burkholder showed in 1947 inhibited both Gram-positive and Gram-negative bacteria. An antibiotic, isolated from this soil organism, later named Streptomyces venzuelae, was shown to be active against not only a wide range of bacteria, but also against Rickettsiae, and the agent responsible for psittacosis (Erhlich et al, 1947).

The range of activity against micro-organisms, low toxicity in animals, and effective intestinal absorption led to early clinical trials of this new antibiotic named chloramphenicol, which indicated that it might be the first drug effective in the treatment of Rickettsial infections and typhoid fever.

At about this time workers at the University of Illinois independently isolated a streptomyces from which they produced an antibiotic which proved to be identical to chloramphenicol from Parke Davis and Company (Gottlieb et al, 1948).

Elucidation of the structure of chloramphenicol led to its chemical synthesis and this is now the usual method of commercial production. The synthetic compound is identical physically, chemically and therapeutically with the natural fermentation product.

PHARMACOLOGY

Chloramphenicol is a bitter white crystalline substance, slightly soluble in water and very soluble in ethanol, methanol and ethyl ether. It is very stable, being unaffected over a wide range of pH, and it resists boiling. Chemically it contains a nitrophenyl group, a propanediol moiety, and a dichloracetamide side chain.

Chloramphenicol is well absorbed from the gastro-intestinal tract: it can be detected in the blood thirty minutes after an oral dose of 1 g, peak levels occurring in about two hours. After a dose of 4 g by mouth, the maximum plasma concentration ranges from 40 to 60 μg/ml. Conjugated forms, detectable by chemical but not microbiological methods are present in blood, but the active form predominates. The drug is about 60% protein bound.

Its relatively small molecular size allows chloramphenicol to diffuse effectively across many membranes into a wide variety of tissues. Animal studies indicate highest concentrations in the kidney and liver, and lowest in the brain and the cerebrospinal fluid. Concentrations in the cerebrospinal fluid of normal adults may approximate to half the plasma concentration. It is present in bile and milk, and penetrates well into the tissues of the eye. The drug crosses the placental barrier, reaching concentrations in the foetal circulation at least 30% of the simultaneous maternal plasma concentration.

Chloramphenicol is conjugated in the liver and excreted in the urine; small quantities are excreted in the bile and faeces. Up to 90% of an oral dose is excreted in the urine within twenty-four hours, but the antibiotic activity of urinary metabolites accounts for only 10% of the administered dose. Active chloramphenicol is excreted by the glomeruli, and the inactive conjugates are excreted by tubular mechanisms. Probenecid does not affect excretion of the active form of the drug.

ADMINISTRATION: DOSE

Chloramphenicol may be administered orally, intramuscularly or intravenously. Capsules containing 250 mg of the drug is the usual preparation for oral administration. The daily adult dose varies between 1.5 to 3 g. There is a suspension — chloramphenicol palmitate — for paediatric use containing 125 mg in 4 ml. The daily dose ranges from 50-100 mg per kilogramme; absorption of the palmitate is less effective than the crystalline form. The preparation for parenteral use is chloramphenicol sodium succinate, provided in vials containing 1 g. This is useful for treating children, the usual dose being 50 mg/kg/day in divided doses; **premature and newborn infants should not receive more than a total daily dose of 25 mg/kg.**

Ophthalmic preparations are available as drops (0.5%), ointment (1.0%) and aplicaps (1.0%).

Preparations and doses are tabulated at the end of the chapter.

MODE OF ACTION OF CHLORAMPHENICOL

Chloramphenicol inhibits protein synthesis by interacting with ribosomes, but the precise mechanism of ribosomal binding is not yet clear (Weisberger & Wolfe, 1964; Vasquez, 1964). Because of the known toxic effects of chloramphenicol on bone marrow, a good deal of effort has been used in trying to relate the mechanism of inhibition of protein synthesis to mammalian cells. A low concentration of chloramphenicol present for prolonged periods has been found to block protein synthesis in human bone marrow cells (Djordjevic & Szybalski, 1960), and to inhibit antibody synthesis (Ambrose & Coons, 1963).

These observations led to the suggestion that chloramphenicol interferes with the function of m RNA in both mammalian and bacterial cells, the difference in susceptibility of protein systems in the two cells being a function of stability of their respective m RNAs.

Chloramphenicol is, in conventional doses, both bacteriostatic and Rickettsiostatic.

RESISTANCE TO CHLORAMPHENICOL

Some bacteria, but not Rickettsiae, may show in vitro resistance to chloramphenicol when cultured in increasing concentrations of the drug. This type of resistance occurs in stepwise manner similar to the development of penicillin resistance.

In clinical use there is an impressive consistency in the antibacterial effects of chloramphenicol when compared with the frequent variations which are encountered with many other antibiotics. This may be related to its restricted use. Resistance during therapy is not a common problem; cross resistance may occur between chloramphenicol and the tetracyclines with regard to Gram-negative, but rarely with Gram-positive, organisms.

IN VITRO RANGE

Chloramphenicol is active against a wide range of micro-organisms, conspicuously Gram-negative bacteria such as Haemophilus influenzae and Bord. pertussis, many Salmonellae including S. typhi, E. coli, Neisseria, Klebsiella pneumoniae and some strains of Proteus. Corynebacterium diphtheriae, Clostridia, Listeria and Leptospira are sensitive to moderate concentrations; Gram-positive organisms such as streptococci and staphylococci are also sensitive in this range.

Chloramphenicol is effective in treating experimental infections due to Rickettsiae; it is also effective against Mycoplasma and the agents responsible for psittacosis and lymphogranuloma venerum.

Chloramphenicol is inactive against fungi and yeasts and virtually all strains of pseudomonas.

CLINICAL APPLICATION

Because of a small though definite incidence of serious bone marrow effects chloramphenicol therapy should be reserved for those infections where it has been shown to be clearly advantageous, and for infections which have failed to respond to other antibiotics. Efforts should be made not to prolong therapy unnecessarily, and to avoid repeated courses of the drug.

SALMONELLA INFECTIONS

Salmonellae cause infections which differ markedly in their severity, ranging from a mild illness with little vomiting and diarrhoea to a severe blood born infection, which may be life-threatening, as is sometimes seen in typhoid fever. The treatment of these infections must be judged individually for each patient, the vast majority requiring no antibiotic; not all patients with typhoid fever merit antibiotic therapy. Some patients with other salmonella infections, especially if there is evidence of blood stream infection, as with *S. cholerae-suis*, will require chemotherapy.

Chloramphenicol is the antibiotic of choice in typhoid fever. In vitro many drugs have been shown to have an inhibitory effect on *S. typhi*, but of these only two have achieved any practical importance: ampicillin and chloramphenicol. The latter drug has proved effective, and despite the risk of toxicity, and occasional therapeutic failure, chloramphenicol is preferred in typhoid fever. Giving both chloramphenicol and ampicillin together does not achieve a better result than chloramphenicol alone.

Sulphamethoxazole-trimethoprim has shown considerable promise in treating typhoid fever. It will almost certainly have some place in the acute stage of the illness but is unlikely to replace chloramphenicol (see page 139).

Oral therapy with chloramphenicol is usually satisfactory except in severely ill or shocked patients. A large initial dose should be avoided, as there is some evidence that symptoms may be made worse. A convenient regime in adults is to give 1 g on the first day, 1.5 g on the second, 2.0 g on the third and 3.0 g daily thereafter to a total of about 35.0 g. Many different regimes have been used including interrupted courses; whatever regime is followed, patients should be treated for at least 14 days and an adult should receive at least 30 g of the drug. For children a daily dose of 25-100 mg/kg is used.

Pyrexia usually takes between two and five days to return to normal; if a more rapid response is required corticosteroids may be used in conjunction with chloramphenicol. When large doses of both drugs are used a marked fall in body temperature may be precipitated. In treating very toxic patients with high fever, combined therapy would appear to offer a definite advantage; 15 to 20 mg of prednisolone per day is given orally for three or four days and the dose is then gradually reduced. Haemorrhage, perforation and other complications do not appear to be more common with combined therapy.

The antibiotic treatment of paratyphoid infection is similar to typhoid fever; the patients on average will be less ill and chloramphenicol less frequently indicated. The clinical response to treatment with chloramphenicol, or indeed any other antibiotic, of many patients with paratyphoid infection is frequently disappointing. Chloramphenicol has no place in the treatment of the carrier state in salmonella infections.

MENINGITIS

Haemophilus influenzae is a common cause of meningitis, the incidence being virtually confined to children under three years of age. There are no specific clinical features of this meningitis which suggest the diagnosis other than the age group, and that some infants have an upper respiratory illness preceding the meningeal infections. The organism — H. influenzae type B — is sensitive to chloramphenicol usually in concentrations of 0.1 to 5.0 μg/ml. This sensitivity, together with the fact that chloramphenicol obtains cerebrospinal fluid concentrations approximately half that of the plasma, makes this antibiotic the drug of choice in H. influenzae meningitis. Clinical usage confirms this belief. Combination with other drugs is not usually required and intrathecal therapy unnecessary. Treatment with a combination of sulphonamide, and streptomycin given intrathecally and parenterally offers an alternative regime which can produce excellent results but which is more difficult to manage and more technically demanding.

The dose of chloramphenicol for H. influenzae meningitis is, when capsules can be taken, 125 mg/kg/day. Absorption of the palmitate is less satisfactory than chloramphenicol in capsular form, and for this reason it may be wise in young children to use the succinate intramuscularly, in doses of 100 mg/kg/day. Intravenous therapy may be used, calculated on the basis of 75 to 150 mg/kg/day. Treatment should be continued for ten days.

In patients with meningitis who have turbid cerebrospinal fluid in which no organism is identified on Gram-stain chloramphenicol with penicillin should be prescribed, while awaiting the results of culture. This is not ideal treatment and is open to theoretical objections; in practice it is useful, the combination of drugs being active against the majority of the common bacteria responsible for meningitis.

KLEBSIELLA PNEUMONIAE INFECTION

Klebsiella pneumoniae, Friedlander's bacillus, is responsible for less than 5% of all bacterial pneumoniae. However it causes a severe infection often with cavitation and destruction of lung tissue; chloramphenicol combined with streptomycin is the treatment of choice, both drugs being given in full doses.

CHLORAMPHENICOL NOT DRUG OF CHOICE

There is no doubt that chloramphenicol is effective in treating Rickettsial infections; epidemic, murine and scrub typhus, Q fever and Rocky Mountain spotted fever all respond well. The tetracyclines are also highly effective and because of less risk of serious side effects are therefore preferred. Similarly in mycoplasma infections, psittacosis, lymphogranuloma venerum and bubonic plague, though active chloramphenicol takes second place to the tetracyclines. In urinary tract infections chloramphenicol is at a disadvantage in that 90% of the drug in the urine is in an inactive form. Despite this occasionally chloramphenicol may be useful when other antibiotics have failed against such organisms as H. influenzae and Proteus vulgaris.

Claims have been made for chloramphenicol in pertussis; the drug may well have some action if given early in the infection, but is best avoided.

Before the introduction of the penicillinase-resistant penicillins, a combination of chloramphenicol and erythromycin proved effective against many strains of staphylococci. This combination offers an alternative to the recent compounds to which some patients may be hypersensitive.

H. influenzae is a common pathogen in exacerbations of chronic bronchitis and it is tempting to offer chloramphenicol in severe attacks. However, it is in this type of patient that chloramphenicol should be avoided, for repeated courses, or continued prophylaxis may lead to severe bone marrow toxicity. Occasionally in a severe attack in selected patients a single course of chloramphenicol may be justified.

SIDE EFFECTS: TOXICITY

Chloramphenicol divides doctors into those who use it freely and those who use it reluctantly, some perhaps who do not use it at all. This division results from different interpretations of the reports of bone marrow toxicity of the drug.

First, bone marrow toxicity occurs. This simple statement is difficult to substantiate for it must be admitted it can never be proved that any single case of marrow aplasia is incontrovertibly caused by chloramphenicol or indeed any other drug. All the evidence is circumstantial; however, the great weight of evidence, some of which will be examined, indicates that chloramphenicol causes a small number of fatal bone marrow reactions.

Two years after its introduction the first fatal case of aplastic anaemia related to chloramphenicol was reported (Rich et al, 1950), this was soon followed by others indicating that in some patients the drug exerts a serious depression on bone marrow.

In 1952 the US Food and Drug Administration organised a survey to obtain information on all cases of aplastic anaemia, granulocytopoenia and other blood dyscrasias observed since 1949. This investigation was carried out in about 60 cities with a population of more than 100,000. Data were collected from hospitals and individual doctors. This report (quoted by Welch, 1954) revealed a total of 539 cases; of these 55 implicated chloramphenicol alone, 142 related to chloramphenicol and other drugs and 341 cases in which chloramphenicol was not involved. Of the 55 cases associated with chloramphenicol alone 23 developed aplastic anaemia and all died. In these 55 cases there was a preponderant incidence and fatality rate in women.

As a result of these findings various warnings were given to doctors and the manufacturers of the drug were required to include warnings on bottle labels and medical literature describing chloramphenicol. The publicity given to these warnings led to a marked drop in the amount of chloramphenicol prescribed, and the quantities of the drug certified by the US Government showed a precipitous drop.

A second survey (Welch et al, 1954) was carried out in 1953 to determine if the warnings and labelling of chloramphenicol were adequate and safe. A total of 1448 case reports of various blood dyscrasias was collected and in 29 of these chloramphenicol was the only drug known to have been prescribed. There were 269 cases of aplastic anaemia of which 137 (13%) were considered idiopathic. Of the 29 cases ascribed to chloramphenicol 22 had received all their drug before the warnings resulting from the first inquiry. If the blood dyscrasias resulting from the use of chloramphenicol alone uncovered by both surveys are combined, a total of 84 cases is obtained. This is 4.9% of the total 1,706 cases reviewed. A disturbing feature of the second survey was that over 60% of these dyscrasias were shown to occur in children under ten years of age.

Cases of chloramphenicol marrow toxicity continue to occur. Having seen four cases of aplastic anaemia due to chloramphenicol within one month Dameshek issued a new warning, and again emphasised that the drug should not be used for trivial infection (Dameshek, 1960).

In January 1967 the Committee on Safety of Drugs circularised all doctors in the National Health Service pointing out that in the previous two years 24 fatal cases of blood dyscrasias following the administration of chloramphenicol had been reported to the Committee. These reports accounted for 80% of all fatal blood dyscrasias reported to have occurred in patients who received an antibiotic.

With some reservations, arising from the difficulty of obtaining accurate data, it is accepted that chloramphenicol is capable of causing fatal bone marrow toxicity; even more difficult is assessing how frequently this fatal reaction occurs. Underlying all attempts to reach a conclusion on this subject is the incidence of fatal marrow reactions in those who have received no drugs or therapy.

During the period 1956-1958 there was a total of 20 deaths due to aplastic anaemia and agranulocytosis ascribed to chloramphenicol in England and Wales. Of the 20, 13 were female. This increased female sex incidence is also reflected in the number of deaths in the same period due to marrow reactions from all forms of drugs and therapy. There were 55 males and 91 females (Registrar General's Survey 1958). Examination of the surveys for the years 1958 to 1962 gives the total number of deaths ascribed to chloramphenicol and the totals due to all adverse drug reactions and therapy. These data are presented in Table VI.

Unfortunately full details of the amount of chloramphenicol prescribed in any period are virtually impossible to obtain. However, the estimated number of prescriptions for chloramphenicol for the years 1961 - 1965

Table VI. Deaths in England and Wales due to Chloramphenicol and other therapy 1958 - 1962

	1958	1959	1960	1961	1962	1963
Chloramphenicol	13	6	8	14	13	6
Other Therapy	132	136	150	188	220	181

(Extracted from Registrar General's Statistical Surveys - 1958 - 1963)

supplied by the Ministry of Health (personal communication) gives an indication of the quantity of the drug used in each year. Information from other sources tends to corroborate the Ministry's figures. These have been plotted in Figure 4, and together with them are shown the number of deaths ascribed to chloramphenicol in the Registrar General's statistical reviews for the appropriate years.

Realising the inaccuracies of death certification and the incompleteness of the data the two curves indicate a decline both in the amount of chloramphenicol prescribed and in the number of yearly deaths, which is probably more than an interesting coincidence.

Estimates of the frequency of fatalities have varied between 1 in 500 to 1 in 100,000 treated cases (see Today's Drugs, 1964), but no indication is

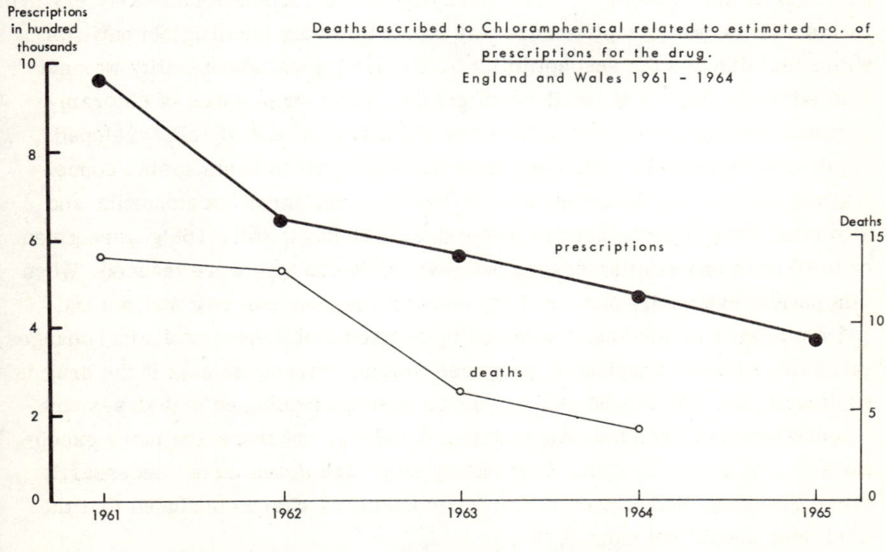

Figure 4. Deaths ascribed to Chloramphenicol related to estimated number of prescriptions for the drug. England and Wales 1961 - 1964.
(Data for the estimated number of prescriptions kindly supplied by the Ministry of Health)

given as to the source of evidence on which these assessments are made. Fatal marrow aplasia has been described after as little as two days therapy when 250 mg was given four times a day, that is two grams total dose (Cone et al, 1952).

PREDICTABLE HAEMATOLOGICAL ABNORMALITIES

When chloramphenicol is prescribed the majority of investigators agree that some haematological abnormality can be detected. Thus Jiji and associates described vacuolation of the proerythroblasts preceded by elevation of the serum iron in eight of ten healthy men given 45-68 mg/kg of chloramphenicol for 13 to 42 days (Jiji et al, 1963); McCurdy was able to correlate increased plasma levels of free chloramphenicol in patients who developed reticulocytopoenia and vacuolated blasts in the marrow (McCurdy, 1963). Total exposure to chloramphenicol, defined as the product of plasma concentration and duration of therapy, was distinctly greater in patients who developed bone marrow toxicity than in those without it. None of these patients developed aplastic anaemia. Gussoff and Lee (1966) studied the haematological effects in ten patients given chloramphenicol, compared with seven who were given tetracycline. These were chronically ill patients, many with liver and renal disease; both antibiotics were given for 21 days in a dose of 3 g/day. No abnormality was noted in the group given tetracycline. Five of the ten patients given chloramphenicol were shown to develop reticulocytopoenia and an average drop in haemoglobin of 2.7 g/100 ml occurring at a mean of 11.2 days, a rise of serum iron (mean 64 μg/100 ml) and cytoplasmic vacuolation of early erythroid forms. There was complete recovery on withdrawing the drug. In patients with renal disease the susceptibility to haematological abnormality was not related to the degree of renal insufficiency. Very large doses of chloramphenicol were given to four patients by Krakoff et al (1955), all developed significant reversible reticulocytopoenia, and a fall in haemoglobin concentration; one patient developed severe leucopoenia, thrombocytopoenia and anaemia. This patient received 184 g during 22 days; later 168 g were given over 20 days and similar severe but reversible changes were induced. When this patient eventually came to post mortem the bone marrow was normal.

Opinion is divided as to whether these predictable haematological changes, inevitably or even frequently, progress to fatal marrow aplasia if the drug is continued. All that can be said is that on average prolonged high doses are frequently found when aplastic anaemia develops, but there are many exceptions to this generalisation. Conversely very high doses do not necessarily cause disaster. Hodgkinson (1954) in reviewing 31 cases concluded that the total dose should not exceed 26 g.

THE GREY SYNDROME

Chloramphenicol therapy in neonates and young infants has led to a number

Table VII. Chloramphenicol

Preparations: Dosage

Drug	Preparation	Dose (Adult)	Dose (Child)
Chloramphenicol (Chloromycetin; Alficetyn)	Capsules 250 mg	1.5 - 3.0 g/day in divided doses	25 - 50 mg/kg/day **Neonates: not more than 25 mg/kg/day**
Chloromycetin Palmitate	Suspension 125 mg/5 ml	-	50 - 100 mg/kg/day
Chloromycetin	Vials (I.M.) 2 g in 4.6 ml	1.0 g/6-12 hrly	100 - 150 mg/kg/day
Chloromycetin Sodium succinate	Vials (I.M.) or S.C.) 250 mg: 1 g	1.0 g/6-8 hrly	50 - 100 mg/kg/day **Neonates: not more than 25 mg/kg/day**
Chloromycetin	Ophthalmic 1. Drops, Vials 25 mg 2. Ointment, 1% 3. Aplicaps, 1%	Twice or more daily	

of deaths (Sutherland, 1959; Burns, 1959). The drug was given in large doses from 100 to 160 mg/kg daily by injection. After two days therapy, vomiting occurred with refusal to suck, irregular rapid respiration and abdominal distention. Flaccidity and an ashen grey colour were noted; hypothermia and circulatory collapse were soon followed by death.

Failure of infants to conjugate chloramphenicol due to deficient glucuronic-conjugating mechanism in the liver is thought to be the cause of this toxic effect (Weiss et al, 1960); inadequate renal excretion of the unconjugated drug may also contribute to the very high blood levels which have been recorded. From these reports it seems clear that high doses of unconjugated drug are responsible for the fatal reactions and not a hypersensitivity state. If the drug is stopped early enough survival is the rule.

CONCLUSIONS

1. Chloramphenicol causes a small number of fatal bone marrow reactions. Unknown host responses are the major factors; other responsible factors are hypersensitivity, and total exposure to the drug.

2. Patients with liver disease, and young infants, should be given the drug in low doses, if at all.

3. During therapy, a reduction in the reticulocyte count or an increase in the serum iron warrant further blood studies. If the reticulocytes are reduced on further examination treatment should be stopped.

OTHER SIDE EFFECTS

Hypersensitivity reactions, although uncommon with chloramphenicol, may result in various skin eruptions; sore mouth and glossitis are relatively common, especially when large doses are used. Nausea, and other gastro-intestinal upsets, while they may occur, are less frequent than with the tetracyclines. Herxheimer-like reactions may be observed if large doses are used initially in treating typhoid fever. Occasionally optic neuritis may occur which can apparently be prevented by large doses of vitamin B_6 and B_{12}. As with all wide spectrum antibiotics, superinfection due to resistant bacteria, or candida may result.

REFERENCES

Ambrose, C. T. and Coons, A. H. (1963) Studies on antibody production, VIII Inhibitory effect of Chloramphenicol on synthesis of antibody in tissue culture. J. exp. Med., **117**, 1075

Burns, L. E., Hodgman, J. E. and Cass, A. B. (1959) Fatal circulatory collapse in premature infants receiving Chloramphenicol. New Engl. J. Med., **261**, 1318

Cahill, K. M. (1962) Chloramphenicol hypersensitivity. A severe haemorrhagic reaction. Lancet, **ii**, 277

Cone, T. E. and Abelson, S. M. (1952) Aplastic anaemia following two days of Chloramphenicol therapy. Case report of a fatality in a 6-year old girl. J. Ped., **41**, 340

Dameshek, W. (1960) Chloramphenicol - a new warning. J. Am. med. Ass., **174**, 1853

Djordjevic, B. and Szybalski, W. (1960) Genetics of human cell lines. III. Incorporation of 5-bromo and 5-iododeoxyuridine into deoxyribonucleic acid of human cells and its effect on radiation sensitivity. J. exp. Med., **112**, 509

Erhlich, J., Bartz, Q. R., Smith, R. M., Joslyn, D. A. and Burkholder, P. R. (1947) Chloromycetin, a new antibiotic from a soil actinomycete. Science, **106**, 417

Gottlieb, D., Bhattachryya, P. K., Anderson, H. W. and Carter, H. E. (1948) Some properties of an antibiotic obtained from a species of Streptomyces. J. Bact., **55**, 409

Gussoff, B. D. and Lee, S. L. (1966) Chloramphenicol induced haematopoietic depression: a controlled comparison with tetracycline. Amer. J. Med. Sec., **251**, 8

Hodkinson, R. (1954) Blood dyscrasias associated with Chloramphenicol. An investigation into the cases in the British Isles. Lancet, i, 285

Jiji, R. M., Gangarosa, M. D. and Fernando de la Macorra (1963) Chloramphenicol and its sulphamoyl analogue. Arch. intern. Med., **3**, 70

Krakoff, I. H., Karnofsky, D. A. and Burchenai, J. H. (1955) Effects of large doses of Chloramphenicol on human subjects. New Engl. J. Med., **253**, 7

McCurdy, P. R. (1963) Plasma concentration of Chloramphenicol and bone marrow suppression. Blood, **21**, 363

Registrar General's Statistical survey of England and Wales. Commentary Vol. III 1958 - 1962. HM Stationery Office, London

Rich, M. W., Ritterhoff, R. J. and Hoffman, R. J. (1950) A fatal case of aplastic anaemia following Chloramphenicol (Chloromycetin) therapy. Ann. intern. Med., **33**, 1459

Sutherland, J. M. (1959) Fatal cardiovascular collapse of infants receiving large amounts of Chloramphenicol. J. dis. Ch., **97**, 761

Today's Drugs (1964) Brit. Med. Ass., Page 27

Vasquez, D. (1964) Uptake and binding of Chloramphenicol by sensitive and resistant organisms. Nature, **203**, 257

Weisberger, A. S. and Wolfe, S. (1964) Effects of Chloramphenicol on protein synthesis. Fed. Proc., **23**, 976

Weiss, C. F., Glazko, A.J. and Weston, J. K. (1960) Chloramphenicol in the newborn infant. A physiological explanation of its toxicity when given in excessive dose. New Engl. Med. J., **262**, 787

Welch, H. (1954) Principles and Practice of Antibiotic Therapy.

Welch, H., Lewis, C. N. and Kerlan, I. (1954) Blood dyscrasias: a nationwide survey. Antibiot. and Chemo., **4**, 607

7. Neomycin and Kanamycin

INTRODUCTION

Four antibiotics, similar to streptomycin, isolated from actinomycetes, have found use clinically. They are, neomycin, kanamycin, paromomycin and framycetin; only the former two will be described. Paromomycin has similar use to neomycin, but is active in amoebic dysentery (Courtney et al, 1960). Framycetin is identical with neomycin B, differing slightly from commercial neomycin, which is a mixture of several compounds.

NEOMYCIN

Neomycin was isolated in 1949 from a strain of Streptomyces fradiae (Waksman & Lechevalier, 1949). It consists of two active compounds, neomycin B and C. Neomycin A was later found to be a degradation product. Commercial preparations consist mostly of Neomycin B sulphate.

PHARMACOLOGY

For practical purposes neomycin sulphate may be considered a single chemical entity with the following characteristics: it is highly water soluble, with low solubility in common organic solvents; it is stable over a wide range of pH; at 37°C in the dry form it is stable for two years, and for at least three months in aqueous solution. Solutions may darken on standing.

Absorption from the gastro-intestinal tract is very limited, about 97% is excreted unchanged in the faeces. The drug is well absorbed after intramuscular injection, 1 g giving plasma levels of 20 μg/ml. Neomycin, after parenteral injection is widely distributed in the tissues, but little reaches the cerebrospinal fluid, and up to 50% is excreted in the urine. Renal insufficiency limits the use of the drug parenterally, for nephrotoxicity and ototoxicity are common. Oral administration, or topical application is associated with a low incidence of toxic reactions.

MODE OF ACTION

The mode of action of neomycin and kanamycin is similar to that of streptomycin, that is they interfere with protein synthesis, by altering ribosomal binding.

RESISTANCE TO NEOMYCIN

Resistance to neomycin develops less quickly than to streptomycin; resistance by staphylococci, though relatively uncommon, may increase when neomycin is widely used to treat nasal carriers of staphylococci. Strains of bacteria which develop resistance to neomycin or kanamycin are also resistant to streptomycin, but the reverse is not always true.

ADMINISTRATION: DOSAGE

The drug is available as tablets of 0.5 g, as a sterile powder in 0.5 g vials for use intramuscularly, and as dermatological or ophthalmic ointments often combined with corticosteroid drugs. It is also available as powder, in a pressurised container, for spraying on the skin, combined with polymyxin B and bacitracin.

Large oral doses, 4-8 g are given daily in divided doses in the treatment of hepatic coma; similar doses have been used in preparation of the bowel for surgery. If given intramuscularly, and there is now very little indication for this, the dose is 0.25 g/6 hourly, provided renal function is normal.

IN VITRO RANGE

Neomycin is a wide spectrum antibiotic, being active against many Gram-positive and Gram-negative organisms, and <u>Myco. tuberculosis</u>. Gram-negative organisms usually sensitive to concentrations of up to 10 μg/ml include <u>Escherichia coli</u>, <u>Klebsiella pneumoniae</u>, <u>Salmonella</u>, <u>Shigella</u>, <u>Proteus vulgaris</u>, <u>Haemophilus influenzae</u>, <u>Neisseria meningitidis</u> and <u>Bordetella pertussis</u>. Gram-positive organisms, also sensitive, include <u>Corynebacterium diphtheriae</u>, <u>Bacillus anthracis</u>, <u>Staphylococcus aureus</u> and <u>Listeria monocytogenes</u>. Neomycin is active against the tubercule bacillus, even though the organism may be insensitive to streptomycin. Streptococci of many groups, including Group A, pneumococci, bacteroides and some staphylococci are relatively insensitive to the action of neomycin.

CLINICAL APPLICATION

Neomycin has a small though useful place in therapy. Given orally it has a definite, but empirical position in the treatment of hepatic failure (Dawson et al, 1957). This use has arisen because resistant strains do not develop very readily to neomycin. The drug may have to be given for prolonged periods in the prevention of portal systemic encephalopathy, and is part of the routine therapy of established hepatic coma. Doses of 4-8 g/day are used unless there is impairment of renal function (Last & Sherlock, 1960). Similar doses are used in preparing the bowel for abdominal surgery; as evidence that this procedure may be beneficial is lacking, it is not recommended. Infections due to <u>E. coli</u>, Salmonella and Shigella, when confined to the gastro-intestinal tract, usually clear spontaneously; neomycin should not be prescribed.

Neomycin is valuable in the local treatment of wounds, and superficial skin and mucous membrane infections due to susceptible organisms such as staphylococci. It is usually given in combination with other antibacterial agents such as polymyxin, bacitracin or chlorhexidine, or with corticosteroid drugs.

In serious systemic infections where other antibiotics have failed and where the responsible organisms are susceptible, neomycin may be given parenterally with justification. Renal function should be normal, the daily dose not exceeding 1 g, and treatment should not be continued for more than 7 to 10 days. To exceed this dose is to invite toxic effects.

SIDE EFFECTS: TOXICITY

The most serious toxic effect of neomycin is on the eighth cranial nerve; deafness occurs during, or occasionally after treatment, is common when the drug is given parenterally and rare when given orally. Renal insufficiency increases the risk of deafness.

Renal tubular necrosis may occur; azotaemia and abnormal urine deposit is common in patients taking parenteral neomycin.

Oral administration of neomycin may result in steatorrhoea; there is reduced absorption of xylose and carotene. A gluten-free diet produced

Table VIII. Neomycin

Preparation	Dose (Adult)	Dose (Child)	Route
Tablets 0.5 g	2-8 g/day divided	1-4 g/day	Oral
Suspension with Kaolin: contains 0.3g neomycin/ 30 ml		5-20 ml 4 times/day	Oral
Neomycin Sulphate powder 0.5 g	0.25 g/6 hrly (when renal function is normal)		I.M.
Cream and ointment with betamethazone Neomycin 0.5% Betamethazone 0.1%	1-3 applications per day	1-3 applications per day	Local application to skin; occlusive dressing may be used
Ophthalmic Drops or ointment Neomycin Sulph. 0.5%	Apply several times/day	Apply several times/day	

inconstant effects on faecal fat output in two subjects with neomycin-induced steatorrhoea (Asatoor et al, 1967). These changes have been attributed to histological alteration, clubbing of jejunal villi (Jacobson et al, 1960) and to a defect of hydrolysis of triolein, which may result either from the intestinal cellular damage or inhibition of lipase action by neomycin (Rogers et al, 1966). These changes are apparently reversible when the drug is stopped.

When injected into body cavities such as the pleura or peritoneum neomycin may cause a curare-like effect, which is reversible by the administration of neostigmine.

Oral administration may result in superinfection causing acute staphylococcal enterocolitis; intestinal candidiasis is occasionally seen.

Neomycin applied to the skin and infected wounds is usually well tolerated, causing no irritation. Occasionally skin eruptions are caused; some of these may well be due, not to hypersensitivity, but a localised monilia infection; neomycin is responsible for a higher incidence of such localised superinfection than other topically applied antibiotics (Waksman, 1950).

KANAMYCIN

INTRODUCTION

Kanamycin, derived from a species of streptomyces found in Japan, was isolated in 1957 (Umezawa, 1957).

PHARMACOLOGY

Chemically, kanamycin is related to neomycin, consisting of two amino sugars linked to a deoxystreptamine. This polybasic water soluble antibiotic in commercial preparations consists of two substances, kanamycin A and B, the latter representing only 3% of the total. It is a white crystalline powder dissolving easily in water to give a solution of pH 6-7.5; solutions may turn dark on exposure to the air, but this has no effect on potency.

Kanamycin is poorly absorbed from the bowel. Intramuscular injection of 1 g gives a peak plasma level of 20 to 35 μg/ml at about one hour; detectable levels persist for up to twelve hours. Higher plasma concentrations occur in older people; very high levels may occur when there is renal insufficiency. Kanamycin is not protein bound. It diffuses into pleural, ascitic, synovial and peritoneal fluids, very little crosses the intact meninges.

The drug is excreted primarily by the renal glomeruli, though some excretion may result from tubular mechanisms. Probenecid does not influence renal clearance. Most of the drug is excreted in the first six hours after injection, urine concentrations in this period ranging from 20 to 100 μg/ml.

RESISTANCE TO KANAMYCIN

Strains of staphylococci and E. coli may develop resistance to kanamycin.

The situation with regard to staphylococci varies widely from region to region and does not seem to be related solely to the frequency with which the drug is used. In Japan where very large quantities of the antibiotic are prescribed, only 0.6% of the strains tested were insensitive to kanamycin, whereas in the United States the figure has been put as high as 30% (Finland, 1966). Pseudomonas strains have developed resistance to a marked degree: of 101 strains examined by Griffith only 22.8% were sensitive to kanamycin (Griffith, 1966).

Resistance of M. tuberculosis to kanamycin may develop; in one series resistance in patients who had previously received the drug, rose from zero in 1960 to 5% in 1965 (Dye, 1966). Organisms which are resistant to streptomycin are frequently sensitive to kanamycin.

ADMINISTRATION: DOSAGE

Kanamycin is available in vials containing 1.43 g kanamycin sulphate, equivalent to 1 g of the base; vials of half this amount are also available. For oral use there are capsules of 250 mg.

The usual adult dose is 0.25 to 0.5 g 6 hourly by the intramuscular route. Total doses greater than 10 g should be avoided. If the drug is used in the presence of azotaemia the dose must be reduced, the object being to achieve plasma concentrations in uraemic patients similar to those in patients with normal renal function. It has been suggested that oliguric patients be given an initial dose of 1 g intramuscularly; this is followed by 0.5 g by the same route at intervals of 2 to 4 days (Kunin, 1966). Clearly the severity of the uraemia will dictate the frequency and size of dose. The dose of kanamycin related to the degree of renal insufficiency is considered in more detail in Chapter 22 (page 259). Blood levels greater than 25 μg/ml should be avoided.

The drug may be given intravenously, and the dose is the same as when the intramuscular route is used.

For children the usual daily dose is 15 mg/kg body weight, given intramuscularly in equally divided doses.

If given orally, the adult dose is 4-6 g/day.

Kanamycin has been given intraperitoneally. The dose recommended is 250 mg in 500 ml of saline twice daily for not more than 3 days (Murdoch, 1966). Doses greater than this may cause a curare-like paralysis.

Kanamycin can be given intrathecally in the following doses: neonatal and premature infants should receive not more than 5 mg in 2 to 3 ml of saline; 25 mg in 10 ml saline for children of 1 year; 50 mg in 10 ml saline for older children; adults may receive 100 mg in 10 ml saline. Intrathecal administration should be carried out not more frequently than once in 24 hours.

IN VITRO RANGE

Kanamycin has a wide range of activity against many Gram-positive and Gram-negative organisms. The useful action of this antibiotic occurs for the most part at concentrations well below plasma concentrations of 30 μg/ml. Concentrations of this order produce toxic effects.

Sensitive bacteria include E. coli, Kl. pneumoniae, Alk. aerogenes, Salmonella, Shigella, M. tuberculosis, atypical mycobacteria, and Staph. aureus.

Most strains of Staph. aureus are sensitive to less than 3.0 μg/ml. Tubercule bacilli are inhibited by concentrations in the range of 2.5 to 10 μg/ml. Some strains of Proteus may be sensitive; Pseudomonas strains are usually insensitive.

It should be remembered that this general guide to in vitro activity may vary from hospital to hospital and may alter with time.

CLINICAL APPLICATION

Kanamycin is a drug effective against a wide range of Gram-negative bacteria, and has some use in the treatment of tuberculosis. It is usually bactericidal; the drug has considerable, though largely predictable ototoxicity: its clinical application is therefore confined to those patients who have serious infections due to Gram-negative organisms, and in certain cases of tuberculosis.

SERIOUS GRAM-NEGATIVE INFECTIONS

i. Septicaemia

Patients in whom Gram-negative septicaemia develops usually have serious underlying disease. This type of infection frequently complicates cholangitis, or surgery on the biliary tract; it is often seen when an infected diverticulum of the colon ruptures, following septic abortion and after multiple injuries. A marked degree of hypotension, not directly attributable to blood loss is a feature of this septicaemic state. Kanamycin is a good drug in this context provided the limitations of reduced renal function are fully appreciated. Treatment may be, indeed will almost invariably have to be, started before the bacteriological cause has been identified. Infections due to the majority of strains of E. coli, Alk. aerogenes, Kl. pneumoniae and Proteus will respond satisfactorily and usually promptly. Even in the presence of renal failure, good results without ototoxicity, can be achieved provided the dose is suitably reduced. This requires that plasma concentrations of the drug can be estimated. If pseudomonas infection is suspected, kanamycin should not be used. Infection with Pseudomonas aeruginosa may be suspected if the patient has suffered widespread burns, if characteristic skin lesions are observed, and sometimes when leukaemia or lymphoma is present.

ii. Neonatal Meningitis

Meningitis in the newborn is difficult to diagnose and very difficult to treat. Organisms responsible for meningitis in this age group include Aerobacter aerogenes, E. coli and salmonella. Any antibiotic which is likely to be effective, with the possible exception of ampicillin, may cause serious side effects. Kanamycin is perhaps the one most useful drug. Given intramuscularly in daily doses of 10-15 mg/kg, adequate cerebrospinal fluid concentrations seem to be obtained. If the response is not considered satisfactory it is justified to give several intrathecal injections of kanamycin at 48 hour intervals. The dose is 1-5 mg in 0.5-1 ml saline according to the size of the infant (Smith, 1966).

It should be remembered that in treating these severe septicaemias and meningeal infections, the ultimate prognosis is dependent for the most part, not on the effectiveness or otherwise of the antibiotic treatment, but is frequently determined by the course of the underlying disorder.

TUBERCULOSIS

There are some dozen drugs now available for treating tuberculosis; kanamycin is by no means the drug of first choice, usually being considered a 'second-line' drug.

Donomae (1958) compared the effect of kanamycin-PAS combination with streptomycin-PAS, and concluded that kanamycin was almost as therapeutically effective as streptomycin. However, these findings were not confirmed by a survey in US Armed Forces (Schwartz, 1959). Kanamycin-resistant strains were common, sputum conversion rare and there was a high incidence of deafness. Many of these cases had failed to respond to previous drug therapy.

Recent work from several sources has suggested a more hopeful if still cautious note. Reports from workers in Japan, Europe and the United States conclude that kanamycin is a useful second-line drug, which can be prescribed with other anti-tuberculous agents, and that its chief application is in retreatment, or in treatment of tuberculous patients undergoing surgery; occasionally it may be useful as a first line drug in those allergic to streptomycin (Kreis, 1966; Kass, 1966; Kitamoto, 1966).

The drug is best given five days per week for four months in doses of 15-20 mg/kg/day, either as a single or in split doses. The plasma level six hours after injection is optimally 20 μg/ml.

Because of the distinct danger of eighth nerve damage Kass (1966) recommends that the drug be given cautiously if the patient is over 50 years old, if the six hour serum level is greater than 25 μg/ml, if the patient has reduced renal function, if there are audiometric changes prior to starting therapy and if more than 20 mg/kg/day is required to achieve the desired six hour serum level.

TOXICITY: SIDE EFFECTS

HYPERSENSITIVITY

Fever, eosinophilia, rashes occurring during treatment with kanamycin have been attributed to hypersensitivity. Anaphalaxis has been described.

Local reactions include pain at the site of injection, sterile abscess, ecchymosis. Diarrhoea and other gastro-intestinal upset may occasionally occur, but is rare during parenteral therapy. Staphylococcal enterocolitis and other superinfections occur.

NEUROTOXICITY

i. Cranial Nerve Damage

The most important toxicity resulting from kanamycin therapy is damage to the cochlea; vestibular damage also occurs, and there is one report of temporary impairment of the ninth cranial nerve resulting in hypertension, tachycardia and loss of taste in the posterior third of the tongue (Corcoran et al, 1960).

Auditory damage is usually bilateral and irreversible; hearing loss does not often progress after stopping treatment unless renal damage prolongs raised plasma levels of the drug. Ototoxicity is directly related to the height and duration of plasma levels and to cochlear susceptibility. Deafness is therefore to some extent predictable. Damage to the outer hair cells of the cochlea is thought to be responsible for this auditory toxic effect.

Certain factors predispose to hearing loss: (i) perceptive deafness whether or not due to previous treatment with ototoxic drugs; (ii) age: ototoxicity occurs earlier in the course of treatment with older patients; (iii) impaired renal function, causing raised blood levels of the drug; (iv) total dose of the drug. If audiometric examinations are carried out, hearing loss may be demonstrated frequently — in one report the incidence was as high as 87% in those given kanamycin parenterally (Frost et al, 1960). If the drug is stopped as soon as there is audiometric evidence of change, conversation hearing loss may be prevented.

Vestibular damage may also occur; vertigo is the common symptom and this usually disappears when the drug is withdrawn.

ii. Curare-like effect

Neuromuscular blockade which can lead to paralysis of respiration may occur particularly after intraperitoneal administration, but it has also followed intravenous therapy. Reversal of the blockade does not always follow a consistent pattern of response. Calcium gluconate is usually recommended but this failed in at least one case where neostigmine succeeded (Ream, 1963); alternatively in another case when edrophonium had not produced a response calcium gluconate was effective (Mullett & Keare, 1961).

Paresthesiae, often circumoral, headaches, restlessness and nervousness are sometimes found in patients receiving the drug.

NEPHROTOXICITY

Nephrotoxicity during kanamycin therapy is primarily of importance because it may predispose to cranial nerve damage, it may occasionally be significant in its own right. Many patients, especially at high dosage, show proteinuria; hyaline and granular casts are frequently found in urine samples and haematuria and cylindruria may occur. These changes, though undesirable, are not significant and usually disappear when the drug is stopped. Azotaemia and oliguria may occur, and rarely acute tubular necrosis results. Older patients, and those with pre-existing renal damage have an increased susceptibility to renal toxicity from kanamycin.

Table IX. Kanamycin

Preparation	Dose (Adult)	Dose (Child)	Route
Capsules 250 mg	4-6 g/day		Oral
Vials 0.5 g/2 ml 1.0 g/3 ml	0.25-0.5 g 6 hrly Total dose NOT to exceed 10.0 g	15 mg/kg/day divided 5 days	I.M.
Vials 0.5 g/2 ml 1.0 g/3 ml	25 mg in 10 ml saline once per day	i. Neonate: 1-5 mg in 0.5-1 ml saline once per day ii. 1-10 years 12.5 mg in 10 ml saline once per day	Intrathecal
Vials 0.5 g/2 ml 1.0 g/3 ml	250 mg in 500 ml saline twice daily Maximum 3 days		Intraperitoneal

REFERENCES

NEOMYCIN

Asatoor, A. M., Chamberlain, M. J., Emmerson, B. T., Johnson, J. R., Levi, A. J. and Milne, M. D. (1967) Metabolic effects of oral Neomycin. Clin. Sci., **33**, 111

Courtney, K. O., Thompson, P. E., Hodgkinson, R. and Fitzsimmons, J. R. (1960) Paromomycin as a therapeutic substance for intestinal amoebiasis and bacterial enteritis. Antibiotic Annual 1950-1960. 304

Dawson, A. M., McLaren, J. and Sherlock, S. (1957) Neomycin in the management of hepatic coma. Lancet, ii, 1263

Jacobson, E. D., Chodos, R. B. and Faloon, W. W. (1960) An experimental malabsorption syndrome induced by Neomycin. Amer. J. Med., **28**, 524

Last, P. M. and Sherlock, S. (1960) Systemic absorption of orally administered neomycin in liver disease. New Engl. J. Med., **262**, 385

Rogers, A. I., Vloedman, D. A., Bloom, E. C. and Kalser, M. H. (1966) Neomycin induced steatorrhoea. A preliminary report on the in vitro

hydrolysis of long-chain unsaturated fat. J. Amer. med. Ass., 197, 117
Waksman, S. A. (1950) 'Neomycin'. Rutgers University Press. Page 193
Waksman, S. A. and Lechevalier, H. A. (1949) Neomycin a new antibiotic, active against streptomycin-resistant bacteria, including tuberculosis organisms. Science, **109**, 305

KANAMYCIN

Corcoran, A. C., Imperial, E. S. and Smith, H. E. (1960) Neurogenic hypertension. A sequel of Kanamycin intoxication. J. Amer. med. Ass., **174**, 1838
Donomae, I. (1958) Clinical studies of Kanamycin treatment of pulmonary tuberculosis. Ann. NY Acad. Sci., **76**, 166
Dye, W. E. (1966) Bacteriology of tuberculosis with special reference to Kanamycin and related drugs. Ann. NY Acad. Sci., **132**, 901
Finland, M. (1966) Summary of the conference on Kanamycin appraisal after eight years of clinical application. Ann. NY Acad. Sci., **132**, 1045
Frost, J. O., Hawkins, J. E. and Daly, J. F. (1960) Kanamycin. II Ototoxicity. Amer. Rev. resp. Dis., **82**, 23
Griffith, L. J. (1966) Development of resistance to Kanamycin. Ann. NY Acad. Sci., **132**, 796
Kass, I. (1966) Kanamycin in the therapy of pulmonary tuberculosis in the United States. Ann. NY Acad. Sci., **132**, 892
Kitamoto, O. (1966) Kanamycin: its therapeutic record in pulmonary tuberculosis in Japan. Ann. NY Acad. Sci., **132**, 905
Kreis, B. (1966) Kanamycin: its therapeutic record in France and other European countries. Ann. NY Acad. Sci., **132**, 912
Kunin, C. M. (1966) Absorption, distribution, excretion and fate of kanamycin. Ann. NY Acad. Sci., **132**, 811
Mullett, R. D. and Kears, A. S. (1961) Apnoea and respiratory insufficiency after intraperitoneal administration of kanamycin. Surgery, **49**, 530
Murdoch, J. McC. (1966) Dangers of Antibiotic Therapy. In 'Therapeutic use of antibiotics in hospital practice'. (Ed) M. Ridly and L.Phillips. E. & S. Livingstone, Edinburgh. Page 79
Ream, C. R. (1963) Respiratory and cardiac arrest after intravenous administration of Kanamycin with reversal of toxic effects by neostigmine. Ann. intern. Med., **59**, 384
Schwartz, W. S. US Veterans' Bureau Trans. 18th Conf. Chemotherapy Tuberc. Page 343
Smith, M. H. D. (1966) Kanamycin: appraisal after eight years of clinical application. The status of kanamycin therapy in the newborn and in infancy. Ann. NY Acad. Sci., **132**, 1030
Sørenen, A. W. S., Szabo, L., Pedersen, A. and Scharff, A. (1967) Correlation between renal function and its application to dosage adjustment. Postgraduate Med. J. Suppl. May, 1967. Page 37
Umezawa, H., Ueda, M., Maeda, K., Yagishita, K., Kondo, S., Okami, Y., Utahara, R., Osato, Y., Nitta, K. and Takeuchi, T. (1957) Production and isolation of a new antibiotic, Kanamycin. J. Antibiotics (Tokyo), Ser. A, **10**, 181

8. Erythromycin and Oleandomycin

INTRODUCTION

Erythromycin and the related oleandomycin belong to a group of antibiotics which have been named 'macrolides' because their chemical structure contains a macrocyclic lacton ring. These compounds have a complicated structure, a molecular weight of more than 700 and have unusual nitrogen containing sugars. Erythromycin was discovered in 1952 in the metabolic products of a strain of Streptomyces erythreus waksman, from soil obtained in the Phillipines.

PHARMACOLOGY

Erythromycin is a whitish, faintly yellow crystalline substance, soluble in water to a limited extent, but readily so in ethanol and other organic solvents. In acid solution erythromycin is unstable, but is stable in neutral solution for weeks at refrigerator temperatures. At room temperature there is loss of activity after a few days.

Erythromycin base is absorbed in the small intestine, but its activity is reduced due to the action of acid in the stomach. This fact, together with the finding that food in the stomach delays absorption, leads to irregular, unpredictable plasma levels. To avoid these difficulties, tablets of erythromycin coated with acid-resistant material, or better absorbed esters of erythromycin, are used.

Erythromycin estolate, the propionyl ester in the form of the lauryl sulphate, is better absorbed in the fasting state, and is more resistant to the action of gastric acid than the parent compound.

Oral administration of erythromycin base, or stearate which is broken down in the intestine liberating the base, gives peak plasma levels in one to four hours. After a single dose of 250 mg in 20 fasting subjects, Griffith found a mean 4 hour plasma level of 0.15 μg/ml when erythromycin base was prescribed in capsules: given as coated tablets of the base the concentration was 0.54 μg/ml, and 1.06 μg/ml when propionyl erythromycin was used (Griffith, 1959).

Administered orally or parenterally erythromycin diffuses well into body fluids and tissues with the exception of the brain. It tends to be retained in liver and spleen. It enters into the pleural and peritoneal cavities and the concentration in prostatic fluid is in the region of one third the plasma concentration. Very little erythromycin crosses the normal meninges into the cerebrospinal fluid. When meningitis is present sufficient erythromycin may get into the cerebrospinal fluid to be therapeutically useful. In a small series of patients with bacterial meningitis Romansky and associates found cerebrospinal fluid erythromycin concentrations in the range 0.3-2.5 μg/ml when the simultaneous plasma concentrations varied from 5-20 μg/ml (Romansky et al, 1956).

Erythromycin crosses the placental barrier, foetal blood levels being up to 20% of the maternal plasma concentration.

The drug is excreted chiefly in bile where the concentrations reached may be up to 1000 times that of the blood when erythromycin is given as base. Bile concentration after administering the propionyl ester is considerably lower.

Urine concentrations are low — about 5% of an oral dose being excreted in the urine in active form.

MODE OF ACTION

The precise mode of action of erythromycin is not clear. It inhibits protein synthesis in E. coli (Brock & Brock, 1959) and has been shown to compete for ribosomal binding sites with radioactive chloramphenicol (Vasquez, 1963). As chloramphenicol binds to the 50s ribosomal subunit it is inferred that erythromycin also binds at this site. Erythromycin may be either bactericidal or bacteriostatic depending on the organisms and the concentration of the drug.

RESISTANCE TO ERYTHROMYCIN

Resistance of staphylococci to erythromycin develops more quickly than to any other antibiotic except streptomycin. When the drug is used frequently in hospital, resistant staphylococci become much commoner; this spread of resistant strains may occur rapidly (Lepper et al, 1954). Resistance has been produced in vitro by strains of Str. pneumoniae, Str. pyogenes, Str. viridans, and enterococci.

Erythromycin-resistant organisms are not known to elaborate any drug-destroying enzyme; resistant staphylococci often produce colonies that are deficient in pigment and coagulase production may be reduced.

During a short course of erythromycin, resistance is seldom encountered; it is common during long term treatment. There is almost complete cross-resistance between erythromycin and oleandomycin in vitro; erythromycin-resistant staphylococci obtained from patients are not necessarily resistant to oleandomycin.

ADMINISTRATION: DOSE

Erythromycin is usually administered orally; it is available as the base or stearate in tablets of 100 mg and 250 mg, or as erythromycin estolate (lauryl sulphate salt of proprionic acid of erythromycin) in capsules (pulvules) of 125 mg or 250 mg. For oral use in children there is a suspension of erythromycin base or stearate containing 100 mg/5 ml. Erythromycin lactobionate is available in ampoules of 300 mg, or the glucoheptonate in ampoules of 250 mg for intravenous administration. For intramuscular use there is erythromycin ethyl succinate in ampoules of 2 ml containing 50 mg erythromycin per ml.

The oral dose of erythromycin for adults is 1 to 2 g/day in divided doses: usually at 6 hour intervals. For infants weighing up to 25 lbs the oral dose is 5 mg/kg every 6 hours; children over 25 lbs are given 125 mg 6 hourly, and over 50 lbs 250 mg 6 hourly.

Intramuscular injections are painful and are not recommended. Intravenous injection in severe infections may be used in doses of 250 to 1 g 6 hrly. Severe thrombophlebitis at the site of injection is common.

IN VITRO RANGE

Erythromycin has an antibacterial range similar to penicillin G. It is most active against Gram-positive cocci such as Group A haemolytic streptococci and enterococci, Staph. aureus and pneumococci. The pathogenic Neisseria, C. diphtheriae, some strains of H. influenzae, and some Rickettsiae are inhibited by low concentrations. Coliform bacteria are insensitive.

CLINICAL APPLICATION

ALTERNATIVE TO PENICILLIN G

In patients hypersensitive to penicillin G, erythromycin is an acceptable alternative in a number of infections. Thus, infections due to Group A haemolytic streptococci such as tonsillitis, erysipelas and scarlet fever respond satisfactorily. It is also useful in the treatment of diphtheria carrier state.

STAPHYLOCOCCAL INFECTIONS

In the treatment of staphylococcal infections erythromycin has a place in management of infections due to Staph. aureus whether penicillin sensitive or resistant. It was common practice in many hospitals to restrain the prescribing of erythromycin and use the drug only for severe penicillin-insensitive staphylococci. Staphylococci quickly become resistant to erythromycin. Now that penicillinase-resistant penicillins and cephalosporin derivatives are available one is much less dependent on erythromycin. It is none the less a useful alternative in what can be a difficult situation.

MISCELLANEOUS INFECTIONS

Erythromycin has been used in the treatment of syphilis and gonorrhoea. Pneumococcal meningitis, in patients hypersensitive to penicillin has been treated successfully by intravenous erythromycin without intrathecal injection.

SIDE EFFECTS: TOXICITY

Untoward effects resulting from the use of erythromycin and its salts are rare. Hypersensitivity manifestations such as fever, eosinophilia and skin eruptions occur. Erythromycin estolate may cause jaundice which is often severe but reversible. This usually occurs after the patient has taken the drug for more than 10 days; there is upper abdominal pain, fever and possibly nausea and vomiting. Leucocytosis and eosinophilia occur; there is increase in the serum bilirubin and transaminase levels. The cholecystogram is normal and liver biopsy shows periportal infiltration mostly with eosinophils. The whole picture suggests an acute jaundice of the cholestatic type, almost certainly a hypersensitivity phenomenon. It is not clear how frequently this toxic reaction is likely to occur.

Gastro-intestinal upset may occur from the use of erythromycin in any form. Diarrhoea sometimes results, more troublesome than dangerous for the relatively narrow spectrum of erythromycin causes less change in the intestinal flora than is expected with wide spectrum drugs such as tetracyclines or ampicillin. Superinfections, especially with Candida, may occasionally occur.

OLEANDOMYCIN

This antibiotic and the related triacetyloleandomycin are similar to erythromycin. They have the same antibacterial range, and probably have similar mechanisms of antibacterial action. Better absorption is obtained with triacetyloleandomycin than with the parent compound, but the ester can cause jaundice.

Erythromycin is at least twice as active as oleandomycin against Staph. aureus when in vitro comparison is made; against Str. pyogenes there is an even greater differential effect in favour of erythromycin.

Oral administration of 250 mg of oleandomycin gives maximum plasma concentrations of about 3 μg/ml in 3 hours. After absorption the drug is distributed throughout the body tissues: appreciable quantities may reach the cerebrospinal fluid, even in the absence of meningitis.

Oleandomycin phosphate is available in capsules of 250 mg; the usual daily dose is 1-2 g in divided doses for an adult; children may be given 6-10 mg/kg every 6 hours.

Table X. Erythromycin. Oleandomycin

DRUG	PREPARATION	DOSE (Adult)	DOSE (Child)
Erythromycin Base	Tablets 100 mg 250 mg		Up to 12 kg: 25 mg/kg/6 hrly
Erythromycin Stearate	Tablets 100 mg 250 mg		12 to 25 kg: 125 mg/6 hrly over 25 kg: 250 mg/6 hrly
Erythromycin estolate (laurylsulphate of Proprionic acid)	Capsules 125 mg, 250 mg (pulvules)	1-2 g/24 hr divided doses usually at 6 hourly intervals	
Erythromycin base or stearate	Suspension 100 mg/5 ml		
Erythromycin i. lactobionate ii. glucoheptonate	Amps. 300 mg I.V. Amps. 250 mg I.V.	250 mg- 1 g 6 hourly	30 mg/kg/24 hr
Erythromycin ethyl succinate	Amps. 2 ml 50 mg/ml I.M. (painful)	100 mg 8 hourly	3-4 mg/kg/8 hrly
Oleandomycin phosphate	Capsules 250 mg		
Triacetyloleandomycin	Caps. 250 mg Suspension 125 mg/5 ml	250-500 mg 6 hourly	30-40 mg/kg/day
Sigmamycin	Caps. oleandomycin 83 mg tetracycline 67 mg	1 to 2 caps. 4 times/day	
Sigmamycin	Syrup oleandomycin 41.7 mg Tetracycline 83.3 mg in each 5 ml	10-20 ml 4 times/day	5-10 mg 4 times/day

A combination of oleandomycin and tetracycline hydrochloride, Sigmamycin (Pfizer) has been used; it is doubtful if there is any synergism between these antibiotics.

SIDE EFFECTS: TOXICITY

Allergic reactions are mild, intestinal upsets may occur with oleandomycin. Triacetyloleandomycin can cause jaundice. Super-infections may occur.

REFERENCES

Brock, T. D. and Brock, M. L. (1959) Similarity in mode of action of Chloramphenicol and Erythromycin. Biochim. biophys. Acta, **33**, 274

Griffith, R. S. (1959) Laboratory and clinical studies with Erythromycin Propionate. Antibiotic Annual 1958-1959, 364

Lepper, M. H., Moulton, B., Dowling, H. F., Jackson, G. G. and Kofman, S. (1954) Epidemiology of Erythromycin-resistant Staphylococci in a hospital population; effect on therapeutic activity of erythromycin. Antibiotic Annual 1953-1954, 308

Romansky, M. J., Nasou, J. P., Davis, D. S. and Ritts, R. E. (1956) The treatment of one hundred and seventy-one patients with Erythromycin, including one hundred and thirty-two with Bacterial Pneumonia. Antibiotics Annual 1958-1959, 48. Med. Enc. Inc., New York

Vasquez, D. (1963) Antibiotics which affect protein synthesis: the uptake of ^{14}C-chloramphenicol by bacteria. Biochem and Biophys. Res. Commun., **12**, 409

9. Miscellaneous Antibiotics

POLYMYXINS

Five polymyxins, A, B, C, D and E have been described; they all have similar antibacterial activity, but differ in their toxicity for animals and man. Only two, polymyxins B and E are commercially available, polymyxin E being identical to colistin.

These antibiotics are obtained from various strains of a soil organism Bacillus polymyxa. They are basic polypeptides whose salts are stable at low pH and withstand heating to 100°C for up to one hour. They are readily soluble in water and methanol.

POLYMYXIN B

Polymyxin B is poorly absorbed when given orally; similarly, little of the drug gets into the circulation when it is applied to the conjunctivae or to extensive areas of mucous membrane. Plasma levels after intramuscular injection are usually low, and this is explained on the basis of the in vitro finding that 50% of the activity of the drug is lost immediately on mixing with serum. When doses of 2-4 mg per kg per 24 hours were given serum levels in the range of 1 to 8 μg/ml were found. If the injections were given at 6 hourly intervals a peak level of 30 μg/ml was reached after the fourth injection (Pulaski et al, 1949). Assay of polymyxin is difficult, and serum levels may not always be reliable. Excretion is mainly by the kidneys, but is delayed, very little being found in the urine twelve hours after treatment, but excretion continues for up to three days after the drug is withdrawn. Renal insufficiency results in high blood levels. Very little polymyxin B enters the cerebrospinal fluid.

MODE OF ACTION

Polymyxin B appears to act on the lipoprotein protoplast membrane, causing its disruption resulting in the escape of cell contents.

There is complete cross resistance between the various polymyxins, but not between polymyxin B and any other antibiotic. Because of impurities the dose of polymyxin B is often given in units: 1 mg of the pure base being equal to 10,000 units.

The antibacterial action of the polymyxins is confined to Gram-negative organisms. Many strains of Gram-negative bacilli are inhibited by concentrations of 2.0 μg/ml; most strains of Ps. aeruginosa can be inhibited by concentrations up to 8.0 μg/ml. Many strains of Proteus, E. coli, Aerobacter and some Neisseria are resistant.

Polymyxin B sulphate is available as tablets of 25 or 50 mg, as an ophthalmic ointment (2 mg/g) and as a topical powder or optic solution. For intramuscular use the sulphomethylated derivative is less painful than the parent compound. It is available in rubber-capped vials each containing 500,000 units equivalent to 50 mg. Doses are given in the table at the end of this section.

CLINICAL APPLICATION

Polymyxins B and E have been widely used, and may continue to be used in treating infections due to Ps. aeruginosa and occasionally other Gram-negative bacilli. Gentamicin has similar antibacterial range and toxicity and possesses some advantages, but these three drugs may well become redundant if carbenicillin proves to be as beneficial as early trials indicate.

URINARY TRACT INFECTIONS

Urinary tract infections due to Ps. aeruginosa are difficult to treat, but may respond to polymyxin B. From 2 to 2.5 mg/kg/day is often effective in acute pyelonephritis in adults. Hawetz reported permanent cure in four patients with acute pyelonephritis when polymyxin B was given in doses of 1.5-2.8 mg/kg/day intramuscularly for 6-8 days. However, in eight patients with chronic pyelonephritis treated with similar doses for 6-11 days the same author reported only temporary suppression of organisms with later relapse in all patients (Jawetz, 1952). In a group of patients with severe renal disease polymyxin B and colistin were well tolerated in reduced dosage in the treatment of Gram-negative infections (Atuk et al, 1964).

MENINGITIS

Meningitis due to Ps. aeruginosa may be treated with polymyxins. They are also useful when Gram-negative organisms, resistant to other antibiotics, are responsible for meningeal infection. This situation is most likely to arise in patients ill in hospital who have received a number of antibacterial agents or in patients with extensive infected burns; it may sometimes occur as a complication of neurosurgical procedures, lumbar puncture, or after genito-urinary manipulations.

Hayes and Yow (1950) describe the case of a 17-year old girl who developed meningitis after spinal anaesthesia. Three days after the anaesthetic the cerebrospinal fluid was examined, but it was not until two months later that Ps. aeruginosa was grown from it. After nine weeks treatment with penicillin, dihydrostreptomycin, sulphadiazine and chlortetracycline, polymyxin was started. It was given in 80 mg doses intramuscularly every 6 hours and 2 mg intrathecally every 12 hours, for three injections. Within 24 hours of starting treatment the cerebrospinal fluid was sterile, but 10 days later Ps.aeruginosa was again cultured. This patient showed side effects of nausea, vomiting and albuminuria, but normal health was eventually regained after six months. A similar type of case was reported by Tomlin (1951) in a patient who had an endoscopy following renal colic. Treatment was with intramuscular injections of polymyxin B — 3.2 mg/kg/day given four hourly and intrathecal injections of 5 mg/day for three days. Pain in the legs after intrathecal injections and other severe side effects occurred. Eventually the patient recovered. Jawetz (1952) reported two patients treated with 5 mg intrathecally daily for four days and then every two days for 2-3 weeks. There was permanent cure with sequelae in one patient and in the second the cerebrospinal fluid was sterilised, but hydrocephalus developed; treatment had been started too late. In treating Ps.aeruginosa meningitis (Mead, 1963) recommends polymyxin B 2-4 mg/day intrathecally and 2.5 mg/kg/day intramuscularly in four equally divided doses.

MISCELLANEOUS INFECTIONS

Polymyxin B is indicated in the treatment of infections of the skin, external otitis and burns. In these situations local application is frequently successful in eradicating Ps.aeruginosa, but is less effective against Proteus vulgaris and E.coli. Farrar (1954) reported good results in 10 of 11 patients with external otitis treated with 10% polymyxin B sulphate in propylene glycol acidified with acetic acid. No sensitisation reaction was noted in any patient. Combining polymyxin with an antibiotic effective against Gram-positive organisms has also led to good results. Graves (1952) used a cream containing 0.8 mg polymyxin and 400 units of bacitracin per g and found this highly effective in 100 consecutive cases of external otitis.

Ps.aeruginosa is a frequent cause of corneal ulceration; polymyxin B either applied locally or injected subconjunctivally in amounts up to 20mg/day may be curative.

Pseudomonas pulmonary infection and bacteraemia can often be successfully treated provided deep tissue infections can be drained. As Ps.aeruginosa is an opportunist pathogen frequently manifesting itself late in the course of serious illness the outcome is often fatal. Pseudomonas endocarditis does not respond in the majority of cases.

Table XI. Polymyxin B

PREPARATION	ROUTE	DOSE	PRECAUTION
1. Polymyxin B (Sulphate BP) (Aerosporin)	Local application ointment: cream 0.1 - 1%	Application as indicated	
2. "	Aerosol	1-2 ml sol containing 1,000 to 10,000 IU 4-6 times/day	
3. " Vials of 500,000 IU (containing not less than 6,500 IU/mg)	I.V. infusion	2,000 IU/kg/hrly for 5 doses 25,000 IU/kg/24 hr Total dose, not to exceed 2,000,000 IU, can be given in 500 ml 5% Dextrose in 60 to 90 min	Beware Respiratory depression; doses refer to patients with NORMAL renal function
4. "	Intrathecal	Adults: up to 100,000 IU Children: 20,000 to 40,000 IU in 1-2 ml once or twice daily	
5. Sulphomethylated Polymyxin B (Thiosporin) Vials equivalent to 500,000 IU polymyxin B sulphate	I.M.	Adults: 1,000,000 to 1,500,000 IU/day, as 2-4 injections. Children: 1. Newborn: (5 kg) 80,000 IU/24 hr as 2-4 injections 2. 5 yrs: (15 kg) 250,000 IU/day 3. 10 yrs: (30 kg) 500,000 IU/day	
6. "	subconjunctival injection	5000,000 IU in 1 ml water	

SIDE EFFECTS: TOXICITY

As very little polymyxin B is absorbed from skin and mucous membranes, even prolonged topical application is safe. Hypersensitivity reactions are uncommon. When the drug is given parenterally manifestations of hypersensitivity such as fever or rashes may be noted.

Parenteral therapy may result in nephrotoxicity. Proteinuria, haematuria, cylindruria, can follow doses of 2.5 mg/kg/day; increasing the dose may cause reduction in glomerular filtration rate. These effects are reversible when the drug is withdrawn. In treating 28 patients for 7 days with daily intramuscular doses of 1.5 to 2.8 mg/kg Jawetz (1952) found a slight and transient increase in proteinuria in 7 associated with a significant increase in the white cells and epithelial cells in the urine in 3 patients. No other abnormality was noted, indeed in four cases an initial high serum creatinine or blood non-protein nitrogen level returned to normal during therapy.

In patients with established renal insufficiency the drug must be used with care. Two injections of the usual dose followed either by sharp reduction of withdrawal of the drug has been suggested in the treatment of uraemic patients (Kunin & Finland, 1959).

Neurotoxic symptoms may also result from polymyxin therapy. These consist of peripheral and circumoral paraesthesiae, flushing of the face, drowsiness and ataxia. These subjective symptoms are not accompanied by objective signs, and disappear within 48 hours of withdrawing the antibiotic.

Pain at the site of injection is common. Meningeal irritation may occur after intrathecal injection.

COLISTIN

Colistin is a cyclic polypeptide antibiotic probably identical to polymyxin E, obtained from the soil micro-organism Bacillus polymyxa. The antibiotic has been separated into two fractions, Colistin A and B, occasionally a third fraction Colistin C is present.

In antibacterial range colistin is similar to polymyxin B, being active against Gram-negative bacilli and particularly useful for its bactericidal action against Pseudomonas aeruginosa.

Colistin is very poorly absorbed from the gastro-intestinal tract except, possibly in very young children. After injection the methane sulphonate salt is hydrolysed, producing colistin in the tissues; this gives a depot effect with slow release of antibiotic into the circulation. After intramuscular injections of 1,500,000 units of colistin sulphomethate (12,500 units - 1 mg) serum levels of 14 μg/ml (175 units/ml) were found at two hours; three hours after injecting 3,000,000 units the level was 25 μg/ml (McMillan et al, 1962). A single injection of 1,000,000 units gave serum levels of 8 μg/ml (100 units/ml) one hour after injection, and these levels persisted for seven hours in three of five patients injected (Colley & Frankel, 1963).

After parenteral injection there is distribution throughout the body fluids. Polymyxin E, in common with other polymyxins tested, was not found in the cerebrospinal fluid of rabbits (Brownlee et al, 1952) and it has been thought that colistin does not cross the blood brain barrier. In studies on children, however, Gomirato Sandrucci (1958) found cerebrospinal fluid concentrations one third to one half the plasma level, and when meningeal inflammation is present the cerebrospinal level of the drug approached that in the plasma.

After parenteral injection a large proportion of the drug is excreted in the urine, high urine levels of the drug are obtained up to twelve hours after administration. The drug has been detected in bile, and in the milk of nursing mothers.

Colistin sulphate is available as tablets containing 1,500,000 units or 250,000 units or in syrup form, an 80 ml bottle containing 4,000,000 units. Colistin sulphomethate sodium is issued in vials of 500,000 units and 1,000,000 units. For topical use there are 1 g and 5 g vials of colistin sulphate. The nomenclature used in Europe and America differs. The unit of colistin was defined in 1957 as being the minimum amount of that substance capable of inhibiting a standard strain of E.coli in 1 ml of broth culture at pH 7.2. The standard preparation of colistin sulphomethate sodium BP contains 12,500 units per mg, and the standard preparation of colistin sulphate BP contains 19,500 units per mg. Colistin base is not used therapeutically, 1 mg of which approximates 30,000 units, but blood levels and minimum inhibitory concentrations are often expressed in terms of the base in American publications. The process of purification of the drug is different in Europe and the US. The result of the American process for purifying colistin sulphomethate sodium is an antibiotic which requires the addition of dibucaine, a local anaesthetic in order to produce a painless injection. This American preparation is **not** suitable for intrathecal injection.

CLINICAL APPLICATION

Clinical indications for the therapeutic use of colistin are similar to those for polymyxin B. In practice this is nearly confined to treating infections due to Ps.aeruginosa, but there is some application in the treatment of infections due to other Gram-negative species such as Klebsiella and Escherichia.

URINARY TRACT INFECTIONS

In urinary tract infections Marsden and Hyde (1962) reported good results in treating ten cases in children; the organisms responsible were Pseudomonas in four, Aerobacter in four, E.coli and mixed Aerobacter and E.coli in one. Colistin sulphomethate was administered intramuscularly in doses ranging from 150,000 - 1,500,000 units daily according to age. The organisms were eliminated in all but one case. Colley and Frankel (1963) had good results in 13 of 18 male paraplegic patients with persistent Klebsiella infection of the urinary tract. In 26 long-standing urinary tract infections Fekety et al (1962) reported good immediate response, but 22 relapsed after withdrawing the drug. A comparison was made between 21 patients treated with colistin, and 17 treated with other antibiotics to which pseudomonas, present in every case, was reported to be sensitive. In all these patients there were either urinary tract abnormalities or recent surgical procedures. Eradication of the organism was obtained in 62% of the colistin-treated group compared with 29% of those given other antibiotics (Brumfitt et al, 1966).

MENINGITIS

Colistin has been used to treat meningitis due to Gram-negative infections. In young children intrathecal injections may not be necessary. The series by Marsden and Hyde (1962) includes two infants, one infected with Ps. aeruginosa the other with E. coli; although both children had meningocoeles, both responded to intramuscular therapy alone. Carroll and Malette (1962) treated three infants suffering from pseudomonas meningitis with four intramuscular injections per 24 hours to a total of 1,000,000 units of colomycin. Recovery occurred with negative cerebrospinal fluid, blood and urine cultures. In adults, a daily intrathecal injection of 500 to 1,000 units per kg may be necessary combined with intramuscular treatment (MacLean, 1962).

MISCELLANEOUS INFECTIONS

There have been several reports of success in treating septicaemia due to pseudomonas (Murdoch, 1964; Holloway & Scott, 1963; Jones et al, 1966). Speirs et al (1963) report an interesting case of an 11-year old boy, previously healthy, with congenital hypogamma-globulinaemia who was successfully treated with colistin.

In treating pseudomonas eye infections colistin has a clear indication (Gordon & McLean, 1960). Hessburg et al (1964) comment on the increase in incidence of pseudomonas keratitis following the use of contact lenses. They treated six cases with a combination of colistin sulphate and sulphacetamide given by continuous corneal lavage via a subpalpebral tube. No eyes were removed; three of the infected eyes had useful vision without further therapy, but three later required corneal transplants.

In skin infections, and especially in burns colonised by pseudomonas, colistin is indicated.

SIDE EFFECTS: TOXICITY

Side effects from colistin appear to be less than with polymyxin B, but they are by no means negligible. Transient oral paraesthesiae, and reversible

Table XII. Coliston (Polymyxin E)

PREPARATION	ROUTE	DOSE
1. Colistin Sulphate BP Tablets 1,500,000 or 250,000 units Syrup. 80 ml bottle containing 4,000,000 units	Oral	Adults: 3,000,000 u 8 hrly Children: Newborn (5 kg): 250,000 u 8 hrly (30 kg): 1,500,000 u 8 hrly
2. Colistin Sulphomethate Sodium BP Vials 500,000 u and 1,000,000 u	I.M.	Adults: 50,000 u/kg/24 hr in 2-4 injections. Five days' treatment usual. Children: Newborn (5 kg): 250,000 u/24 hr 2-4 injections (15 kg): 750,000 u/24 hr 2-4 injections (30 kg): 1,500,000 u/24 hr 2-4 injections
3. "	I.V. by repeated injection	Same dose as for I.M.
4. "	Intrathecal	500-1,000 u/kg one injection daily
5. Eye preparations	1. Drops 1% W/V Colistin Sulphomethate Sodium or Colistin Sulphate in water or saline 2. Subconjunvtival injection 1% Sol. Colistin Sulphomethate Sodium in 0.5% lignocaine	as required

ataxia have been documented after intramuscular colistin sulphomethate. One case of apnoea has been reported. There was weakness with difficulty in breathing three days after starting colistimethate therapy, and three hours after a dose of the drug the patient became unresponsive. The patient finally recovered when the drug was withdrawn (Perkins, 1964).

Azotaemia may be found after large doses. There is one report of the use of very high doses of colistin sulphomethate (10 mega units by intramuscular injection, 10 mega units by intravenous injection and 6 mega units by aerosol inhalation each day) in 14 patients (Price & Graham, 1970). All 14 patients developed acute renal failure and acute tubular necrosis was found in some. Leucopoenia and granulocytopoenia may possibly be associated with the use of colistin. Rashes and superinfection occur.

GENTAMICIN

Gentamicin is a broad spectrum antibiotic, chemically related to streptomycin, isolated from an actinomycete Micromono-spora-purpurea in 1963.

This antibiotic consists of two compounds called gentamicin C and gentamicin C_2 which have similar chemical structure and antibacterial action. Gentamicin is a white powder, water soluble and is usually provided as the sulphate.

This antibiotic is not absorbed in significant quantities from the gastrointestinal tract and is usually given parenterally. A single intramuscular dose of 0.8 mg/kg gives average peak serum concentrations of 4.7 μg/ml. Approximately 30% of an administered dose of gentamicin becomes bound to serum proteins.

Gentamicin is almost completely excreted by glomerular filtration; high concentrations of the drug are found in the urine; renal insufficiency can result in prolonged high plasma levels which increases the risk of eighth nerve toxicity. A small amount of the drug is excreted in the bile.

In antibacterial activity gentamicin has a similar range to kanamycin, excepting that strains of Staph. aureus and Ps. aeruginosa are usually inhibited. Plasma concentrations up to 4 μg/ml will usually inhibit most strains of E. coli, Proteus vulgaris, Klebsiella, and Staph. aureus. Ps. aeruginosa may require concentrations up to 8 μg/ml; the activity of gentamicin against this organism is similar to that of the polymyxins, and these two antibiotics may have an additive effect against strains of pseudomonas (Bulger & Kirby, 1963). In concentrations two to three times the MIC gentamicin is bactericidal.

Gentamicin is available in vials containing 40 mg of base per ml. The intramuscular dose for an adult is 0.8 - 1.2 mg/kg/day given as three equal doses. A total daily dose of 2 mg/kg should not be exceeded. However, Darrell and Waterworth (1967) point out that initial doses of 80 mg are required to produce realistic peak levels (5.4 μg/ml - 10.15 μg/ml and that estimation of plasma concentrations may be required if toxicity is to be avoided.

CLINICAL APPLICATION

Because of its action against Gram-negative organisms especially Ps. aeruginosa and the high urine concentrations obtainable, gentamicin is most likely to be effective in infections of the urinary tract. Barber and Waterworth (1966) were impressed by the in vitro activity of the drug against Ps. aeruginosa and it has had considerable, though not unqualified, success in clinical use. Jao and Jackson (1964) for instance gave 66 courses of the drug to 57 patients in doses of 0.8 mg/kg body weight every 8 hours for the first day and thereafter 0.4 mg/kg every 8 hours for 5-7 days. Urinary infections without obstruction were cured in 15 of 28 patients; patients with bacteraemia and non-urinary infection did not respond well. No failures were noted in Klebsiella or Aerobacter infections; half the patients with pseudomonas infection were cured. Nearly all these patients had severe renal disease and five developed serious labyrinthine disturbance.

Newman and Holt (1967) successfully treated three cases of Gram-negative meningitis (one caused by Ps. aeruginosa and two by Klebsiella aerogenes) in infants operated on for spinal cord defects. These authors gave initially intramuscular doses of 1 mg/kg per day, but later used double this dose; gentamicin was also given intraventricularly in doses of 0.5 to 1.0 mg daily.

Pines et al (1967) used gentamicin in patients with chronic bronchitis in which Ps. aeruginosa or Kl. pneumoniae had been repeatedly isolated in profuse growth. Gentamicin given by intramuscular injection or by inhalation or a combination of these produced results that were not impressive.

Recent assessment of gentamicin has to a large extent confirmed earlier experience, Louria and colleagues (1969) considered gentamicin quite effective in pulmonary infections due to many Gram-negative species particularly when there was no previous underlying disease and Martin and associates (1969) concluded that gentamicin with or without the addition of cephaloridine was one of the most reliable ways of treating serious acute infections presumed to be caused by Gram-negative rods. In children and infants Nunnery and Riley (1969) used gentamicin successfully in the treatment of eleven children with meningitis due to various Gram-negative species. They gave 0.4 mg/kg eight hourly by intramuscular injection; eight of eleven patients responded satisfactorily.

The main indication for the use of gentamicin is therefore in urinary tract infections due to sensitive organisms; meningitis or septicaemia caused by Gram-negative organisms can be successfully treated. It is becoming clear that success in using this antibiotic will depend on administering doses that are close to the toxic range. Another unfortunate disadvantage is that resistance to the drug may occur during treatment.

SIDE EFFECTS: TOXICITY

The chief toxic effect of gentamicin is on the eighth nerve. Both vestibular and auditory branches may be affected, but the former is more susceptible. Because high plasma levels of the drug predispose to toxicity and occur in renal insufficiency the drug should be prescribed in those with severe renal disorders only after careful consideration. (For dose in renal disease see page 260.) Proteinuria, azotaemia and possibly uraemia may be produced. Maculo-papular rashes, urticaria and transient elevation of serum transaminase has been described. To date there have been no reports of serious hypersensitivity phenomena or blood dyscrasias.

BACITRACIN

Bacitracin is a polypeptide antibiotic first produced from an organism found in the contaminated wounds of a patient named Tracy. It exists as three separate compounds, bacitracin A, B and C, the chief constituent of commercial bacitracin being compound A.

The antibacterial range of bacitracin is very similar to that of penicillin G. Resistance is uncommon and develops slowly. Many penicillinase-producing staphylococci are sensitive to this antibiotic, but occasionally staphylococci not exposed to the drug are resistant to its action.

MODE OF ACTION

Bacitracin acts as a cell wall inhibitor in a manner similar to penicillin; uridine nucleotides accumulate, protoplasts are formed and staphylococci are lysed.

The antibacterial activity of bacitracin is defined as the amount which when diluted 1 in 1,024 will inhibit the growth of a strain of Str. pyogenes. To comply with the British Pharmacopoeia, preparations must contain not less than 50 units per mg.

Very little bacitractin is absorbed when it is administered orally; Prigal and Furman (1949) showed that giving the drug as an aerosol led to detectable levels in the urine, but not in the plasma — some absorption presumably having occurred. There is good absorption after intramuscular injection, maximum levels being reached in 1 to 2 hours, and the drug is widely distributed in the tissues. Excretion is by glomerular filtration: 10% to 40% of an intramuscular dose is recovered from the urine within 24 hours.

CLINICAL APPLICATION

Although bacitracin may be administered orally or intramuscularly its present day indications are virtually confined to topical application. It is available as a powder and as dermatological or ophthalmic ointment. The majority of preparations combine bacitracin with another topically useful drug such as polymyxin or neomycin; some preparations contain all three antibiotics and hydrocortisone is sometimes added.

Local application of bacitracin alone, or in combination with other antibiotics, to infected wounds and skin lesions may have limited success. Superficial infection may be cleared, but as the application does not reach the deeper tissues, failures are common. The same rather unpredictable results were reported in ocular infections by Bellows and Farmer (1948); they found that 11 out of 16 patients with acute conjunctivitis responded satisfactorily, and had success in two of three cases with acute kerato-conjunctivitis, but only 6 of 18 cases of chronic conjunctivitis responded. Eggers (1951) reported enthusiastically on the effect of local application of solutions or ointment in the treatment of 400 patients with a variety of ocular infections. Occasionally bacitracin may be instilled into the pleural sac or into infected cavities as in chronic osteomyelitis.

As there is now a number of active drugs, such as the penicillinase-resistant penicillin compounds and cephalosporin derivatives to treat resistant staphylococcal infection there is virtually no indication for parenteral use of the more toxic bacitracin.

If the drug is given parenterally renal toxic effects are common. Proteinuria, cylindruria and haematuria are found; high doses may lead to azotaemia and uraemia.

Hypersensitivity reactions following topical applications are uncommon.

NOVOBIOCIN

Novobiocin was obtained from Streptomyces spheroides or niveus found in Vermont, USA: the original isolations were made simultaneously in several laboratories which led to some confusion. The Food and Drug Administration called the new antibiotic 'novobiocin' in 1956.

It is a dibasic substance usually supplied as the calcium or monosodium salt. The calcium salt is poorly soluble in water; the sodium salt freely soluble in water is less stable than the calcium salt.

In its antibacterial range novobiocin is similar to penicillin but staphylococci and pneumococci are usually more sensitive than Str. pyogenes. The majority of strains of Staphylococci and Pneumococci are inhibited by concentrations up to 1 μg/ml; some staphylococci require concentrations up to 5 μg/ml and a few strains are completely resistant. Concentrations of 1-16 μg/ml will usually inhibit most strains of Group A streptococci, Str. viridans and Str. faecalis. Similar concentrations will inhibit some strains of Proteus mirabilis and Proteus vulgaris.

Novobiocin is well absorbed from the gastro-intestinal tract, especially in children, peak plasma levels are reached in about two hours. There is some accumulation of the drug with the first few doses; an oral dose of 500 mg every six hours provides a plasma concentration frequently above 100 μg/ml.

Novobiocin is widely distributed in the body tissues, although quite a high proportion is protein bound and very little of the drug reaches the cerebrospinal fluid. Almost one third of an orally administered dose is excreted in the faeces in active form, about 3% is passed in the urine, and high concentrations are reached in bile.

MODE OF ACTION

Although novobiocin causes accumulation of cell wall nucleotides in some bacteria it does not induce protoplast formation and it has been assumed that this is not the primary mechanism of action of the drug, which at the moment is unknown.

The drug is available as tablets, each containing 250 mg; the usual adult oral dose is 1-2 g daily in divided doses. For parenteral use vials containing 500 mg novobiocin are available; this is prepared for use by dissolving the contents in 5 ml of the accompanying solvent. If administered intramuscularly the preparation should be used immediately; it is usually a painful injection. For intravenous use the concentrated solution is best diluted in 500 ml to 1000 ml of sterile saline solution and infused by the drip method. The intramuscular or intravenous dose for an adult is usually 0.5 g every six hours.

CLINICAL APPLICATION

Although novobiocin has in the past been used effectively in treating staphylococcal infections, it has little place in therapy today. Staphylococci readily become resistant and side effects are relatively common. The drug has been superseded by more effective and less toxic agents. Combinations of novobiocin with other antibiotics do not seem to offer any advantages.

SIDE EFFECTS: TOXICITY

Skin eruptions and hypersensitivity phenomena are common. More than 10% of patients may show these manifestations which are frequently observed during the second week of treatment, especially if doses are high. Rashes usually disappear quickly when the drug is withdrawn. High fever, eosinophilia, leukopoenia, agranulocytosis, thrombocytopoenia, and Stevens-Johnson syndrome occur. Mild gastro-intestinal upset is common with oral therapy.

Yellow discolouration of the skin and sclerae may be due, either to a lipochrome pigment which is a degradation product of the antibiotic or to a failure of excretion of bilirubin as a result of inhibition of glucuronyltransferase by the drug.

VANCOMYCIN AND RISTOCETINS

These antibiotics have much in common; they have been used chiefly in treating staphylococcal infections, are administered intravenously, and occasionally cause deafness. Ristocetin is no longer available.

Vancomycin, isolated from Streptomyces orientalis in 1956 is a white solid amphoteric substance freely soluble in water. Its mode of action, not fully understood, is probably by inhibition of cell wall mucopeptide with secondary suppression of RNA.

Ristocetin was isolated from Nocardia lurida in 1957. It contains two microbiologically active compounds, ristocetins A and B; ristocetin is soluble in water at pH 5 or higher.

Both vancomycin and ristocetin are poorly absorbed from the intestinal tract and cause pain or even necrosis on intramuscular injection; both are therefore administered intravenously. Vancomycin is available in vials of 10 ml, containing 50 mg/ml of solution; ristocetin is presented as a dry powder in vials containing 500 mg of ristocetin A activity. The usual adult dose of vancomycin is 1 g every 12 or 8 hours; each dose is best given diluted in 100 ml saline or dextrose solution and infused intravenously in 30 minutes. Similarly ristocetin may be given in the adult dose of 0.5 to 1 g every 12 or 8 hours as a 100 ml infusion in 30 minutes.

Both drugs diffuse into body tissues, but only very small quantities reach the cerebrospinal fluid. Excretion is chiefly by the kidney and renal insufficiency leads to persisting high levels of vancomycin.

Vancomycin and ristocetin are active against the majority of species of Gram-positive cocci, the former being about twice as active as the latter. Ristocetin has some antituberculous action. Bactericidal and bacteriostatic concentrations are very similar for each individual drug. Cross resistance between these two antibiotics and others in common use is not observed.

CLINICAL APPLICATION

The production of newer effective antistaphylococcal drugs such as cloxacillin and the cephalosporin derivatives has made vancomycin and ristocetin virtually obsolete. There must be very few occasions when either of these drugs are selected as the first choice in treating staphylococcal infection. None the less they are effective antistaphylococcal agents, and within fairly rigid limitations, a case can be made against discarding them altogether, vancomycin being preferred to ristocetin.

Reports in the literature (Ehrenkranz, 1959; Kirby et al, 1960; Spears & Koch, 1960) indicate that vancomycin is capable of curing various forms of staphylococcal infection including severe conditions such as septicaemia, endocarditis and osteomyelitis. Resistance during treatment has not been a problem; this fact alone probably makes the drug worth retaining.

SIDE EFFECTS: TOXICITY

Thrombophlebitis may occur at the site of intravenous injection of either vancomycin or ristocetin. The former, if given rapidly, causes a sensation of warmth and generalised tingling; rigors and drug fever may be produced.

With vancomycin the most serious toxic effects encountered are deafness and nephrotoxicity. Deafness which may become permanent can progress even when treatment is stopped. High blood levels and renal insufficiency are thought to encourage deafness.

Deafness may also occur with ristocetin; agranulocytosis and thrombocytopoenia are definite hazards when this drug is used.

LINCOMYCIN

Lincomycin, an antibiotic introduced in 1963, was isolated from an organism in soil obtained from Lincoln, Nebraska. It is a monobasic substance isolated as a white crystalline solid, stable in the dry state for at least one year and in aqueous solutions for nine months in both acid and basic solutions. Lincomycin is readily soluble in water.

This antibiotic has a narrow range of antibacterial activity similar to erythromycin, being most active against Gram-positive cocci. Concentrations of up to 0.5 μg/ml inhibit most strains of Str. pneumoniae, group A haemolytic streptococci, Str. viridans; Staph. aureus varies in its sensitivity, the majority of strains being inhibited by concentrations of 2 μg/ml, but some strains survive a concentration of 5 μg/ml (Daikos et al, 1963).

Lincomycin is rapidly absorbed after oral or intramuscular administration; after an oral dose of 500 mg levels above the MIC of most Gram-positive organisms are maintained for about six hours; intramuscular injection of a 600 mg dose gives peak serum levels at 30 minutes and detectable levels are maintained for up to 24 hours. Intravenous infusion of 600 mg lincomycin in 500 ml of 5% glucose in distilled water provides useful plasma levels for 14 hours. After oral, intramuscular or intravenous administration the biological half life is about five hours.

Lincomycin is distributed throughout body tissues; in subjects with normal meninges entry into the cerebrospinal fluid is minimal. The drug is excreted in the urine and in bile. Urinary excretion is very variable, but may account for up to 30%; the mean urinary excretion after a single 500 mg oral dose in a 24 hour period is 4%.

This antibiotic acts by interfering with protein metabolism; the formation of DNA is suppressed.

Lincomycin is available as capsules, each containing 500 mg lincomycin hydrochloride monohydrate, in ampoules of 2 ml sterile solution each containing 600 mg or in syrup form, 5 ml containing 250 mg of the drug. The adult dose is 500 mg three or four times daily orally or up to 600 mg intramuscularly every 12 hours. Larger doses can be used in severe infections. The oral dose in children is from 15-30 mg/lb given in three or four doses during a 24 hour period.

CLINICAL APPLICATION

Although chemically unrelated to other antibiotics lincomycin has many similarities to erythromycin, having essentially a narrow antibacterial range confined for the most part to Gram-positive pathogens.

STREPTOCOCCAL AND PNEUMOCOCCAL INFECTIONS

In infections due to β haemolytic streptococci (Group A) and pneumococci lincomycin is generally effective. In one study (Jackson et al, 1965) patients diagnosed as having streptococcal pharyngitis were divided into two groups with more than 400 patients in each group. One group received oral penicillin and the other lincomycin – an average sized adult was prescribed 500 mg eight hourly by mouth. Results indicated that both drugs were almost equally effective. Holloway and Scott (1965) also comment on the effectiveness in streptococcal and in pneumococcal infections.

STAPHYLOCOCCAL INFECTIONS

MacLeod et al (1964) presented an assessment of lincomycin as an antistaphylococcal agent over an 18 month period. Sensitivity tests on 1,055 unselected cultures of Staphylococcus pyogenes showed that 95% were sensitive to lincomycin, 100% sensitive to methacillin and oxacillin, but only 17% to penicillin G. Of six patients with severe staphylococcal infections (four with septicaemia) three survived: the dose of lincomycin in this group ranged from 15 to 64 g over 5 to 15 days. Seven patients were treated for osteomyelitis by surgical debridement followed by lincomycin therapy. Three had excellent results, one died from pulmonary embolism and three had persisting lesions which, however, were free from pathogenic staphylococci. Good results in osteomyelitis were also reported by Grondin et al (1965) who were impressed with the effectiveness of the drug in chronic cases.

Ability to penetrate into avascular infected bone may prove to be one of the most useful attributes of this antibiotic. Two uses of lincomycin which have been given in preliminary reports will require clarification, namely, its effect on diphtheria and in the diphtheria carrier state (Harnecker et al, 1965), and in its action on L form variants of staphylococci (Kagan et al, 1964).

The restricted antibacterial range of lincomycin imposes certain limitations on its use; within these limitations it may prove to be a useful and relatively non-toxic agent.

SIDE EFFECTS: TOXICITY

The only common side effect is gastro-intestinal upset and diarrhoea. This may occur in 10-20% of patients and is found when the drug is given either orally or intramuscularly. Its cause is not clear.

Jaundice and abnormal liver function tests without jaundice may occur especially with large doses. There have been a few instances of leucopoenia.

The use of lincomycin in pregnancy, in neonates and in patients with liver and kidney disorders should be avoided until further assessment establishes its safety in these situations.

Table XIII. Lincomycin

PREPARATION	ROUTE	DOSE (Adult)	DOSE (Children)
Caps. (500 mg)	Oral	500 mg 3 to 4 times per day	15-30 mg/lb/day in 3 or 4 equal doses
Ampoules (2 ml: 600 mg)	I. M.	600 mg twice daily	5 mg/lb every 12 or 24 hours
Ampoules (2 ml: 600 mg)	I. V.	Infusion 250 ml 5% glucose in water with 600 mg 8-12 hrly	5-10 mg/lb/day in 2 or 3 doses as infusion at 8-12 hr intervals
Syrup (250 mg/5ml)	Oral		15-30 mg/lb/day

CLINDAMYCIN

Clindamycin is a semisynthetic derivative of lincomycin produced by chemical substitution of the 7(R) hydroxyl group of lincomycin by a chloro group in the 7(S) position. It is a white crystalline solid, stable in the dry state, water soluble at room temperature in concentrations up to 100 mg/ml at pH 6.0 and is insoluble in most organic solvents.

Clindamycin and lincomycin have similar ranges of antibacterial action, though clindamycin is considerably more active against the common Gram-positive cocci — including both penicillin G sensitive and resistant strains of Staph. aureus. All of the strains of these organisms tested by Meyers and colleagues (1969) were inhibited by concentrations of 0.015 to 0.3 μg/ml of clindamycin. Enterococci are usually resistant and there seems to be considerable doubt about the sensitivity of Haemophilus influenzae; other Gram-negative species are usually resistant with the exception of Bacteriodes.

Cross-resistance with lincomycin hydrochloride occurs; antagonism has been demonstrated with erythromycin in vitro.

Clindamycin is extremely well absorbed after oral administration; peak serum levels of 1.9 μg/ml were present one hour after an oral dose of 150 mg and this was independent of whether food was taken simultaneously. About 2.4% of the drug was excreted in the urine in a 24 hour period (Meyers et al, 1969). Clindamycin acts by inhibition of protein synthesis.

CLINICAL APPLICATION

Clindamycin like the parent compound lincomycin is indicated in the treatment of infections due to susceptible Gram-positive cocci. Infections of the respiratory tract usually respond satisfactorily and some severe infections such as septicaemia and osteomyelitis have been satisfactorily treated, though many would be reluctant to use an orally administered drug as the sole therapy in these situations. It should also be recalled that resistance during treatment to Staph. aureus can occur and that the drug cannot be administered with erythromycin.

Full assessment of this drug has not yet been carried out; it may well be that its most acceptable place in therapy will be as an alternative to penicillin G in the management of upper respiratory infections, including those due to group A streptococci.

SIDE EFFECTS: TOXICITY

Side effects of clindamycin are few though loose stools occur quite commonly. Other effects occasionally noted include vomiting, nausea, abdominal cramp or pain, rashes, pruritis and hypersensitivity reactions. Abnormal liver function tests and some cases of leucopoenia have been recorded.

Clindamycin may be given to patients with severe uraemia in approximately half conventional doses. Neither peritoneal nor haemodialysis effectively remove clindamycin from the blood.

ADMINISTRATION: DOSAGE

Clindamycin is available as capsules containing either 150 mg or 75 mg and the usual adult dose is 150-300 mg every six hours.

In children a dose of 8-16 mg/kg/day in three or four equal doses is used.

FUCIDIN

Fucidin is the sodium salt of fucidic acid, an antibiotic with a steroid structure chemically related to helvolic acid and cephalosporin Pl. It was isolated from a fungus, Fusidium coccineum in 1962.

The drug is well absorbed from the gastro-intestinal tract: a single oral 0.5 g dose gives plasma levels averaging 17 μg/ml within one hour. Plasma levels are higher if the drug is given in the fasting state. It is widely distributed in the tissues, a large proportion becomes protein bound and only minimal quantities enter the cerebrospinal fluid. It is excreted mainly in bile; 2% of an oral dose may be recovered in the faeces. Very little fucidin is excreted by the kidney.

Fucidin is highly active against most species of Staph. aureus, the minimum inhibitory concentration for the majority of strains being 0.1 μg/ml. It has some action against Neisseria and Mycobacteria, but its main use is as an anti-staphylococcal agent. An acid pH increases in vitro activity of fucidin. In some circumstances fucidin and penicillin combined may have an enhanced action against certain penicillinase-producing staphylococci. Provided that the organism is not a very active penicillinase producer fucidin delays inactivation of penicillin so that the latter may kill the staphylococci. Fucidin-resistant staphylococci can be quickly produced in vitro and they also occur in vivo.

ADMINISTRATION: DOSAGE

Fucidin is available in capsules of 250 mg; the adult dose is 500 mg three times daily. For paediatric use a suspension is available, the usual dose being 20-30 mg/kg per day given in three equal doses.

For topical application fucidin ointment contains sodium fusidate 2% in a neutral base. There is also a wound dressing — Intertulle Fucidin which is impregnated with 2% sodium fusidate ointment.

INTRAVENOUS FUCIDIN

Recently a preparation has been introduced for intravenous use which is issued in two ampoules — one containing diethanolamine fusidate BPC as dry powder (580 mg) equivalent to 500 mg sodium fucidate BP. The second ampoule contains 50 ml sterile phosphate - citrate buffer (pH 7.4-7.6). The diethanolamine fucidate powder is dissolved in the 50 ml of phosphate buffer and is then further diluted to 250-500 ml with physiological saline or other suitable intravenous infusion (not Aminosol). The fucidin infusion is then given over a period of 2-4 hours, and this dose in adults may be given three or four times in 24 hours. The maximum daily dose should not exceed 2 g (4 ampoules). In children the intravenous dose has been calculated on the basis of the oral paediatric dose, 20 mg/kg in three divided doses over 24 hours.

Experience with intravenous fucidin is limited and assessment of possible side effects of this therapy in patients ill with systemic staphylococcal infections is necessarily difficult. The following points should be kept in mind. Venospasm and thrombophlebitis may occur. In some experimental animals when fucidin given intravenously resulted in plasma levels of over 300 μg/ml a slight haemolytic effect was noted. In one patient a rise in 'free' haemoglobin was noted and jaundice occurred in several. It is not certain that these effects were related to intravenous fucidin therapy.

CLINICAL APPLICATION

Fucidin has been used almost entirely as an anti-staphylococcal agent; there are many reports of its effectiveness in severe staphylococcal infection, sometimes improvement occurs dramatically. This antibiotic has now established itself as an important antistaphylococcal agent in the treatment of systemic infection. Good absorption and minimal side effects after oral administration combined with an impressive penetration in deep-seated infections gives fucidin an important place in the management of staphylococcal infections. Although the question of antagonism between fucidin and some other antibiotics has not been finally resolved there is at the moment insufficient evidence to claim that antagonism presents serious practical difficulties.

Applied locally to skin lesions fucidin is sometimes effective. Combined oral and local administration is perhaps the most helpful antibiotic measure available at the moment in dealing with staphylococcal wound infections. An important property of the drug is its ability to penetrate into tissues. There are good reports of high concentrations obtained in burn crusts (Sorenson et al, 1966) and in bone (Hierholzer et al, 1966). Unfortunately when fucidin or indeed any other antibiotic is applied locally in open general wards resistant organisms must be expected to flourish and to spread.

SIDE EFFECTS: TOXICITY

Although fucidin has a steroid structure whose fate in the body is not fully known, no untoward metabolic effects have so far been described. It has been shown to have a mild protein catabolic effect, and to lower urinary calcium excretion (Wynn, 1965).

The drug is usually well tolerated, side effects being virtually confined to mild gastro-intestinal upset; there is one report of drug fever. There are as yet no reports of serious toxicity.

NALIDIXIC ACID

Nalidixic acid is a napthyridine derivative synthesised in 1962. It is a pale yellow crystalline powder slightly soluble in water and readily soluble in alkaline solutions. Solutions are stable and do not require refrigeration.

After oral administration the drug is well absorbed. Excretion is almost entirely by the kidney, 80% can be recovered in the urine, the major part of an oral dose being excreted within eight hours, although the drug and its metabolites can be detected after 12-24 hours. Usual plasma levels are less than those obtained in the urine and the drug is to some extent selectively concentrated in the kidneys. Only traces enter the cerebrospinal fluid.

Nalidixic acid is available as tablets of 500 mg or as a suspension containing 60 mg in each ml. The usual adult dose is 4 g daily in divided doses for at least one week; chronic infections may require treatment for much longer periods when the daily dose may be halved. Children over one month may be given 25 mg per pound body weight per day in divided doses. Nalidixic acid in a concentration from 1 to 25 μg/ml is effective against most strains of E.coli, Proteus mirabilis, Proteus vulgaris; other Gram-negative bacteria such as Klebsiella, Aerobacter and Brucella also show in vitro sensitivity. Pseudomonas aeruginosa strains are generally resistant to the drug. The mode of action of nalidixic acid is by blocking of DNA synthesis, but the precise mechanism is unclear.

CLINICAL APPLICATION

The major use of nalidixic acid is in the treatment of urinary tract infections; it has been used in the treatment of shigella infections and in brucellosis, but these reports are difficult to evaluate. It does not seem to be effective in the treatment of non-gonococcal urethritis.

In using this drug for the treatment of urinary tract infections two facts emerge. First, that the dose for an adult must be at least 4 g/day; with lower doses the failure rate increases. Secondly, that resistance occurring during the course of treatment is relatively common. Another unfortunate, though not unexpected feature, is the extremely high failure rate in patients with abnormality in the urinary tract. Sleet and associates, for instance, found that 15 of 22 patients with abnormal pyelograms failed to respond to treatment (Sleet et al, 1964).

SIDE EFFECTS: TOXICITY

Nalidixic acid is usually well tolerated, the most frequent side effects being nausea, vomiting and other gastro-intestinal upset. Drowsiness and a feeling of weakness may occur. Itching, urticaria and other skin eruptions, sometimes accompanied by fever and eosinophilia have been noted early in treatment. Photosensitivity has been reported in a number of patients.

As the drug is mainly metabolised in the liver and excreted by the kidney care should be taken when prescribing nalidixic acid in patients with advanced renal or hepatic disease. There is also a suggestion that respiratory depression was increased by the drug when given to two patients with advanced pulmonary infection and respiratory insufficiency.

The urine of patients taking nalidixic acid contains a metabolite which gives a positive result with Benedicts reagent, with 'clinitest' paper but not 'clinistix'. There is one report of a 14-year old child who admitted taking thirteen 500 mg tablets. She had headache, vomiting and convulsions, the urine contained albumin and sugar; the white blood cell count was 23,300 per c.mm and blood glucose 240 mg per 100 ml. With intravenous infusion therapy recovery was complete (Islam et al, 1965).

NITROFURANTOIN

Derivatives of the cyclic compound furan were shown by Dodd and Stillman (1964) to possess antibacterial properties. The presence of a nitro group at the five position and a side chain at the two position impart this activity and, of the many compounds synthesised, nitrofurantoin (N-(5 nitro-2 furfury lidine)-1 amino-hydantoin) was selected as the most promising. This substance forms yellow crystals, bitter to taste, and is only slightly soluble in water.

Nitrofurantoin is rapidly absorbed from the gastro-intestinal tract; antibacterial concentrations are not reached in the blood, and about 40% of an oral dose is excreted in the urine. Concentrations in the urine of the order of 100-200 μg/ml are frequently achieved and capable of suppressing the growth of a large number of both Gram-negative and Gram-positive organisms. Thus the majority of strains of E.coli, Proteus, Bact. aerogenes, Staphylococci and Str. faecalis are inhibited; most strains of Pseudomonas are now probably resistant to the action of nitrofurantoin. This compound is thought to act by inhibition of acetyl co-enzyme A leading to breakdown of the Krebs cycle. Resistance which emerges slowly is usually not encountered during treatment.

The drug is available as tablets containing either 50 or 100 mg, and as a suspension each 3.5 ml of which contains 25 mg nitrofurantoin. The usual adult dose is four 100 mg tablets, calculated as 5 to 8 mg/kg body weight each 24 hours. Doses of up to 10 mg/kg may be given. Children can be given either the tablets or the suspension – a 20 kg child for instance may receive either one teaspoonful (3.5 ml) of the suspension, or half a 50 mg tablet four times daily, and either three teaspoonfuls of the suspension or one and a half ($1\frac{1}{2}$) 50 mg tablets four times daily can be administered to a 35 kg child. Nitrofurantoin is best taken with food.

CLINICAL APPLICATION

It must be remembered that nitrofurantoin has a bacteriostatic action which is confined to the urine. It might be classified as a broad spectrum and fairly effective urinary antiseptic. Nitrofurantoin cannot be expected to kill bacteria which are deep in the substance of the kidney; indeed cure of this type of pyelonephritis may not be possible, but suppression of superficial urinary tract infection is often possible with this drug. Paradoxically in chronic pyelonephritis symptoms may often be lessened and urine bacterial counts reduced when nitrofurantoin is administered. Thus an important indication for its use is in continued treatment of patients who are considered to have parenchymatous renal lesions after courses of other antibacterial agents have been prescribed.

SIDE EFFECTS: TOXICITY

Nausea and vomiting are common, but reduction of the daily dose by as little as 50 mg often produces marked improvement in tolerance. Hypersensitivity may be manifest as skin eruption, sometimes accompanied by eosinophilia, fever or rigors. Rarely, bronchospasm dyspnoea and chest pain occur and these can be associated with transitory pulmonary infiltration or pleural effusion.

Peripheral neuritis may occur. Prolonged therapy especially in patients with renal insufficiency is often a contributory factor. As excretion is entirely by the urine nitrofurantoin should not be prescribed in those with a marked degree of azotaemia.

Nitrofurantoin may induce haemolysis when there is a deficiency of glucose-6-phosphate dehydrogenase in the red cells.

Patients who are taking nitrofurantoin may produce urine of brown colour due to presence of inactive metabolites of the drug. Crystalluria does not occur. In pregnancy urinary tract infections may be treated with nitrofurantoin and there is no evidence linking the drug with congenital malformation.

THE RIFAMYCINS

The rifamycins are a group of antibiotics obtained from *Streptomyces mediterranei* with a novel molecular structure. Three clinically interesting derivatives have been produced.

RIFAMYCIN SV

This, the first of the family of rifamycin antibiotics, is very poorly absorbed after oral administration but therapeutically useful concentrations are present in blood for up to eight hours after intramuscular injection of 250 mg. Antibacterial activity is predominantly against Gram-positive cocci (at concentrations less than 1 μg/ml) and mycobacteria; concentrations of 10 to 100 μg/ml are required for activity against Gram-negative bacteria.

Excretion of rifamycin like all the related compounds is predominantly in bile; there is an entero-hepatic circulation and high concentrations are found in faeces. Significant amounts do not appear in cerebrospinal fluid, amniotic fluid, placenta or foetal blood.

RIFAMIDE

Similar in pharmacology and antibacterial range rifamide is excreted chiefly in bile, some 80% of the injected dose being cleared by this route. Bile concentrations in excess of 1000 μg/ml are achieved and at this level Gram-negative pathogens as well as the more susceptible Gram-positive pathogens may be inhibited. Cavenagh (1969) has demonstrated in vitro activity at a concentration of 1 μg/ml against a number of strains of Myco. tuberculosis but not against atypical mycobacteria. In clinical use this drug has proved useful in biliary infections (Kahn & Scott, 1967).

RIFAMPICIN

Unlike rifamycin SV and rifamide rifampicin is well absorbed after oral administration; a 600 mg dose produces blood levels of 32 and 2 μg/ml after two and 12 hours respectively (Begg, 1967). Although many Gram-positive species including staphylococci are inhibited by concentrations of less than 1 μg/ml and the minimum inhibitory concentration for Gram-negative bacteria ranges between 1 and 10 μg/ml the main interest in this drug lies in its marked activity against mycobacteria. The MIC for Myco. tuberculosis is about 0.5 μg/ml; some of the atypical mycobacteria, including Myco. kansasii are inhibited by similar concentrations but Myco. avium, Myco. fortuitum and Battey strains are less sensitive. Rapid growing anonymous mycobacteria are resistant to rifampicin.

CLINICAL APPLICATION

In four patients with multi-resistant mycobacteria there was conversion within three months (Pines et al, 1967) and Verbist et al (1967) treated ten multiresistant cases with a mean conversion time of seven weeks. Nitti and colleagues (1967) treated 27 new cases of tuberculosis chiefly with rifampicin in doses of 600 mg daily for two to four months. There was rapid sputum conversion in over 60% of cases though rifampicin-resistant organisms were cultured from the sputum of some patients who did not convert.

At present rifampicin is used mainly as a second line antituberculous agent combined with other agents such as ethambutol, capreomycin or pyrazinamide. Pines and associates (1970) consider rifampicin in combination with ethambutol and capreomycin as the treatment of choice at the present time for patients with cultures resistant to the standard anti-tuberculous drugs. Animal studies have suggested that rifampicin combined with isoniazid sterilises tuberculous lesions more effectively than any other drug combination and it may be that this combination will prove of value in the initial treatment of human tuberculosis. Full assessment must await results of further trials.

SIDE EFFECTS: TOXICITY

Rifampicin may produce a reddish colouration of urine, sputum and lacrimal fluid and it may cause an overestimation of the serum bilirubin in patients taking the drug. Occasional cases of jaundice or, abnormal liver function tests without jaundice, have been reported. Developmental abnormalities have been noted in the progeny of rats given high doses and it is recommended that rifampicin is not given to women in pregnancy, certainly not during the early months.

There has been one case report of rifampicin-induced immune thrombocytopoenia (Blajchman et al, 1970) but no other major haemotological effects have been reported. The drug is usually well tolerated but rashes and intestinal upsets may occur.

MODE OF ACTION

The rifamycin group of antibiotics act by inhibiting the formation of m RNA from the RNA-polymerase/DNA complex. Some animal studies suggest that rifampicin may have antiviral activity; the drug is capable of reducing multiplication of virus in cells infected with vaccina, cow pox and some other pox viruses.

Cross resistance between rifampicin and other antituberculous drugs has not been demonstrated.

ADMINISTRATION: DOSAGE

In treating tuberculosis rifamycin should be used in conjunction with other antituberculous agents.

It is available as capsules (Rifadin) containing either 150 or 300 mg rifampicin.

In adults a single daily dose, preferably before meals, is given based on a schedule ranging from 8-12 mg/kg daily as below:

kg	Daily dose mg
38 - 50	450
50 - 77	600
77 - 90	750
90 and over	900

Children: a single daily dose of up to 20 mg/kg which should not exceed 600 mg per day

REFERENCES

POLYMYXINS

Atuk, N. O., Mosca, A. and Kunin, C. (1964) The use of potentially nephrotoxic antibiotics in the treatment of Gram-negative infections in uraemic patients. Ann. intern. Med., **60**, 28

Farrar, D. A. T. (1954) Use of Polymyxin B in the external ear. Brit. med. J., **2**, 629

Graves, J. W. (1952) Otitis externa, and its treatment with a new antibiotic preparation. Eye, Ear, Nose & Throat Monthly, **31**, 32

Hayes, E. R. and Yow, E. (1950) Meningitis due to Pseudomonas aeruginosa treated with Polymyxin B. Amer. J. med. Sci., **220**, 633

Jawetz, E. (1952) Infections with Pseudomonas aeruginosa treated with Polymyxin B. Arch. intern. Med.. **89**, 90

Kunin, C. M. and Finland, M. (1959) Restrictions imposed on antibiotic therapy by renal failure. Arch. intern. Med., **104**, 1030
Mead, R. H. (1963) Treatment of meningitis. J. Amer. med. Ass., **185**, 1023
Pulaski, E. J., Baker, H. J., Rosenberg, M. W. and Connell, J. F. Jr. (1949) Laboratory and clinical studies of Polymyxin B and E. J. clin. Invest., **28**, 1028
Tomlin, C. E. (1951) Pseudomonas meningitis. Report of a case with recovery after Polymyxin B therapy. Arch. intern. Med., **87**, 863

COLISTIN

Brownlee, G., Bushby, S. R. M. and Short, E. I. (1952) The chemotherapy and pharmacology of the Polymyxins. Brit. J. Pharmacol., **7**, 170
Brumfitt, W., Black, M. and Williams, J. D. (1966) Colistin in Pseudomonas pyocyanea infections and its effect on renal function. Brit. J. Urol., **38**, 495
Carroll, G. and Malette, W .F. (1961) Use of Colymycin in chronic urinary infections due to the Pseudomonas aeruginosa. J. Urol., **85**, 86
Colley, E. W. and Frankel, H. L. (1963) 'Colomycin' treatment of Klebsiella aerogenes infection of urinary tract in paraplegia. Brit. med. J., **2**, 790
Fekety, F. R. Jr., Norman, P. S. and Cluff, L. E. (1962) The treatment of Gram-negative bacillary infections with Colistin. Ann. intern. Med., **57**, 214
Gomirato, Sandrucci (1958) Quoziente emato-liquorale e colimicina. Minerva med. (Torino), **49**, 4538
Gordon, D. M. and McLean, J. M. (1960) Colistin in Pseudomonas infection. Amer. J. Ophthal., **50**, 33
Hessburg, P. C., Truant, J. P. and Penn, W. P. (1964) Pseudomonas corneal ulcers in animals and man. Antimicrob. Agents Chemother. American Society for Microbiology, Michigan. Page 752
Holloway, W. J. and Scott, E. G. (1963) Colistimethate sodium: a clinical study. J. Urol (Baltimore), **89**, 264
Jones, R. J., Jackson, D. McG. and Lowbury, E. J. L. (1966) Antiserum and antibiotics in the prophylaxis of burns against Pseudomonas aeruginosa. Brit. J. plast. Surg., **19**, 43
MacLean, K. S. (1962) 'Medical Treatment'. 2nd Edition. Page 362. Churchill, London
McMillan, M., Price, T. M. L., MacLaren, D. M. and Scott, G. W. (1962) Pseudomonas pyocyanea infection treated with Colistin Methane Sulphonate. Lancet, **ii**, 737
Marsden, H. B. and Hyde, W. A. (1962) Colistin methane sulphonate in childhood infections. Lancet, **ii**, 740
Murdoch, J. McC. (1964) The treatment of severe Pseudomonas pyocyanea infections with Colistin. Proceedings of Third International Congress of Chemotherapy, 319. (Stuttgart)
Perkins, R. L. (1964) Apnoea with intramuscular Colistin. J. Amer. med. Ass., **190**, 421
Price, D. J. E. and Graham, D. I. (1970) Effects of large doses of Colistin Sulphamethate Sodium on renal function. Brit. med. J., **4**, 525
Speirs, C. F., Selwyn, S. and Nicholson, D. N. (1963) Hypogammaglobulinaemia presenting as Pseudomonas septicaemia. Lancet, **ii**, 710

GENTAMICIN

Barber, M. and Waterworth, P. M. (1966) Activity of Gentamicin against Pseudomonas and hospital Staphylococci. Brit. med. J., **1**, 203
Bulger, R. J. and Kirby, W. M. M. (1963) Gentamicin and Ampicillin: synergism with other antibiotics. Amer. J. med. Sci., **246**, 717
Darrell, J. H. and Waterworth, P. M. (1967) Dosage of Gentamicin in Pseudomonas infections. Brit. med. J., **2**, 535

Jao, R. L. and Jackson, G. G. (1964) Gentamicin Sulphate. New antibiotic against Gram-negative bacilli. Laboratory, pharmacological and clinical evaluation. J. Amer. med. Ass., **189**, 817

Louria, D. B., Young, L., Armstrong, D. and Smith, J. K. (1969) Gentamicin in the treatment of pulmonary infections. J. infect. Dis., Suppl. 1969, page 483

Martin, C. M., Cuomo, A. J., Geraghty, M. J., Zager, J. R. and Mandes, T. C. (1969) Gram-negative Rod Bacteremia. J. infect. Dis., Suppl. 1969, page 506

Newman, R. L. and Holt, R. J. (1967) Intrathecal Gentamicin in treatment of ventriculitis in children. Brit. med. J., **2**, 539

Nunnery, A. W. and Harris, D. R. Jr. (1969) Gentamicin. Pharmacologic observations in newborns and infants. J. infect. Dis., Suppl. 1969, page 402

Pines, A., Raafat, H. and Plucinski, K. (1967) Gentamicin and Colistin in chronic purulent bronchial infections. Brit. med. J., **2**, 543

BACITRACIN

Bellows, J. G. and Farmer, C. J. (1948) Use of bacitracin in ocular infections: bacitracin therapy of experimental and clinical ocular infections. Amer. J. Ophthal., **31**, 1211

Eggers, H. (1951) Clinical ophthalmic experience with Bacitracin. Amer. J. Ophthal., **34**, 1706

Prigal, S. J. and Furman, M. L. (1949) Use of Bacitracin, new antibiotic in aerosol form; preliminary observations. Ann. Allergy, **7**, 662

VANCOMYCIN

Ehrenkranz, N. J. (1959) The clinical evaluation of Vancomycin in treatment of multi-antibiotic refractory staphylococcal infections. Antibiotics Annual, 1958-1959. Pages 587-594

Kirby, W. M., Perry, D. M. and Bauer, A. W. (1960) Treatment of Staphylococcal Septicaemia with Vancomycin. New Engl. J. Med., **262**, 49

Spears, R. L. and Koch, R. (1960) The use of Vancomycin in paediatrics. Antibiotics Annual, 1959-1960. Pages 798-803

LINCOMYCIN

Daikos, G. K., Kontonichalon, P., Papdoyannakis, N. and Tourkantonis, A. (1963) Clinical and laboratory experience with Lincomycin. Antimicrob. Agents Chemother., 197

Grondin, C., St. Martin, M. and Potvin, A. (1965) Lincomycin and Staphylococcal infections: a clinical study of 18 cases. Canad. med. Ass. J., **92**, 1062

Harnecker, J., Contreras, J., Gilabert, B. and Ubilla, V. (1963) Bacteriological and clinical studies of Lincomycin Hydrochloride. Antimicrob. Agents Chemother., 204

Holloway, W. J. and Scott, G. E. (1965) Clinical experience with Lincomycin. Amer. J. med. sci., **249**, 691

Jackson, H., Cooper, J., Mellinger, W. J. and Olsen, A.R. (1965) Group A β Haemolytic Streptococcal Pharyngitis — results of treatment with Lincomycin. J. Amer. med. Ass., **194**, 1189

Kagan, B. M., Zolla, S., Busser, R. and Liepnieks, S. (1964) Sensitivity of coccal and L forms of <u>Staphylococcus aureus</u> to five antibiotics. J. Bact., 88, 630

MacLeod, A. J., Ross, H. B., Ozere, R. L., Digout, G. and Van Rooyen, C. E. (1964) Lincomycin: a new antibiotic active against Staphylococci and other Gram-positive cocci. Canad. med. Ass. J., **91**, 1056

CLINDAMYCIN

Meyers, B. R., Kaplan, K. and Weinstein, L. (1969) Microbiological and pharmacological behaviour of 7-Chlorolincomycin. Applied Microbiology, **17**, 653

FUCIDIN

Hierholzer, G., Knothe, H., Rehn, J. and Koch, F. (1966) Fucidic acid concentrations in chronically inflamed tissue. Investigations in chronic post-traumatic osteomyelitis. Arzneim-Forsch, **16**, 1549 (in German)
Sorensen, B., Sejrsen, P. and Thomsen, M. (1966) Fucidin, Pro-staphlin, and Penicillin concentration in burn crusts. Acta chir. scand., **131**, 423
Wynn, V. (1965) Metabolic effects of the steroid antibiotic Fucidic Acid. Brit. med. J., **1**, 1400

NALIDIXIC ACID

Islam, M. A. and Sreedharan, T. (1965) Convulsions, hyperglycaemia, and glycosuria from overdose of Naladixic Acid. J. Amer. med. Ass., **192**, 1100
Sleet, R. A., Gray, W., Calder, M. and Murdoch, J. McC. (1964) Treatment of urinary tract infections with Nalidixic Acid: Clinical Trial. Chemotherapia, **8**, 137

NITROFURANTOIN

Dodd, M. C. and Stillman, W. B. (1944) The in vitro bacteriostatic action of some simple furan derivatives. J. Pharmacol. exp. Ther., **82**, 11

RIFAMYCINS

Begg, K. J. (1967) Rifamide: addendum on serum levels. Tubercle, **48**, 149
Blajchman, M. A., Lowry, R. C., Pettit, J. E. and Strading, P. (1970) Rifampicin-induced immune thrombocytopoenia. Brit. med. J., **3**, 24
Cavenagh, P. (1969) Sensitivity of some mycobacteria to Rifocin-M. Brit. med. J., **1**, 317
Kahn, G. A. and Scott, A. J. (1967) The place of Rifamycin-B-diethylamide in the treatment of cholangitis complicating biliary obstruction. Brit. J. Pharm. Chemo., **31**, 506
Nitti, V., Catena, E., Bariffi, F. and Delli Veneri, F. (1967) Arch. Tisiol., **22**, 417
Pines, A., Aafat, H. R. and Bundi (1967) The Rifamycins with other drugs in the treatment of pulmonary tuberculosis: a report of nine cases. Tubercle, **48**, 281
Pines, A., Siddiqui, G. M. and Aafat, H. R. (1970) Rifampicin and Ethambutol in the treatment of drug resistant and far advanced pulmonary tuberculosis. J. Irish med. Ass., **63**, 82
Verbist, L., Gyselen, A., Cosemans, J. and Priguot, J. (1967) Vth Int. Cong. Chemotherapy, Wien **2**, 2, 591

10. The Sulphonamides

INTRODUCTION

Historically the sulphonamides occupy a unique position in relation to bacterial infections, for they were the first effective compounds to be used systematically in their treatment. The widespread use of these drugs was soon reflected in a marked decline in mortality and morbidity for those infections susceptible to treatment with the sulphonamide compounds.

The azo dyes were being investigated in Germany and in 1935 Domagk reported that one of them, the red dye prontosil, protected mice from streptococcal infection. Other workers soon showed that the dye was broken down in the body to -aminobenzene sulphonamide, or sulphonilamide, which was responsible for the antibacterial activity of prontosil. Sulphonilamide was found to be effective in puerperal sepsis and meningococcal infection. Then followed a period when many sulphonamide compounds were synthesised, tested and made available for clinical use. Sulphapyridine, particularly active against the pneumococcus was introduced, sulphathiazole and sulphadiazine less toxic and generally more active became available. These compounds were followed by others of low solubility, which were for practical purposes not absorbed and whose site of action was confined to the bowel. Further modification in recent years has produced compounds which are highly bound to protein and are therefore 'long acting', requiring infrequent doses.

The introduction of antibiotics with a broader and more certain action against many micro-organisms has displaced the sulphonamides from their unique position; today they are one of many agents available to the physician which may be selected for a special purpose, such as ease of entry into the cerebrospinal fluid.

PHARMACOLOGY

Sulphonamides, excepting bowel active insoluble compounds, are well absorbed from the gastro-intestinal tract. Most absorption occurs in the small intestine, but some takes place in the stomach. Approximately 70% of an oral dose reaches the blood; within an hour of administration sulphonamide may be found in the urine. After absorption the sulphonamides become bound to protein, are to some extent acetylated, and excreted chiefly by the kidney. There are wide variations in the behaviour of different sulphonamides in these three respects.

PROTEIN BINDING

Variations in protein binding partially account for the characteristics of a particular sulphonamide in its clinical behaviour. The rate of excretion, and therefore the frequency of dosage, is to some extent at any rate determined by the degree of protein binding. Sulphadiazine, for instance, being protein bound to the extent of about 55% is readily excreted in the urine and enters the cerebrospinal fluid within four hours of a single dose. Sulphamethoxypyridazine is approximately 90% protein bound and has a half life probably five times longer than most 'soluble' sulphonamides. It is slowly excreted by the kidneys and cerebrospinal fluid concentrations are only 5% to 10% of the plasma levels. Because plasma levels are persistently high the absolute concentration in the cerebrospinal fluid may also be high despite the marked degree of protein binding.

ACETYLATION

Acetylation and glucuronide formation are changes which occur in the metabolism of the sulphonamides. Both reactions result in the formation of inactive compounds, and acetylation which is common may produce compounds poorly soluble in urine which are likely to produce crystalluria and blockage of renal tubules.

EXCRETION

Excretion of absorbed sulphonamides is almost entirely renal; the relatively insoluble compounds are excreted in the faeces. In bile the concentration is usually extremely low but may reach 5% when long acting derivatives are used.

Glomerular filtration is the principal excretory mechanism, modified in most cases by tubular reabsorption and in some instances by tubular secretion. Each sulphonamide is handled in a characteristic way, protein binding and metabolism by the liver resulting in fairly predictable behaviour for individual drugs. Urine concentrations are high and this has led to frequent use of sulphonamides in urinary tract infection; crystalluria and ureteric blockage can, unfortunately, also occur. These undesirable sequelae are less likely to occur when fluid intake is high and when the urine is kept alkaline.

MODE OF ACTION

Micro-organisms which require folic acid for their metabolism, but are unable to utilise preformed acid, most therefore synthesise it; in so doing para-amino benzoic acid (PABA) is incorporated into the molecule. Sulphonamides act by competitively denying PABA for this purpose. It follows that only those organisms which necessarily synthesise folic acid are sensitive to sulphonamide action. The action of sulphonamide is therefore purely bacteriostatic.

Resistance to the action of the sulphonamides may occur both in vitro and in vivo, and is related to the ability of the organism to produce PABA or similar sulphonamide inhibitors. Within ten years of the introduction of these drugs many species originally susceptible became resistant. This was perhaps most noticeable with the gonococcus, but extraordinarily, resistance of the meningococcus was delayed a further twenty years and is still a rarity. A few strains of group A streptococci and Pneumococci are resistant, and resistance is usual in the coliform group, especially Shigella sonnei.

IN VITRO RANGE

Most strains of the following organisms are highly susceptible to sulphonamide action: Group A streptococci, Pneumococci, Corynebacterium diphtheriae, Haemophilus influenzae, Bacillus anthracis, and the agents responsible for trachoma, lymphogranuloma venereum, and inclusion conjunctivitis. Gonococci, in which resistance was widespread have now in many areas regained sensitivity. Most strains of the meningococcus are highly sensitive; a few are totally resistant — this phenomenon has not at the time of writing been recorded in the UK. Sulphadiazine resistance is defined as those organisms with a minimum inhibitory concentration greater than 10 mg per 100 ml (Leedom et al, 1966). Some strains of E. coli and Shigella are sulphonamide-sensitive as also is Clostridium welchii.

ADMINISTRATION: DOSAGE

The sulphonamides are usually administered orally, occasionally intravenously, rarely subcutaneously, never intrathecally. The dose varies widely depending on the particular drug used, the site and severity of infection. Only a brief guide will be given here; examples will be found in the section on clinical application and further details are in the table at the end of the chapter.

Sulphonamides are available as tablets of 0.5 g or as suspension; several soluble sulphonamides are available in ampoules, usually containing 1 g for intravenous or subcutaneous use.

SOLUBLE SULPHONAMIDES

These compounds include sulphadimidine, sulphadiazine, sulphamerazine and sulphathiazole and are usually prescribed with an initial loading dose, equivalent to half the daily dose, and followed by four hourly administration.

Thus in serious infection in an adult an initial 'loading' dose of 3 to 6 g sulphadiazine is given; thereafter 4 hourly doses of 1 to 2 g are prescribed. If the patient is vomiting, as frequently occurs in meningitis, initial therapy at least, is best given intravenously in a dose not exceeding 4 g. Oral and intravenous priming doses may be combined. Adequate hydration must be ensured. When clinical response is obvious the dose can be reduced to 3-6 g per 24 hours and this should be continued for 7 to 10 days.

In urinary tract infections the 'loading' dose may be omitted and daily doses of 2-3 g are sufficient. There appears to be little to choose between the various soluble sulphonamides in treating urinary infection. In simple acute infections of the urinary tract the drug should be given for at least 6 weeks.

TRIPLE SULPHONAMIDES

Combining three sulphonamides in approximately equal proportions allows each compound to retain its distinct solubility characteristics, and therefore reduces the risk of renal complications. Lower plasma concentrations of the individual components may possibly lead to less risk of sensitisation. Sulphatriad (sulphathiazole; sulphadiazine; sulphamerazine) the first of these mixtures is a useful combination.

INSOLUBLE SULPHONAMIDES

These compounds are very poorly absorbed and very high concentrations are obtained in the bowel. They have therefore been used in prophylaxis of infection in abdominal surgery, in specific bowel infections such as bacillary dysentery and in non-specific diarrhoea. As there is no good evidence that they are effective in these conditions they are not recommended. Succinylsulphathiazole (sulphasuxidine), phthalylsulphathiazole (sulphathalidine) and sulphaguanidine are the compounds usually employed in oral doses of 10-20 g per 24 hours.

LONG-ACTING SULPHONAMIDES

Sulphonamides in this group are most commonly used for long term therapy. Being highly protein bound and slowly excreted relatively high blood levels can be maintained on doses as low as 0.5 g daily. Most commonly prescribed include sulphamethoxy-pyridazine (Lederkyn; Midicel), sulphamethoxydrazine (Durenate) and sulphaphenazole (Orisulf).

CLINICAL APPLICATION

The number of antibacterial agents is now so great that sulphonamides are first choice in few situations: meningococcal infection being the clearest indication for their use. This includes those forms of disease with acute and chronic septicaemia, whether meningitis is present or not. In epidemics these drugs may be used prophylactically. In circumstances where the choice of agent is limited, usually because of cost, sulphonamides continue to have an important role, as they possess the great advantages of cheapness and ease of administration.

MENINGITIS

The sulphonamides have been used to treat various forms of meningitis including pneumococcal and that due to H. influenzae, but the major use and clearest indication, is in treating meningococcal infection.

The sulphonamide usually recommended is sulphadiazine, but there appears to be little to choose between any of the soluble sulphonamides, sulphamethazine and sulphathiazole also being effective. The author has most frequently used sulphatriad, if necessary treatment being initiated by an intravenous dose, usually 3-6 g of either sulphadiazine or sulphamerazine. It is important to ensure adequate hydration when patients are receiving full doses of sulphonamides, especially when the drug is given by the intravenous route. Treatment should be continued for 7 to 10 days.

Children tolerate sulphonamides well, indeed the younger the patient the higher should be the dosage in relation to body weight; adults can be given 1 g per 20 lbs body weight, whereas infants will tolerate 1 g per 5 lbs body weight in a 24 hour period.

In recent years there have been reports from American military establishments of sulphonamide-resistant meningococci. These have nearly all been Group B meningococci; the subject is reviewed by Eickhoff and Finland (1965) and Feldman (1966). As a result of this experience sulphonamides in America now take second place to penicillin in the treatment of meningococcal infection. In the UK sulphonamide resistance has not yet been encountered, but penicillin is frequently prescribed in conjunction with sulphonamide in treating acute meningococcal infection and this practice is recommended.

If resistant meningococci are prevalent in the community sulphonamides are not effective in prophylaxis and clearance of the carrier state with penicillin is difficult to achieve.

URINARY TRACT INFECTIONS

Sulphonamides are most likely to be effective in urinary tract infections when they are of recent origin, when abnormality of the urinary tract is not present, and when the responsible organisms are either E. coli or Gram-positive cocci, other than enterococci. The presence of catheters or other drainage apparatus reduces the prospects of success.

Sulphonamides, being bacteriostatic will succeed when the drug concentration is high and the bacterial population relatively small. Infections deep within the renal parenchyma or very severe infections may therefore show poor response. Conversely these drugs may suppress infection or keep urine bacterial counts at a low level, when they are prescribed over a long period.

Symptoms from acute urinary tract infections settle so rapidly, and bacteriological 'cure' of chronic infections is so inconstant, that true assessment of the function of any drug, including sulphonamide, is extremely difficult.

BOWEL INFECTIONS

In the treatment of specific bowel infections the sulphonamides are of little use. Initially Shigella infections may have responded, but today resistant strains are so common that treatment is almost invariably without avail. This is particularly true of strains of Sh. sonnei encountered in the United Kingdom; infections due to Sh. flexneri may respond to treatment with sulphonamides.

The sulphonamides are sometimes used in preparation of the bowel for surgery. It is as yet unclear if this is useful, and it is not recommended.

One sulphonamide compound – salicylazo-sulphapyridine (salazopyrin) – has definite indications in patients with ulcerative colitis which is usually considered not to be an infective condition. Initially daily doses of 4 to 8 g per day are given, but doses up to 16 g may be required. When improvement occurs the dose is reduced usually to 1.5-3 g and may be continued for a period of weeks. Remission can be induced and maintained with this regime; corticosteroid therapy may be carried out simultaneously.

MISCELLANEOUS CONDITIONS

OPHTHALMIC DISORDERS

Sodium sulphacetamide, a slightly alkaline salt, which does not precipitate on neutralisation, is frequently used in the treatment of a number of ophthalmic infections. Solution of various concentrations from 5% to 30% or ointment of 2.5%, 6% and 10% are available.

Bacterial conjunctivitis due to various pyogenic organisms including Neisseria gonorrhoea may be treated by local application of sulphacetamide. Keratitis and blepharitis are similarly treated. If these conditions are severe systemic antibiotic therapy, usually with penicillin, will also be required.

Trachoma is treated with sulphonamide both locally and orally. Ten to fourteen days' therapy is frequently successful. Antibiotics are useful in clearing common pyogenic bacteria.

Inclusion conjunctivitis, will respond to tetracycline or chloramphenicol, but topical application of 5% sulphacetamide either as drops or ointment, 6 times daily for 10 days is frequently used with success.

TOXOPLASMOSIS

When this condition requires treatment it is usual to prescribe a sulphonamide in conjunction with pyrimethamine. Sulphatriad 3 g initially is followed by 1 g every 4 hours; pyrimethamine 50 mg is given initially, 25 mg 6 hours later and then 25 mg daily. This combined therapy is continued for 14 days.

DERMATITIS HERPETIFORMIS

This condition characterised by an intensely itchy eruption of groups of vesicles and bullae responds to sulphones and sulphapyridine. The condition may be brought under control with a dose of 3 g of the latter for several days. Thereafter 0.5 to 2 g per day may be continued for months. Sulphapyridine is the only sulphonamide with this action and its mechanism is quite unknown.

CHANCROID

This condition responds well provided suppurative buboes have not formed. Sulphonamide therapy will not mask a co-existing syphilitic infection. Sulphadiazine 1 g four times per day for one week is a suitable method of administration.

NOCARDIOSIS

Sulphadiazine may occasionally be very useful in this condition. Early diagnosis and prolonged treatment is desirable. Hall (1966) reports a case of pulmonary nocardiosis which was treated with 9 g of sulphadiazine daily to a total of 189 g.

SULPHONAMIDE-ANTIBIOTIC COMBINATIONS

Sulphonamide may be used in combinations with parenteral and intrathecal streptomycin in the treatment of H. influenzae meningitis. This may produce good results, but is more demanding than chloramphenicol therapy which is simple and probably equally effective.

Penicillin G is sometimes used, together with sulphonamide, to produce a 'broad spectrum' effect in treating infections of unknown aetiology. Despite some advantages, such as cheapness and lack of inhibitory effect of sulphonamides on the action of penicillin, the results are often unpredictable and the practice is not recommended.

TOXICITY: SIDE EFFECTS

The sulphonamides have been in use for 30 years and this has been long enough for a formidable array of side effects and toxic reactions to be well documented.

HYPERSENSITIVITY

This usually occurs when the drug has been given for at least a week. Fever, a syndrome like serum sickness, and a variety of rashes may occur. Occasionally rashes are severe and exfoliative dermatitis has been described. In recent years the use of long acting sulphonamides has been associated with the Stevens-Johnson syndrome and toxic epidermal necrolysis (Lyell's syndrome).

Vasculitis resulting in a syndrome similar to polyarteritis nodosa has been attributed to sulphonamides. Exposure to sunlight may precipitate these hypersensitivity phenomena.

BLOOD DYSCRASIAS

Haemolytic anaemia may occur either as a sensitisation phenomenon or from red cell deficiency of glucose-6-phosphate dehydrogenase. The letter reaction is not dose related and can occur early in the course of treatment with sulphonamides. Heinz bodies may be present.

Leucopoenia may occur early and usually has little significance; if, however, the white cell count falls suddenly after 10 days the reaction should be regarded with caution. In some cases there may be a progressive neutropoenia, in others the count falls suddenly. Most cases recover spontaneously when the drug is withdrawn, but this may be delayed for weeks or months.

Thrombocytopoenia, causing haemorrhage is rarely seen in sulphonamide therapy. Aplastic anaemia, with complete suppression of the formed elements in the blood, is fortunately a rare occurrence.

RENAL EFFECTS

Crystals of sulphonamide may form in the urine and provided this is not progressive probably little harm is done. However, aggregates of crystals can form in the tubules, in the pelvis and ureter, resulting in obstruction to urine flow. Catheterisation of the ureter may, in some cases, free the obstruction. Crystalluria and obstruction are avoided by ensuring good urine output and maintaining an alkaline reaction in the urine. Special care should be taken when a patient is known to have only one kidney.

Toxic nephrosis, or renal damage as part of a hypersensitivity phenomena may rarely cause death in the absence of haematuria or crystalluria.

MISCELLANEOUS SIDE EFFECTS

Nausea and vomiting are relatively common when large doses of sulphonamide are being taken; reducing the dose will often allow the drug to be continued.

Blue colour of the skin and mucous membranes developed in a number of patients taking sulphonilamide, a drug which was soon discarded for more potent compounds. It has not been clearly established whether this is due to changes in haemoglobin or to a coloured metabolite of the drug. This colour change is very rarely seen with the sulphonamides in common use today.

Sulphonamides compete for binding sites on plasma protein; bilirubin may thus be displaced so that it is present chiefly in the unbound state. This allows bilirubin to cross the blood-brain barrier and in the newborn can result in kernicterus. Sulphonamides should therefore not be prescribed in the first week of life or in the later days of pregnancy.

Local application of sulphonamide to wounds and ulcers is best avoided as there is a high incidence of hypersensitivity reactions.

SULPHONAMIDE / TRIMETHOPRIM

INTRODUCTION

Sulphonamides exert their antibacterial action (see page 132) by inhibiting the formation of dihydrofolinic acid from para-aminobenzone acid. The synthesis of folate, essential for bacterial cells, is prevented; mammalian cells are capable of utilising preformed folic acid and thus a selective action unfavourable to bacteria occurs. A systematic search for substances which would block subsequent steps in folate metabolism carried out by Hitchings and colleagues indicated that the diaminopyrimidines and related structures were capable of inhibiting folate reductases. Further work indicated that 2, 4-diamino-5-(3, 4, 5-trimethoxybenzyl pyrimidine (trimethoprim) had high antibacterial activity and was essentially free of side effects (Hitchings, 1969; Bushby & Hitchings, 1968). Trimethoprim thus inhibits enzymatic conversion of dihydrofolinic acid to tetrahydrofolinic acid. By combining sulphonamide and trimethoprim there is a sequential blockade at two points directed against folates essential for bacterial survival.

Two compounds (Septrin: Bactrim) combining sulphamethoxazole (400 mg) and trimethoprim (80 mg) in single tablet form have been produced. Sulphamethoxazole was chosen because it is absorbed and excreted at approximately the same rate as trimethoprim.

PHARMACOLOGY

Absorption of sulphamethoxazole/trimethoprim by the oral route is rapid; peak plasma levels occur between two and four hours after administration, persist up to seven hours and detectable amounts have been found after 24 hours. Tissue concentrations are high particularly in the lungs and kidneys.

About 50% of ingested trimethoprim is excreted in the urine within 24 hours; sulphamethoxazole is mainly excreted in the urine 60% in the acetylated form. This is the situation in patients with normal renal function on normal fluid intake. Marked alterations in urine pH, urine flow-rate and creatinine clearance may result in urine concentrations and subsequently plasma concentrations of both drugs which are not optimum for antibacterial synergy (Sharpstone, 1969).

IN VITRO RANGE

Trimethoprim has antibacterial activity against many species of bacteria. Combined with sulphonamide there is a synergistic effect which differs from sulphonamide action in being bactericidal. The spectrum of activity ranges widely from common Gram-negative species such as E. coli, Salmonellae, Haemophilus influenzae and Proteus spp, also the common Gram-positive cocci Str. pyogenes, staphylococci (including penicillin-resistant ones) are usually sensitive. There is no activity against Ps. aeruginosa, Myco. tuberculosis, Treponema pallidum.

Cross resistance with other agents has not been described; resistance to the combined action of these two compounds seems unlikely to develop during treatment.

CLINICAL APPLICATION

Trimethoprim/sulphamethoxazole combination has proved useful in treating urinary tract infections. Reeves and colleagues (1969) found the combined therapy more effective than either ampicillin, or sulphamdimadine in urinary tract infections whether assessment was carried out one week or four to five weeks after stopping therapy. Using five day courses of therapy Gruneberg and Kolbe (1969) also reported a high success rate in urinary tract infections.

In treating acute exacerbations of bronchitis it seems probable that sulphamethoxazole/trimethoprim is at least as effective as tetracycline or ampicillin though more controlled trials are necessary before the position with regard to chest infections is settled (Pines et al, 1969; Lal & Bhalla, 1969).

Trimethoprim/sulphamethoxazole appears to be an effective therapy for gonorrhoea both in men and women (Schofield et al, 1969; Csonka, 1969) and does not affect darkground positive lesions of syphilis. It is not effective in non-gonococcal urethritis, and gonococcal proctitis does not respond. In treating venereal infections other disadvantages of this therapy is that oral administration is obligatory and that it is not yet recommended in pregnancy.

Early reports of trimethoprim/sulphamethoxazole in the treatment of small series of patients with typhoid fever were encouraging (Akinkugbe et al, 1968; Pugsley, 1969) and recently two larger series support the original optimism (Kamat, 1970; Farid et al, 1970). In both these series trimethoprim/sulphamethoxazole appeared to be equal to chloramphenicol in the time taken for reducing temperature to normal but the combined therapy was more

Table XIV. Sulphonamide: Dose Scheme

ACUTE INFECTIONS

Preparation	Adult		0 - 3 yr		3 - 10 yr	
	Loading	Subsequent	Loading	Subsequent	Loading	Subsequent
Soluble sulphonamide: e.g. Sulphadiazine Sulphadimidine	3-6 g	1-2 g 4 hrly	0.5 g	0.25-0.5 g 4 hrly	1-2 g	0.5-1 g 4 hrly
MILDER INFECTIONS						
Soluble sulphonamide	2 g	1 g 4 hrly	0.5 g	0.25 g	0.75 g 4 hrly	0.5 g 4 hrly
Long-acting sulphonamide: e.g. Sulphamethoxypyridazine Sulphadimethoxine		0.5-1 g daily				
Bowel-active sulphonamide						
1. Succinylsulphathiazole		10-20 g daily				
2. Salicylazo-sulphapyridine	4-8 g daily					

effective in lessening toxicity. Of particular interest is the good response in the few cases of paratyphoid fever in which this therapy was used. Clearly trimethoprim/sulphamethoxazole has good potential in salmonella infections but its true place is as yet undecided. This combination may also be used in salmonella septicaemia and invasive infections

TOXICITY: SIDE EFFECTS

Side effects of this combination are those relating to the sulphonamide constituent, mainly rashes, and those particular to trimethoprim. Nausea and vomiting may occur but are not particularly troublesome unless high doses are used. After prolonged therapy some alterations in folate metabolism may occur. These have not been associated with any clinical upset and disappeared after cessation of treatment.

These drugs are not recommended during pregnancy.

ADMINISTRATION: DOSAGE

Tablets of Septrin and drapsules of Bactrim each containing trimethoprim 400 mg and sulphamethoxazole 80 mg are available for oral administration. Both preparations are also issued as tablets containing 20 mg trimethoprim and sulphamethoxazole 100 mg or syrup (trimethoprim 40 mg/sulphamethoxazole 200 mg per 5 ml) suitable for paediatric use.

In adults the usual daily dose is one or two tablets or drapsules twice daily. In very severe infections up to 6 tablets in divided doses may be taken.

In children between 6 and 12 years half the adult dose is satisfactory — usually one tablet twice daily. In children between 2 and 6 years the paediatric tablet may be used — one to two tablets twice daily.

In severe renal impairment reduced doses should be administered; estimations of blood levels may be required.

REFERENCES

SULPHONAMIDES

Domagk, G. (1935) Ein Beitrag zur Chemotherapie der bakteriellen Infektionen. Dt. med. Wshr., **61**, 250

Eickhoff, T. C. and Finland, M. (1965) Changing susceptibility of Meningococci to Antimicrobial Agents. New Engl. J. Med., **272**, 395

Feldman, H. A. (1966) Meningococcal Disease (1965) J. Amer. med. Ass., **196**, 391

Hall, G. V. (1966) Case of pulmonary nocardiosis with apparent cure with sulphadiazine. Med. J. Aust., **2**, 455

Leedom, J. M., Ivler, D., Mathies, A. W .Jr., Thrupp, L. D., Fremont, J. C., Wehrle, P. F. and Portnoy, B. (1966) The problem of sulphadiazine-resistant Meningococci; in antimicrobial agents and chemotherapy. Am. Soc. Microbiol. Page 281

SULPHONAMIDE/TRIMETHOPRIM

Akinkugbe, O. O., Lewis, E. A., Montefiore, D. and Okubadejo, O. A. (1968) Trimethoprim and Sulphamethoxazole in typhoid. Brit. med. J., **3**, 721

Bushby, S. R. M. and Hitchings, G. H . (1968) Trimethoprim a sulphonamide potentiator. Brit. J. Pharmac. Chemother., **33**, 72

Csonka, G. W. (1969) Therapeutic trial of some genital infections with trimethoprim-sulphamethoxazole. Postgrad. med. J. Suppl., **45**, 77

Farid, Z., Hassan, A., Wahab, M. F. A., Sanborn, W. R., Kent, D. C., Yassa, A. and Hathout, S. E. (1970) Trimethoprim-sulphamethoxazole in enteric fevers. Brit. med. J., **3**, 323

Gruneberg, R. N. and Kolbe, R. (1969) Trimethoprim in the treatment of urinary infections in hospital. Brit. med. J., **1**, 545

Hitchings, G. H. (1969) Species differences among dihydrofolate reductases as a basis for chemotherapy. Postgrad. med. J. Suppl., **45**, 7

Kamat, S. A. (1970) Evaluation of therapeutic efficacy of Trimethoprim-sulphamethoxazole and Chloramphenicol in enteric fever. Brit. med. J., **3**, 320

Lal, S. and Bhalla, K. K. (1969) Comparison of tetracycline and trimethoprim-sulphamethoxazole in acute episodes of chronic chest infections. Postgrad. med. J. Suppl., **45**, 91

Pines, A., Freenfield, J. S. B., Aafat, H. R., Rahman, M. and Siddiqui, A. M. (1969) Preliminary experiments with trimethoprim and sulphamethoxazole in the treatment of purulent chronic bronchitis. Postgrad. med. J., **45**, 89

Pugsley, D. J., Mwanje, L., Pearson, C. and Blowers, R. (1969) Use of trimethoprim and sulphamethoxazole in tropical Africa: typhoid fever; Sal. typhi carriage and Staph. aureus sepsis. Postgrad. med. J. Suppl., **45**, 95

Reeves, D. S., Faiers, M. C., Pursell, R. E .and Brumfitt, W. (1969) Trimethoprim-sulphamethoxazole: comparative study in urinary infection in hospital. Brit. med. J., **1**, 541

Schofield, C. B. S., Masterton, M. M. and McGill, M. I. (1969) The treatment of gonorrhoea in women with sulphamethoxazole-trimethoprim. Postgrad. med. J. Suppl., **45**, 81

Sharpstone, P. (1969) The renal handling of trimethoprim and sulphamethoxazole in man. Postgrad. med. J. Suppl., **45**, 38

11. Antifungal Agents

INTRODUCTION

Mycotic infection in humans is due to three different groups of fungi, the actinomycetes, dermatophytes responsible for superficial mycoses, and mycoses which involve the deeper structures.

ACTINOMYCETES

These are a heterogeneous group of filamentous micro-organisms, superficially resembling fungi, which grow typically as branched mycelia and break into fragments. Actinomyces israelii (A. bovis) is responsible for actinomycosis which is usually manifest as a hard, non tender swelling with chronic sinus production involving tissues in the neck and jaw, abdominal organs especially the caecum and appendix, or the thorax, when lung abscess and empyema occur. Nocardia asteroides and related species of aerobic actinomyces can cause either a localised granuloma of subcutaneous tissues or bone ('Madura foot'), or systemic infection involving lungs, brain, meninges and other organs.

Treatment in this group is usually carried out by surgical drainage combined with antibiotics, the most useful of which are penicillin, sulphonamides and tetracyclines. Treatment may have to be prolonged, for penetration of these drugs into deep masses of infected tissue is difficult or impossible.

SUPERFICIAL MYCOSES

Dermatophytes, classified into three genera, Epidermophyton, Microsporum, Trichophyton, infect only superficial keratinised tissues, chiefly hair, skin and nails. They have world-wide distribution and some can infect animals as well as man. These dermatophytes are responsible for the various forms of ringworm and treatment has been markedly improved since the introduction of the antibiotic griseofulvin.

DEEP MYCOSES

Candida albicans (Monilia albicans) is an oval budding yeast-like fungus frequently present in the normal mouth and gastro-intestinal tract. It can cause infection of the skin, mucous membranes of the mouth and vagina, and less commonly may infect the nails. The characteristic lesion of candidiasis is thrush, most commonly encountered in the mouths of children. Whitish patches, of varying size, are found on the tongue, cheeks, gums or pharynx, which contain the blastospores and speudomycelia of the fungus. Candidiasis is encouraged by the prolonged use of wide spectrum antibiotics and corticosteroid drugs, the presence of debilitating or chronic diseases such as diabetes mellitus, and is common in patients whose immune response is reduced by disease or drugs. Nystatin is used to treat this form of candidiasis. Occasionally systemic infection occurs, especially in the lungs and pleura; endocarditis and peritonitis may occur in generalised candidiasis.

Other mycoses which are associated with systemic involvement include Cryptococcus neoformans (Torula histolytica), Histoplasma capsulatum, Blastomyces dermatitidis, Sporotrichum schenckii, Coccidioides immitis, and Aspergillus fumigatus.

The treatment of these conditions, which are very rare in this country, is with the antibiotic amphotericin B.

GRISEOFULVIN

This antibiotic was discovered in 1939, but was not introduced for clinical use until 1959. In the intervening years it was used in the treatment of fungus diseases of plants and ringworm in animals. Gentles (1958) showed that given orally the drug could control experimental fungal infection in guinea pigs and later demonstrated its presence in hair keratin. Clinical trials in Europe and America confirmed the usefulness of the drug in humans.

Griseofulvin, a colourless neutral substance produced from Penicillium griseofulvum, is very sparingly soluble in water and is heat stable.

PHARMACOLOGY

Griseofulvin is administered orally and peak plasma levels of 1.5 μg/ml are obtained about four hours after a single dose of 3 g. Factors influencing the degree of absorption are particle size (particles of 2.7 μ in diameter are absorbed about twice as effectively as those of 10 μ) and whether the antibiotic is taken with food. When taken with a meal of high fat content absorption is increased. The majority of orally administered griseofulvin is excreted in the faeces; very small quantities are excreted in the urine.

The unique property of this drug is that it is deposited not only in diseased tissue, but has an affinity for the precursor cells of keratin. New growth of hair and skin is therefore free of infection.

MODE OF ACTION

Present evidence suggests that griseofulvin acts by blocking nucleic acid synthesis. It somewhat resembles colchicine in structure and may block rapidly dividing cells in metaphase.

ADMINISTRATION: DOSAGE

Griseofulvin is available as tablets (coarse particles) containing 250 mg or in tablets of fine particles of 125 mg, which has been accepted for the preparation of griseofulvin tablets BP.

The usual daily dose for an adult is four tablets, that is either 1 g coarse particles or 0.5 g fine particles, given as a single dose or subdivided. For children the recommended dose is 15 mg griseofulvin (fine particles) per kg body weight daily.

ANTIFUNGAL ACTIVITY

Griseofulvin inhibits in vitro growth of various dermatophytes; it is not active against Candida albicans or bacteria and its action against Aspergilli and certain species of Nocardia is only slight.

CLINICAL APPLICATION

This antibiotic is the treatment of choice in ringworm infection of hair, skin and nails. Thus tinea capitis caused by M. canis, M. audouini, T. schoenleini responds well. Clinical cure may be achieved within four to eight weeks. As new uninfected hair grows it is possible to see fungal fluorescence becoming confined to the distal portion of the hair. Infected hair should be removed by shaving and clipping. T. rubrum infection of the nails may require very prolonged treatment; slow growth of toe-nails is partially responsible.

Epidermophytosis, one variety of athlete's foot is usually markedly improved, but mycological cure is more difficult.

It is important to remember in treating fungus infections that reinfection is common, and that final assessment of cure is the absence of fungus from scrapings both microscopically and culturally. It is wise to continue treatment for at least one week after complete clinical cure.

TOXICITY: SIDE EFFECTS

Serious reactions to griseofulvin are few; minor upsets such as headache, epigastric discomfort and rashes can often be minimised by reducing dosage. Transient depression of the white cell count has been described.

Toxicity studies in animals have shown that mice may survive single oral doses of 50 g/kg. Very high doses given intravenously to animals may cause transient arrest of mitosis; such doses may cause disturbance of porphyrin metabolism and hepatic lesions. Patients with porphyria should probably not be given the drug. Photosensitivity may occur.

There is one report of a patient who had taken griseofulvin for two months and who developed disorder of coordination, unrealiable memory and had difficulty in driving a motor care (Fenno, 1960).

NYSTATIN

This antibiotic derives its name from the fact that it was discovered in the laboratories of the New York State Department of Health. It is an amphoteric substance derived from Streptomyces noursei, the exact structure of which is not known. It is very sparingly soluble in water, and quickly decomposes in the presence of water or plasma losing up to 50% of its activity in 6 hours. The preparation of the antibiotic available for therapeutic use is not fully purified and its potency is expressed in units. One milligram of the pure substance being equal to 3, 500 units.

PHARMACOLOGY

After oral administration of conventional doses of nystatin only very small quantities are absorbed, plasma levels being hardly detectable. Local application does not lead to appreciable absorption. When taken orally practically all nystatin is excreted in the faeces.

MODE OF ACTION

The drug penetrates susceptible cells and becomes bound to the cell membrane; a sterol present in the membrane has been postulated as the requirement for binding. The nystatin-sterol combination alters membrane permeability allowing leakage of cell constituents, especially potassium (Kinsky, 1962).

ADMINISTRATION: DOSAGE

Nystatin is available as tablets (500, 000 units), and an oral suspension which is reconstituted by the addition of 22 ml distilled water to give a concentration of 100, 000 units per ml. It is also provided as sterile powder, ointment, and in tablets for insertion into the vagina.

Nystatin is usually administered orally or topically. The adult oral dose is 500, 000 to 1 million units three times per day, and for children 100, 000 units three or four times per day. Suspensions for topical application are usually applied three times per day. Vaginal tablets may be inserted once or twice each day.

ANTIFUNGAL ACTIVITY

Nystatin, which has no action on bacteria is most active against yeast-like fungi (C. albicans), and has some action on filamentous fungi. It is both fungicidal and fungistatic. Strains of Candida albicans are invariably sensitive, but occasionally a slow stepwise resistance develops. Other strains of Candida may become quite resistant when they are repeatedly sub-cultured in nystatin-containing media.

CLINICAL APPLICATION

Nystatin is used principally in the treatment of candidiasis. The typical lesions of thrush and vaginitis usually respond well.

Intestinal and pulmonary candidiasis present several problems; firstly Candida organisms may appear in sputum and stools without causing disease. Their persistence in high numbers favours, but does not necessarily indicate, an aetiological significance; the administration of nystatin will usually result in clearing of candida from cultures. Another difficulty is that claims have been made for the inclusion of nystatin to prevent intestinal candidiasis when a wide-spectrum antibiotic is prescribed. The diagnosis of intestinal candidiasis, as indicated above, is only established with difficulty and the benefits of nystatin are not easily assessed; clear indication for the use of nystatin in this context is lacking.

Pulmonary candidiasis or aspergillosis may be treated with nystatin suspension administered as an aerosol. Nystatin sterile powder (500,000 units) is used; a small quantity of 20% alocohol is added to the powder to form paste. Sterile water is then added to obtain the desired concentration. Usually the concentration aimed at is from 10,000 to 25,000 units/ml. It is claimed that 75% of the particles in nystatin sterile powder are between 2 and 4 microns in diameter. This suspension must be freshly made up and administered two or four times each day.

TOXICITY: SIDE EFFECTS

Nystatin is not a toxic drug and side effects are few. Occasionally nausea, vomiting and diarrhoea may occur after oral administration. Hypersensitivity skin eruptions do not seem to occur even when nystatin is applied locally. Haematological disorders have not been described.

AMPHOTERICIN B

Amphotericin B is a polyene antibiotic produced by a strain of Streptomyces nodosus the precise structure of which is not known. Fractionation of the crude fermentation product yields two chemically related active components named Amphotericin A and Amphotericin B. The latter compound although less soluble than the former is more active in vitro and in vivo.

Amphotericin B is a pale yellow, semicrystalline material, with high molecular weight and is insoluble in water.

PHARMACOLOGY

The drug is very poorly absorbed from the gastro-intestinal tract and blood levels are not detectable after intramuscular injection. Administration is therefore by the intravenous route, usually by infusion. After intravenous administration fungistatic levels persist for prolonged periods and urinary excretion is slow. In one trial, over each 24 hour period approximately 5% of the daily dose was excreted in the urine in the active form.

Cerebrospinal fluid levels of amphotericin B are low even after large intravenous doses; there has been a suggestion that when the protein content of the cerebrospinal fluid is high increased quantities of the drug may enter the cerebrospinal fluid (Seabury & Dascomb, 1958).

MODE OF ACTION

Amphotericin B, like nystatin is dependent on the binding of a sterol present in the cell membrane of sensitive organisms for its antifungal activity.

ADMINISTRATION: DOSAGE

Amphotericin B is available as a 3% lotion for local application, and in vials providing on reconstitution 50 mg of amphotericin B activity. For intravenous infusion an initial concentrate of 5 mg/ml is prepared by addition of 10 ml sterile water, **without bacteriostatic agent**, to the vial. The vial is agitated until the solution is clear. The infusion solution is then obtained by further dilution with 5% dextrose infusion BP of pH above 5.0 to give a concentration of 0.1 mg per ml. Fresh solutions should be prepared for each infusion and during infusion the solution should be protected from light. Containers must be inspected for foreign material or precipitate and if these are present the solutions are discarded.

The initial intravenous dose of amphotericin B is 0.25 mg/kg; this dose is gradually increased over a period of days until a dose of 1.0 mg/kg is given each day. Even in severe infections the total daily dose should not exceed 1.5 mg/kg. When maximum therapy is reached the drug may be given on alternate days. Infusion time for each dose should be approximately six hours.

The length of the period of therapy depends on the nature and severity of the infection. Repeated courses lasting from 6 weeks to 3 months may be required. Fever, chills, headache and vomiting are common when amphotericin B is given intravenously; with this drug one expects side effects. Pre-injection treatment with sedation and aspirin is recommended. A direct injection of 25 mg hydrocortisone into the infusion apparatus when the treatment starts may help to minimise reactions.

Amphotericin B may be given intrathecally in treating fungal meningitis. The technique is as follows: 5 ml of cerebrospinal fluid is withdrawn into a large syringe; 20 mg hydrocortisone is added and the mixture is instilled slowly intrathecally. After some minutes 5 ml of cerebrospinal fluid is again withdrawn, a solution containing 0.5 mg amphotericin B is added and the mixture again instilled carefully. Three intrathecal injections (total 15 mg) separated by several days are usually sufficient.

ANTIFUNGAL ACTIVITY

Amphotericin B is active against all yeast-like fungi; and has some activity against pathogenic species of filamentous fungi. Thus the drug is indicated in infections due to Histoplasma capsulatum, Cryptococcus neoformans, Coccidiodes immitis, Candida albicans, Blastomyces dermatitidis and Sporotrichum schencki. The drug is both fungistatic and fungicidal and has no effect on bacteria, Rickettsiae and viruses.

CLINICAL APPLICATION

Before embarking on treatment with amphotericin B it is well to remember that it is a toxic drug which causes frequent and severe reactions. On the other hand there is no other drug which is likely to benefit patients suffering from systemic mycotic infections. Histoplasmosis, cryptococcosis, coccidiodomycosis, North American blastomycosis, South American blastomycosis and systemic moniliasis are indications for intravenous amphotericin B therapy. Candida endocarditis responds poorly; there is one case report of successful treatment of cryptococcal endocarditis (Colmers et al, 1967). It must be emphasised that these infections may require several courses of treatment and that despite considerable toxicity effort should be made to offer adequate treatment.

TOXICITY: SIDE EFFECTS

Proper technique will reduce side effects and as these are commonest in the early stages of treatment initial doses should be small and increased gradually. Most patients will get troublesome systemic effects such as fever, chills, headache, nausea, vomiting, during or after intravenous infusion of the drug. Premedication with sedative and antihistamine drugs may reduce these reactions. Thrombophlebitis at the injection site is often troublesome. Hydrocortisone injected with the infusion may help.

Azotaemia frequently occurs. This may demand reduction in dosage or even withdrawal of the drug. The precise nature of the renal disturbance is not known but permanent damage is rare. Acute hepatic failure is occasionally seen; the histological picture is similar to that produced by chlorpromazine.

Normochromic normocytic anaemia may occur; the bone marrow shows decreased erythrocyte production.

Hypokalaemia and hypomagnesaemia have been described. Intrathecal injection of Amphotericin B may result in chemical meningitis, paraesthesiae, radiculitis and difficulty with micturition.

Very many other side effects have been recorded. In one patient an infusion of 28 mg was inadvertently given in 40 minutes and this resulted in convulsions, ventricular fibrillation and cardiac arrest, which fortunately responded to a sharp blow on the chest.

FLUOROCYTOSINE

5-Fluorocytosine is an antimetabolite of cytosine in C. neoformans, Candida albicans, and some other fungi but apparently not in man. It inhibits the growth of these fungi but has no antibacterial effect.

Fungistatic concentrations persist in the blood for six to ten hours after single oral doses of 2 g of 5-fluorocytosine, and the drug is excreted unchanged in the urine.

There are few reports of its clinical use and the drug is not generally available. Tassel and Madoff (1968) treated a single case resistant to amphotericin B in which the patient responded to 5-fluorocytosine in an oral dose of 2.25 g daily for 50 days. Watkins and associates (1969) treated a single case with 5-fluorocytosine with the recommended dose of 100 mg/kg per day for a period of 43 days. Marked improvement occurred after five days' treatment. A second course of 53 days' therapy was required as relapse occurred three days after stopping the initial therapy.

Reversible pancytopoenia and altered serum transaminases have been recorded during treatment.

This agent appears promising primarily because of ease of oral administration and relative lack of toxicity. Much more experience with this drug is required before it can be accepted as a suitable alternative to amphotericin B in the treatment of cryptococcal meningitis.

PIMARICIN

This antibiotic is a product of Streptomyces natalenis and has recently been introduced. It is a polyene substance related to nystatin and amphotericin B, which is stable in the dry state, virtually insoluble in water and decomposes on exposure to direct sunlight.

Pimaricin is effective in vitro against Aspergillus, Candida and Mucor, being most active against Aspergillus. The drug is poorly absorbed from the gastro-intestinal tract and successful treatment of pulmonary aspergillosis has been carried out by bronchial inhalation, 2.5 ml of a 2.5% suspension being given two or three times each day.

This is a promising drug but not sufficient is yet known about its therapeutic or toxic effects to make a proper assessment.

Table XV. Fungus Infections

INFECTION	DRUG	DOSE	COMMENT
Actinomycosis	Penicillin G Tetracycline		Prolonged systemic therapy necessary
Nocardiosis	Sulphonamides	Sulphonamide 6-9 g/day 150-200 g may be required	
Superficial Mycoses: (Ringworm)	Griseofulvin	Tablets of 125 mg (fine particle) or 250 mg (coarse particle) Four tablets per day. Children: 15 mg FP/kg/day	
Candidiasis	Nystatin	Tablets (500,000 u) 1 or 2 tablets 3 times/day Children: Suspension 100,000 u 3 or 4 times/day	Tablets for vaginal insertion available. One per day 1 week
	Amphotericin B lotion, 3%	Local application 3 times/day	
Deep Mycoses including systemic candidiasis	Amphotericin B	I.V. infusion - see text for preparation and dose	**Beware side effects and toxicity**

REFERENCES

Colmers, R. H., Irniger, W. and Steinberg, D. H. (1967) Cryptococcus neoformans. Endocarditis cured by Amphotericin B. J. Amer. med. Ass., **199**, 762

Fenno, R. F. (1960) Some effects of griseofulvin. J. Amer. med. Ass., **173**, 1402

Gentles, J. C. (1958) Experimental Ringworm in guinea pigs; oral treatment with Griseofulvin. Nature (Lond.), **182**, 476

Kinsky, S. C. (1962) Nystatin binding by protoplasts and a particulate fraction of Neurospora crassa, and the basis for the selective toxicity of polyene antifungal antibiotics. Proc. nat. Acad. Sci. (Wash.), **48**, 1049

Seabury, J. H. and Dascomb, H. E. (1958) Experience with Amphotericin B for the treatment of systemic mycoses. Arch. intern. Med., **102**, 960

Tassel, D. and Madoff, M. A. (1968) Treatment of Candida Sepsis and Cryptococcus Meningitis with 5-Fluorocytosine. J. Amer. med. Ass., **206**, 830

Watkins, J. S., Campbell, M. J., Gardner-Medwin, D., Ingham, H. R. and Murray, I. G. (1969) Two cases of cryptococcal meningitis: one treated with 5-Fluorocytosine. Brit. med. J., **3**, 29

12. Antiviral Agents

INTRODUCTION

The principle of selective toxicity applies equally to antiviral as to antibacterial agents, but the nature of viruses and their intimate relation to host cells impose difficulties which are far from resolved.

In bacterial infection the sequence of events is such that clinical manifestations are usually conspicuous when micro-organisms are abundant and multiplying; late in untreated bacterial infection physical signs abound. On the other hand by the time there is clinical evidence of viral infection the stage of multiplication of the virus may have passed. Influenza, yellow fever, infective hepatitis and to a lesser extent poliomyelitis and smallpox are examples of diseases in which clinical manifestations usually occur after the most active stage of virus multiplication. To affect the course of such diseases antiviral agents would have to be administered before clinical signs develop, and this implies prophylactic therapy. In fact this approach has been used with some effect in the prophylaxis of smallpox by certain thiosemicarbazone compounds. Not all virus infections behave in this way and those with long prodromal periods such as measles, those with protracted clinical courses such as herpetic keratitis and perhaps chicken pox should prove susceptible, theoretically at any rate, to specific agents administered during the phase of clinical illness. Early diagnosis is clearly of paramount importance.

Another difficulty arises from the intracellular nature of viruses; so closely is the metabolism of the virus bound up with its host cell that agents which, for instance, inhibit protein metabolism in the virus, also act against the cell. Interferons produced by the cell itself should be effective antiviral agents and there may well be a future for substances like helenine and statolon which are capable of stimulating interferon formation in animal cells. These substances are not sufficiently pure for use in man.

Vaccines may prevent virus illness. Major advances have been made in this field in recent years conspicuously in the prevention of poliomyelitis and more recently measles. Gamma globulin, by supplying antibody confers passive immunity and this may modify the clinical course of illnesses such as rubella, infective hepatitis and measles.

At the time of writing the thiosemicarbazones and iododeoxyuridine are the only chemical compounds which have practical application in prophylaxis and therapy of virus infections and will be described in some detail. Interferon, amantadine, guanidine and hydroxybenzylbenzimidazole which undoubtedly possess antiviral properties are not sufficiently clinically useful for discussion here.

THIOSEMICARBAZONES

Prophylaxis of Smallpox

In 1950 Hamre and his associates showed that benzaldehyde thiosemicarbazone was active against vaccinia virus infection in mice and fertile eggs and in 1953 Thompson and co-workers found that isatin β thiosemicarbazone had considerably greater antiviral activity. Bauer and Sadler (1960) synthesised the N-methyl and N-ethyl derivatives which were slightly more active than the parent compound. These related compounds were shown to have prophylactic effect in mice infected with the viruses of both variola major and minor.

In clinical trials thiosemicarbazones have protected contacts of variola major. In Madras there were six cases and two deaths among 2,297 contacts treated with N-methylisatin β-thiosemicarbazone (methisazone), whereas in 2,842 untreated contacts there were 114 cases of smallpox and 20 deaths (Bauer et al, 1965); similar results in variola minor were reported by do Valle and his associates in an outbreak in Brazil (do Valle et al, 1965).

Another thiosemicarbazone (4-bromo-3-methyl isothiazole-5-carboxaldehyde thiosemicarbazone) has also been used in the prophylaxis of smallpox; results showed that there was some protection of contacts though less than with methisazone. Neither of these drugs are of use in the treatment of established cases of smallpox.

There are two other situations in which methisazone may have clinical application, in the treatment of eczema vaccinatum and in protecting patients during primary vaccination carried out in the presence of contraindications.

Eczema Vaccinatum

This condition which has a mortality rate probably in the range of 30-40% may be treated successfully with methisazone, but it is rather difficult to assess the efficacy of the drug, for it is often administered late in the disease, and other measures, especially hyperimmune vaccinial antiserum, are usually in operation. Adels and Oppé (1966) describe two children who received serotherapy and also methisazone in an initial dose of 200 mg per kg followed by 50 mg per kg every four or six hours for 48 hours. Both children survived.

Vaccinia gangrenosa may also be cured by methisazone. There are several reports of its effectiveness, the most impressive by Hansson and Vahlquist (1963) whose patient had not improved four and a half months after vaccination despite serotherapy, antibiotics and surgery. There was dramatic improvement when methisazone was administered, the lesion eventually being successfully skin grafted. Recovery has been obtained in 5 of 10 patients with vaccinia gangrenosa treated with methisazone (Bauer, 1966).

Vaccination in the presence of contraindications

In a trial in Poland Jaroszynska-Weinberger and Meszaros (1966) showed that methisazone was as effective as anti-vaccinal gamma globulin in protecting children from untoward effects when primary vaccination was carried out in the presence of contraindications such as eczema, tuberculosis, or history of previous convulsions. Methisazone was used in the form of a 20% suspension in sucrose syrup and administered orally in an initial dose of 100 mg per kg followed by 50-60 mg per kg daily for 3-6 days.

Clinical Use of Methisazone

In most reported series when methisazone has been used side effects have been chiefly gastro-intestinal; taking of alcohol may make these worse and the drug should not be administered to those with liver and renal disorders. Minor degrees of fluid retention may occur.

In prophylaxis of smallpox the drug has established a position of some usefulness and it is certainly one measure to be considered in protection. The dose recommended by Bauer (1965) is initially 200 mg/kg followed by a further 400 mg/kg in divided doses over the next 48 hours.

Its use in other conditions is less clear, but is probably worth trial both in eczema vaccinatum and vaccinia gangrenosa. Those wishing to use methisazone in these conditions are advised to get in contact with the makers of the drug (Burroughs Wellcome & Co).

IODODEOXYURIDINE (IDU)

Of the halogenated pyrimidine nucleotides with antiviral action 5-iodo-2-deoxyuridine (IDU) has received most attention. This compound inhibits replication of DNA viruses being incorporated in preference to thymidine which eventually results in cessation of cell division. In 1961 Herrmann reported that IDU was active against herpes simpex virus in cell culture and later Kaufman showed that the compound could be used to treat herpetic keratitis in rabbits and man (Kaufman, 1963). There have now been a considerable number of publications on the effectiveness of IDU in the treatment of herpetic keratitis and despite some reservations the overall impression is that this compound is a definite advance over standard treatment with antibiotics. Less satisfactory results have been reported when IDU has been used to treat cutaneous herpes infection; recently there have been several reports of the systemic use of iodoeoxyuridine in the treatment of herpes simplex encephalitis.

Keratitis

In the majority of people antibodies to herpes simplex virus can be demonstrated, and many of these subjects will have had no clinical manifestations of herpetic infection. The primary corneal lesion may be associated with herpetic lesions on the face, or a generalised skin eruption, or there may be involvement of other systems particularly the central nervous system. The commonest ocular herpetic lesion is therefore secondary or recurrent herpes simplex when circulating antibodies are present.

The usual type of recurrent herpes lesion affecting the eye begins in the cornea and consists of small punctate epithelial spots or tiny vacuoles that appear in the epithelium of the cornea. Progression leads to a branching or dendritic figure. If the ulcer widens large irregular areas are involved producing the so-called geographic ulcer, which involves Bowman's membrane and the stroma. Ulcers occurring weeks or months after the initial infection and similar in appearance to geographic ulcers, but from which the virus cannot be isolated are called metaherpetic ulcers. Later the uveal tract may be involved and a hypopyon keratitis may develop. In view of the great variation in herpetic corneal ulceration and the behaviour of individual lesions making accurate diagnosis and prognosis difficult it is not surprising that opinion on the efficacy of IDU is not unanimous.

Kaufman and associates treated 76 patients with dendritic ulcers using IDU. The spread of the ulcers ceased on starting treatment and the patients experienced subjective relief in 12 to 24 hours. One patient failed to improve. Four patients with stromal involvement took more than a week for all grossly visible staining to disappear. There was recurrence in eight patients (Kaufman et al, 1962). There are now many reports confirming these results. Two points emerge, first, healing when it occurs usually occurs early, and second, some apparently typical lesions do not heal.

Luntz and MacCallum (1963) treated eleven cases of dendritic ulcer with IDU and compared the results with eleven neomycin treated patients. These authors were unable to demonstrate any advantage for IDU.

Clinical Use of IDU in Herpes Keratitis

IDU is available as a 0.1% aqueous solution with thiomersal (0.002%) as preservative. The recommended initial dose is one drop instilled into the eye every hour during the day and every two hours at night. When improvement occurs as shown by loss of staining with fluorescin the frequency of dosage is reduced to one drop every two hours during the day and one drop every four hours at night. Treatment should not be continued for longer than 21 days and increasing the frequency of administration does not improve efficiency and may lead to damage of the corneal epithelium.

Side effects are few: photophobia, irritation, pain or oedema of the eyelids may occur. Small defects on the cornea, usually disappearing during continued treatment, may be due to the action of IDU. Rare allergic reactions have been reported.

CUTANEOUS HERPES SIMPLEX

Iododeoxyuridine has been used in the treatment of recurrent cutaneous herpes. Hall-Smith and associates (1962) found considerable relief of symptoms and rapid healing of lesions when IDU was applied as an 0.5% cream, but Juel-Jensen and MacCallum (1964) in a double blind controlled trial found no difference between the active drug and a placebo, and these same authors report that when IDU was applied to the lesions under pressure there was clear advantage over a placebo solution (Juel-Jenson & MacCallum, 1965). A 5% solution of IDU in 100% dimethylsulphoxide (DMSO) brushed three times daily on to oral or cutaneous herpetic lesions assists healing, relieves pain but does not eliminate the virus.

HERPES SIMPLEX ENCEPHALITIS

Herpes simplex encephalitis is a condition which may well be increasing in incidence and it is no longer confined to children. The diagnosis may be suspected clinically when in a patient with encephalitis focal signs emerge and red cells, not explicable on the basis of trauma, are found in the cerebrospinal fluid accompanying the other typical abnormalities. The virus can be cultured from the cerebrospinal fluid and from the brain substance. The prognosis is usually bad, but some patients survive often with considerable brain damage. The only treatments which are likely to be successful are cerebral decompression possibly combined with systemic administration of iododeoxyuridine.

Calabresi used large doses of IDU systemically in treating malignant tumours and was able to show that in these patients jennerian vaccination was suppressed and that there might be some beneficial effect in herpes zoster (Calabresi, 1965). This led others to investigate its use in virus infections of the central nervous system.

Breedon and co-workers (1966) treated a patient with herpes simplex encephalitis by means of surgical decompression and systemic IDU. On the first day post-operatively the drug was begun in a dose of 40 mg/kg/24 hr (3 g) by constant intravenous infusion. During the next 7 days 6 g/24 hr were given by constant intravenous infusion to a total dose of 39 g. Maximum toxicity (fever, thrombocytopoenia, leucopoenia, diarrhoea) was noted 13 days after starting therapy.

Evans et al (1967) treated an eight year old girl with an intravenous infusion of 1.5 g of IDU in dextrose saline given in 8 hours. Four similar infusions were given on alternate days. The total dose of drug was estimated on the basis of 500 mg/kg. There was little improvement in the patient's condition.

Buckley and MacCallum (1967) gave IDU by carotid artery infusion to a 41-year old patient with herpes encephalitis who had marked lateralising signs. A continuous slow perfusion with physiological saline was set up and once daily for 5 days idoxuridine as 0.1% solution was administered. This was prepared in the laboratory and made bacteria-free by filtration through a sintered glass filter. A total of 100 mg was administered over a 2-hour period on the first day, and 100, 200, 300 and 400 mg respectively at the same rate on the four succeeding days. No untoward effects were noted and there was slight but definite improvement in the patient's condition.

It is plain that systemic treatment with iododeoxyuridine should not be undertaken lightly, and that its place in the management of herpetic encephalitis has not been fully explored. However, its use, intravenously or intraventricularly may in the future alter the prognosis in a condition which is at the moment rather gloomy. The real difficulty lies in deciding at what stage the drug should be used, for culture of simplex virus may take about one week, and the early use of the drug is clearly desirable. If the patient's condition deteriorates and the clinical diagnosis appears to be confirmed by the presence of otherwise unexplained erythrocytes in the cerebrospinal fluid or local central nervous system signs, then the drug deserves trial. Brain biopsy is desirable and may provide material for the establishment of a definitive diagnosis.

REFERENCES

Adels, B. R. and Oppé, T. E. (1966) Treatment of eczema vaccinatium with N-methyl-isatin beta-thiosemicarbazone. Lancet, **i**, 18

Bauer, D. J. (1965) Clinical experience with the antiviral drug Marboran. Ann. NY Acad. Sci., **130**, 110

Bauer, D. J. (1966) Antiviral Chemotherapy. In 'The Scientific Basis of Medicine' Annual Reviews 1966

Bauer, D. J. and Sadler, P. W. (1960) The structure-activity relationships of the antiviral chemotherapeutic activity of β thiosemicarbazone. Br. J. Pharmac. Chemother., **15**, 101

Breeden, C. J., Hall, T. C. and Tyler, H. R. (1966) Herpes Simplex encephalitis treated with systemic 5-Iodo-2-deoxyuridine. Ann. int. Med., **65**, 1050

Buckley, T. F. and MacCallum, F. O. (1967) Herpes Simplex encephalitis treated with idoxuridine. Brit. med. J., **2**, 419

Calabresi, P. (1965) Clinical studies with systemic administration of antimetabolites of pyrimidine nucleosides in viral infections. Ann. NY Acad. Sci., **130**, 192

do Valle, L. A. R., de Melo, P. R., de Salles Gomes, L. F. and Proenca, L. M. (1965) Methisazone in prevention of variola minor among contacts. Lancet, **ii**, 976
Evans, A. D., Gray, O. P., Miller, M. H., Verrier Jones, E. R., Weeks, R. D. and Wells, C. E. C. (1967) Herpes Simplex encephalitis treated with intravenous idoxuridine. Brit. med. J., **2**, 407
Hall-Smith, S. P., Corrigan, M. J. and Gilkes, M. H. (1962) Treatment of Herpes Simplex with 5-iodo-2-deoxyuridine. Brit. med. J., **2**, 1515
Hamre, D., Bernstein, J. and Donovick, R. (1950) Activity of p-Amino benzaldehyde 3 - this semicarbazone on vaccinia virus in the chick-embryo and in the mouse. Proc. Soc. exp. Biol. Med., **73**, 275
Hansson, O. and Vahlquist, B. (1963) Vaccinia gangrenosa and compound 33T57. Lancet, **ii**, 687
Herrmann, E. C. (1961) Plaque inhibition test for detection of specific inhibitors of DNA containing viruses. Proc. Soc. exp. Biol. Med., **107**, 142
Jaroszynska-Weinberger, B. and Meszaros, J. (1966) A comparison of the protective effect of methisazone and a hyperimmune antivaccinal gamma-globulin in primary smallpox vaccination carried out in the presence of contraindications. Lancet, **i**, 948
Juel-Jensen, B. E. and MacCallum, F. O. (1965) Treatment of Herpes Simplex lesions of the face with idoxuridine; results of a double-blind controlled trial. Brit. med. J., **1**, 901
Kaufman, H. E. (1963) in 'Perspectives in Virology'. III New York
Kaufman, H. E., Martola, E. L. and Nesburn, A. B. (1962) Use of 5-iodo-2-deoxyuridine (IDU) in the treatment of herpes simplex keratitis. Arch. Ophth., **68**, 235
Luntz, M. H. and MacCallum, F. O. (1963) Treatment of Herpes Simplex Keratitis with 5-iodo-2-deoxyuridine. Brit. J. Ophthal., **47**, 449
Thompson, R. L., Minton, S. A. Jr., Officer, J. E. and Hitchings, G. H. (1953) Effect of heterocyclic and other thiosemicarbazones on vaccinia infection in the mouse. J. Immun., **70**, 229

Part Two

13. Streptococcal Infection

INTRODUCTION

Streptococci comprise a large group of micro-organisms which are Gram-positive, oval or spherical in shape, approximately 1 micron in diameter and tend to grow in chains. Classification of these organisms is based on action on red blood cells, biochemical reactions, and resistance to certain physical and chemical factors. Streptococci which produce β haemolysis on blood agar may be further subdivided according to Lancefield's method into 18 groups designated A to T. This grouping depends upon group-specific cellular antigens, carbchydrate in nature, demonstrable by precipitin reactions, the source of which in Group A streptococci is the bacterial cell wall. The presence of certain surface proteins, designated M and T proteins, in Group A streptococci allows further subdivision into Griffith types. Griffith's typing is chiefly used in epidemiological surveys of outbreaks of streptococcal infections. Group A streptococci cause the majority of streptococcal infections in man, and are also associated with rheumatic fever, glomerulonephritis, and some cases of erythema nodosum.

Streptococci which on blood agar cause incomplete or α haemolysis include many species which turn haemoglobin green and are often designated viridans streptococci. These organisms are prominent normal flora of the respiratory tract and in man only cause disease when they infect heart valves damaged by disease or distorted by congenital defect; occasionally they infect meninges or the urinary tract.

Enterococci belong to Group D, cause variable haemolysis and in man normally inhabit the intestinal tract. They are associated with genito-urinary infection and endocarditis.

Lactic streptococci, commonly present in milk, are often responsible for its coagulation, but do not cause disease in man.

INFECTION DUE TO GROUP A STREPTOCOCCI

Group A β haemolytic streptococci are responsible for about 90% of streptococcal infections in man. These include tonsillitis, erysipelas, scarlet fever, impetigo, cellulitis and puerperal infection. Occasionally invasion of the blood stream occurs, which may be fatal unless treatment is prompt and vigorous.

Fortunately Group A streptococci are always sensitive to penicillin G; in vitro concentrations of 0.02 μg/ml or less will inhibit growth of these organisms. Penicillin G is therefore the drug of choice and rapid improvement is expected, often within an hour or two of the first injection.

TONSILLITIS, PHARYNGITIS, SCARLET FEVER

These are common conditions and their diagnosis is not always easy. Streptococci may be cultured when they are not responsible for infection and sometimes fauces quite clearly infected may produce no growth. Further, other conditions, especially virus infections, may be indistinguishable clinically from streptococcal infection. In acute cases the decision to treat is a clinical one and therefore errors may be expected.

Penicillin should be prescribed for ten days; initially administration is by the intramuscular route and after five days oral therapy with phenoxymethyl penicillin may be substituted. In children oral therapy may be started after an initial injection of a mixture containing penicillin of different solubilities, but the total duration of therapy should be not less than ten days. In more complicated conditions the severity of the infection will dictate the dose and the route of administration — a peritonsillar abscess for instance demands parenteral therapy with high doses, on occasions intravenous therapy being justified. Scarlet fever requires treatment similar to tonsillitis and pharyngitis.

Occasionally patients are seen who continue to complain of sore throat when no obvious clinical infection is present, and who have received apparently adequate chemotherapy. Some of these may be true streptococcal carriers, and careful swabbing of the tonsillar fossae may produce a growth of Group A streptococci. In others no growth is obtained, but a persistently high antistreptolysin O titre may be recorded. It is possible, though adequate data to support the contention is lacking, that these patients have become colonised by L-form variants of streptococci. The implications for therapy are that if symptoms persist after administration of penicillin G an alternative antibiotic, which acts not on the bacterial cell wall, but which inhibits protein synthesis should be tried. Erythromycin or lincomycin are the obvious drugs for trial.

RHEUMATIC FEVER. GLOMERULONEPHRITIS

These conditions, to which may be added some cases of erythema nodosum, are responses, which may be called hypersensitivity responses, to infection with Group A β haemolytic streptococci. There is usually an interval of 1 to

3 weeks between infection and the onset of manifestations of the hypersensitivity state. Confirmation of recent streptococcal infection is suggested by the presence of a raised antistreptolysin O titre.

Although evidence is incomplete that eradication of streptococci will alter the course of these conditions, it is rational to try to remove continuing sources of antigen, realising of course that the major damage will probably have occurred before the patient presents with his illness. Ten days' penicillin therapy is warranted.

PROPHYLAXIS OF RHEUMATIC FEVER

The prevention of recurrent Group A streptococcal infection in those who have suffered an initial attack of rheumatic fever can reduce the likelihood of subsequent attacks and possibly further cardiac damage. This may be done in two ways (1) daily administration of an oral penicillin, such as phenoxymethyl penicillin 250 mg BD, or (2) a monthly injection of 1.5 mega units of benzathine penicillin. The latter method is preferred. Whichever regime is adopted it must be carried on throughout the child's school life and probably to the age of 35 or even longer (see Chapter 23).

It is important to remember that this is prophylaxis of Group A streptococcal infection and that patients receiving this therapy will harbour many organisms, especially Str. viridans which will be resistant to the action of penicillin, and that these resistant organisms can be responsible for endocarditis. During dental or surgical treatment these patients should be protected by an alternative antibiotic such as cephaloridine.

ALTERNATIVE ANTIBIOTICS IN GROUP A INFECTION

If penicillin G is contraindicated because of hypersensitivity, the alternatives are erythromycin, cephaloridine, lincomycin. Tetracyclines should not be used; they may be effective provided the particular strain of streptococcus is sensitive, but in British hospitals between 30 and 50% of Group A streptococci are now resistant to tetracycline.

STREPTOCOCCUS VIRIDANS INFECTIONS

This is a heterogeneous group of organisms, many members of which cause α haemolysis of red blood cells, but some produce no haemolysis. They are common organisms in the mouth and respiratory tract. The most important infection produced by viridans streptococci is subacute bacterial endocarditis; meningitis and urinary tract infection occasionally results.

The bacteriological diversity in this class results in variable resistance to penicillin G which is however, the most effective antibiotic, and the majority of strains will be inhibited by concentrations as low as 0.02 μ/ml. It is important that antibiotic sensitivities be carried out for in treating endocarditis plasma antibiotic levels of several times the bactericidal concentration should be achieved. For the majority of viridans streptococci penicillin G 6 mega units per 24 hours for a period of four to six weeks will suffice. Few strains will require larger doses; some may demand antibiotic combinations to achieve bactericidal effects.

GROUP D STREPTOCOCCAL INFECTIONS

The classification of organisms possessing group D antigen is open to discussion. Organisms in this group are sometimes referred to as enterococci, but this term has never been fully defined. From the clinical standpoint one organism — Str. faecalis — with its two varieties, zymogenes and liquefaciens, is most important. Those seeking further details on nomenclature may find it in Topley and Wilson's principles of bacteriology and immunology (1964). Whatever classification is accepted, one factor which is common to the majority of group D streptococci is their insensitivity to penicillin.

Str. faecalis is normally found in the intestine; most strains are non-pathogenic or their pathogenicity is of a low order. This organism is responsible for genito-urinary infection or endocarditis. Endocarditis due to Str. faecalis tends to occur in young women and older men; it is frequently an insidious, indeed a chronic illness in which fever and cardiac murmurs are the most conspicuous features. Classical findings such as Osler's nodes retinal and skin lesions or other embolic phenomena may be absent or late in appearing.

In treating this form of endocarditis it is vital to obtain the organism on blood culture; only in this way may careful evaluation of antibiotic sensitivity assays indicate the best combination of drugs. Any streptococcus which is resistant to 0.5 units or more of penicillin G per millilitre should from the therapeutic standpoint be regarded in the same class as enterococci as recommended by Lerner and Weinstein (1966). In general penicillin G in large doses combined with streptomycin is most likely to produce effective bactericidal action. Occasionally penicillin G alone may suffice, but very high doses will be required. The author has treated one patient who required 100 mega units of penicillin G daily given intravenously for three months, combined with streptomycin to effect cure (see page 36). In a review of this subject Jawetz and Sonne (1966) found that in 20% of enterococcal strains selected at random the bactericidal effect of penicillin G alone was as good a combination of penicillin and streptomycin; the combination, however, was essential for complete bactericidal action in 40% of strains. For a few strains effective bactericidal activity was only achieved when erythromycin or bacitracin or both were administered in addition to penicillin G.

INFECTION WITH STREPTOCOCCI OF OTHER GROUPS

Occasionally streptococci of unusual groups may be associated with significan illness. Reinarz and Sanford (1965) collected reports of 19 patients who suffered from endocarditis, meningitis, genital tract sepsis, suppurative arthritis and liver abscess and in whom streptococci other than groups A or D were isolated. Antibiotic sensitivity tests were carried out on eleven strains of these organisms. Their results suggest that penicillin G and or erythromycin are the antibiotics of choice.

REFERENCES

Jawetz, E. and Sonne, M. (1966) Penicillin-Streptomycin treatment of enterococcal endocarditis. New Engl. J. Med., **274**, 710

Lerner, P. I. and Weinstein, L. (1966) Infective endocarditis in the antibiotic era. New Engl. J. Med., **274**, 323

Reinarz, J. A. and Sanford, J. P. (1965) Human infections caused by non Group A or D streptococci. Medicine, **44**, 81

Topley and Wilson's 'Principles of Bacteriology and Immunity'. Fifth Edition. Volume II, pages 715-719. Edward Arnold, London

14. Staphylococcal Infection

INTRODUCTION

Staphylococcal infection is common, but considering the ubiquity of these bacteria it is extraordinary that infection is not very much more frequent. They offer proof, if proof were required, that the mere presence of micro-organisms does not constitute infection. Staphylococci are present on the skin, especially in the anterior nares, and the perineal region; they form part of the ambience in which we live and are scattered into the air when clothing, bedding, furniture and such are disturbed. The presence of a large population of pathogenic epidemic-strain staphylococci in hospital wards constitutes a considerable risk to patients and staff.

Staphylococci are Gram-positive spherical cells that tend to grow in clusters. They are readily cultured on various media, are metabolically active and produce pigments that vary from white to deep yellow. Pigment production is used as a basis for classification; two species are recognised, *Staphylococcus aureus* and *Staphylococcus albus* (epidermidis). Both species may produce a variety of toxins and enzymes, but these activities are more conspicuous in *Staph. aureus* and relate to the more obvious pathogenicity of this species. The ability to coagulate plasma is probably the best indication of pathogenicity, but this is not infallible, and on occasions coagulase negative *Staph. albus* can cause disease. Staphylococci produce various haemolysins, leucocidins, fibrinolysin, hyaluronidase, and an enterotoxin which is responsible for the symptoms of food poisoning of staphylococcal origin. Classification of staphylococci is carried out on the basis of antigenic structure, antibiotic sensitivity and phage type. Phage typing is most important in epidemiological studies of staphylococcal infection. Knowledge of prevalent phage types in the community is required for correct assessment of the significance of a single isolation from a particular individual.

LOCALISED STAPHYLOCOCCAL INFECTION

The characteristic and probably the commonest lesions resulting in man from infection with Staph. aureus are local skin lesions. These include pustules, boils (furuncles) and finger pulp infections; carbuncles are more serious manifestations of staphylococcal skin infection, being deeper, tending to spread and usually have several areas where pus exudes to the surface. Subjects who have one such staphylococcal infection frequently develop others; family contacts have a much higher incidence of staphylococci infections than the general population. Some patients have chronic, recurrent furunclosis which may last for months or even years, and the cure of which often bears little relation to any treatment offered.

Other skin manifestations of staphylococcal infection are secondary infection in wounds, burns and superficial skin injury. Staph. aureus is one of the causes of impetigo; septic bullae are frequently found in infants, and sycosis barbae, which is a staphylococcal skin infection difficult to eradicate, affects the beard area in men.

SYSTEMIC STAPHYLOCOCCAL INFECTION

Blood stream invasion by staphylococci causes metastatic focal infection. Favourite sites are the metaphysis of long bones, perirenal tissues, muscles, lungs and brain. Any one of these sites may be involved, but if there is a continuing septicaemia and especially if the heart valves are affected multiple and repeated metastatic foci must be expected and may be found in any organ. There is sometimes an obvious primary staphylococcal infection in the skin or uterus perhaps, but in many cases no portal of entry will be found.

Staphylococcal pneumonia probably occurs with two distinct presentations. Either there are multiple areas of breaking down lung tissue which are in fact abscesses resulting from staphylococcal septicaemia in which metastatic foci appear mainly in the lungs; or primary staphylococcal infections of the lungs occur. This is most commonly seen in infancy, in those with a recent respiratory infection such as influenza or chickenpox, or in those with chronic broncho-pulmonary disease such as bronchitis or mucoviscidosis.

In these situations the responsible organisms are coagulase positive Staph. aureus; in some cases in which the clinical presentation is less florid, a coagulase negative Staph. albus is cultured from lesions or from blood. It is clear that some of these organisms can be responsible for infection, and this is particularly likely to occur when prostheses such as valves are inserted into the heart or the ventricular draining system of the brain. These rather indolent bacteraemic states do not usually respond until the infected prosthesis is replaced (page 42).

STAPHYLOCOCCAL BOWEL INFECTION

Staphylococci cause gastro-intestinal disease in two ways: food poisoning due to ingestion of staphvlococcal enterotoxin, or by overgrowth in the bowel of antibiotic-resistant staphylococci which results in enterocolitis.

STAPHYLOCOCCAL FOOD POISONING

Certain strains of Staphylococcus aureus usually belonging to phage groups III and IV produce substances which are emetic for man and some animals. Attempts to characterise these substances have led to identification of enterotoxin A and B (Casman, 1965) and there are others yet to be identified. Enterotoxin A is probably the commonest found in association with food poisoning; enterotoxin B may be found alone, but is often present with enterotoxin A.

Cooked rather than raw meat is associated with staphylococcal food poisoning. In raw and cooked meat both growth of staphylococci and enterotoxin production occurred easily on the surface of ground beef which was not contaminated, and much less freely when samples were contaminated (Casman, 1965). This suggests that staphylococci are unable to compete in growth when large numbers of other organisms are present.

Food poisoning resulting from ingestion of staphylococcal enterotoxin is usually sudden in onset, vomiting occurring in from one to six hours after eating contaminated food is a result of stimulation of medullary centres. Diarrhoea follows vomiting and prostration can be marked. As routine tests for enterotoxin are not available, diagnosis depends on clinical suspicion combined with the fact that others who have eaten the same food are similarly afflicted, and that the food contains large numbers of coagulase positive Staph. aureus.

STAPHYLOCOCCAL ENTEROCOLITIS

Staphylococcal enterocolitis is characterised by profuse watery diarrhoea of sudden onset in a patient who has been taking wide spectrum antibiotics orally. There is often a history of chronic illness with prolonged periods in hospital and a high proportion of these episodes occur after surgical operations. The diagnosis may be confirmed by finding large numbers of Gram-positive cocci with many leucocytes in a stool smear. These organisms are usually penicillin resistant Staph. aureus belonging to phage types in Group III. Infection combined with rapid loss of water and electrolytes may lead to profound circulatory impairment and death unless treatment is prompt and energetic.

HOSPITAL STAPHYLOCOCCAL INFECTION

Hospital environment has provided a rich source of pathogenic organisms causing local epidemics in general medical, surgical and obstetric wards. In the latter part of the nineteenth century the organism responsible was the haemolytic streptococcus, but in the antibiotic era of the twentieth century streptococci have virtually been replaced by staphylococci, and to some extent in recent years by Gram-negative organisms.

Before 1940 few strains of penicillinase-producing staphylococci were isolated, but in 1945 and thereafter an increasing proportion of penicillin-resistant Staph. aureus was noted and attention was focused on the hospital as a source of endemic staphylococcal infection. It was shown that resistant organisms were spread from patient to patient by cross-infection rather than by individual patients developing penicillin-resistance during therapy (Barber, 1947). Gould (1958) showed that antibiotic dust present in the hospital environment affected nasal bacterial flora, thus explaining how untreated patients and members of the hospital staff became carriers of penicillin-resistant strains of Staph. aureus. New antibiotics caused similar changes. Their introduction led to the appearance in hospital of strains bred from naturally resistant mutants and to their spread by cross-infection.

The prevalence of penicillin-resistant staphylococci in hospitals in many parts of the world has focused attention not only on the epidemiology of staphylococcal infection, but has led to reassessment of control measures and the reasons for their failure. Antibiotic prescribing habits have been examined, in some quarters at any rate, with a view to minimising the rate and extent of antibiotic resistant staphylococcal carriage.

TYPES OF HOSPITAL INFECTION

Many of the problems relating to staphylococcal infection occurring in different hospital units have features in common. Thus the presence of a high proportion of carriers of Staph. aureus, or of those subjects who seem to have special facility for shedding staphylococci in large numbers, will lead to problems just as much in medical as in surgical wards or maternity units. Special problems may relate to the separate environments; mothers colonised by staphylococci may infect their infants, surgical wounds can become infected from organisms present in the surgeon's throat or on the skin of the anaesthetist, or a patient with a tracheostomy may disseminate staphylococci over a wide area.

In most cases the individual clinical manifestations of sepsis are of a minor nature. Pustules and local skin lesions, conjunctivitis or infected wounds are the common findings. It is important to remember that these relatively minor infections merely represent overt manifestations of a much wider and less well understood hazard — what might be called the clinical tip of the cross-infection iceberg. Sooner or later some patients will develop systemic staphylococcal infection, such as pneumonia, septicaemia or meningitis and only then may catastrophe proclaim the high level of endemic minor staphylococcal infection.

TREATMENT OF STAPHYLOCOCCAL INFECTION

SKIN LESIONS

Minor staphylococcal skin infections may require no treatment; recurrent minor lesions suggest a focus which is a constant source of staphylococci and which may be eradicated by local application of hexachlorophane. Boils can be treated with antibiotics, but recurrence is common. Penicillin G, cloxacillin and lincomycin are the most useful drugs.

Major skin lesions such as abscesses and carbuncles will usually require surgery; drainage is the first principle of treatment and antibiotics a useful adjunct.

SYSTEMIC STAPHYLOCOCCAL INFECTION

Treatment of systemic infection has two facets. First, establishing that the infection is staphylococcal in origin, and second, the choice of specific chemotherapy. Inevitably there is some time lag before cultures prove the diagnosis, and selection of therapy will have to be based on clinical assessment perhaps combined with the microscopical appearance of smears made from lesions and stained by Gram's technique. The question which requires answering is, is it justified to treat a patient for staphylococcal infection when the diagnosis is decided by clinical acumen alone, or should antibiotic cover be sufficiently broad to include virtually all possibilities? In the final analysis each clinician will have to make up his own mind on how to proceed; the method adopted by the author is, in the first instance, to treat the patient for staphylococcal infection with large doses of penicillin G and cloxacillin, provided the clinical picture is sufficiently clear. This may lead to much difficulty for what is clear to one clinician may be very unclear to another; to a large extent the choice is therefore subjective and personal. Alternatively, one uses a combination of drugs such as cloxacillin or methacillin effective against penicillin-resistant staphylococci, with a drug like chloramphenicol which will be effective against not only a high proportion of staphylococci, but also most Gram-negative organisms. A good compromise is to use cephaloridine which is an effective bactericidal antibiotic, but its antistaphylococcal action is by no means as certain as the penicillinase-stable penicillins. It must also be emphasised that in treating ill patients with suspected staphylococcal infection, whatever drugs are used they must be given in large doses, preferably by the parenteral route to ensure bactericidal action.

In established staphylococcal infection there is much greater choice. Penicillin G, providing the organism is sensitive, is the most effective single antibiotic; it has been well tried and its limitations are understood. For penicillin G-resistant staphylococci one of the semisynthetic penicillinase-stable compounds is the first choice, cloxacillin or oxacillin have little to choose between them; cephaloridine, lincomycin, erythromycin, fucidic acid and vancomycin are useful alternatives.

The following is a guide to some special infections.

STAPHYLOCOCCAL SEPTICAEMIA OR PNEUMONIA

Penicillin G in doses of 10 to 60 million units per day given intravenously if necessary, and cloxacillin up to 8 g/daily are used. Therapy must be continued for a minimum of two weeks. Superinfection may occur, especially when treating pneumonia, and care must be taken to treat opportunist infections, especially those due to Gram-negative organisms.

ACUTE OSTEOMYELITIS

A few early cases may respond to antibiotics alone, but the majority must be treated by the established surgical principle of open operation to drain pus. Osteomyelitis can be difficult to diagnose and by the time an orthopaedic surgeon sees the patient drilling will almost invariably be required. Another reason for operation is to secure cultures which in the majority of cases yield Staph. aureus. The penicillins should be given in high doses; two antibiotics which may well have application here are fucidic acid and lincomycin because of ability to penetrate bone.

STAPHYLOCOCCAL MENINGITIS

Here antibiotic regimes are similar to those used in septicaemia. Cloxacillin can be given intrathecally if required. Consideration should be given to chloramphenicol because of its ability to reach very high concentrations in cerebrospinal fluid.

PUERPERAL AND POST ABORTUM SEPSIS

In the puerperal period breast abscess and less frequently uterine infection results from Staph. aureus; diagnosis is not usually difficult and the response to antibiotics is satisfactory; occasionally blood stream invasion occurs.

On the other hand in septic induced abortion blood stream infection may present many difficulties. In this context mixed infection with staphylococci, anaerobes especially Clostridium welchii, and Gram-negative organisms such as Escherichia coli are common; clostridia will require massive penicillin therapy (see page 36) and coliforms may not respond at all to the usual antistaphylococcal drugs. As many as five pathogens may be isolated simultaneously on blood culture. In practice if the patient is jaundiced indicating haemolysis produced by toxins from Cl. welchii, she should receive large doses of intravenous penicillin G and hyperbaric oxygen may be required. Unresponsive shock in the absence of jaundice suggests Gram-negative infection.

STAPHYLOCOCCAL INTESTINAL INFECTION
FOOD POISONING

Treatment of staphylococcal food poisoning is directed towards the relief of symptoms and the replacement of water and electrolyte losses. Antibiotics are not indicated.

ENTEROCOLITIS

Three measures are used in treating staphylococcal enterocolitis:

1. Withdrawal of oral broadspectrum antibiotic
2. Electrolyte and water replacement. This may require large volumes of fluid
3. Administration of antistaphylococcal antibiotics

Mild cases respond when the oral antibiotic therapy is stopped, though the majority will require energetic supportive infusion therapy, plasma and blood transfusion may be necessary.

It is wise to give a penicillinase-stable penicillin intramuscularly or intravenously as well as orally – cloxacillin is the drug of choice, but other antistaphylococcal drugs have been used effectively, especially vancomycin.

METHICILLIN-RESISTANT STAPHYLOCOCCI

Three different, though related facets of problems thrown up by methicillin-resistant staphylococci have recently received prominence. The first of these relates to the incidence of these organisms, the second to their pathogenicity, and the third concerns therapy.

INCIDENCE

The incidence of Staph. aureus resistant to methicillin (and cloxacillin) is extremely variable. This variation is noted not only between hospitals but also between different countries. In some hospitals where these organisms are relatively numerous they may persist for a number of years but there are instances where these resistant strains have virtually disappeared from an 'endemic' hospital. The relationship between the incidence of methicillin-resistant staphylococci and the clinical use of methicillin is not very clear; there may be a high incidence where little of the drug is used. Parker (1970) has suggested that the incidence may show a better correlation with the total usage of penicillins than to the use of methicillin alone. In 28 personal cases of staphylococcal septicaemia collected during the period 1965-1970 methicillin resistance was not demonstrated in a single isolate although cloxacillin was widely used during this period.

Methicillin resistance among strains of Staph. aureus tested at the Staphylococcal Reference Laboratory at Colindale showed a gradual increase from 0.06% in 1960 to 0.97% in 1964 and a further increase to 4.11% in 1969 (Parker & Jevons, 1964; Parker & Hewitt, 1970). In parts of Europe methicillin resistance, particularly in Paris and Denmark, has become a major problem but the incidence continues at a remarkably low level in the United States. It should be pointed out that some of these apparent differences may be accounted for by differences in bacteriological technique — for instance the curious behaviour of these organisms cultured at different temperatures in the presence of methicillin may explain some anomalies.

PATHOGENICITY

Because methicillin-resistant strains of Staph. aureus may represent only a proportion of staphylococcal pathogens in an individual patient treatment with methicillin (or cloxacillin) may be effective occasionally. This was sometimes interpreted as indicating that these penicillins were clinically successful even though in vitro resistance to them was reported by the laboratory. Experience now indicates that methicillin-resistant organisms are as virulent as any other 'hospital' strains of staphylococci and that serious invasive infections such as septicaemia will not respond to treatment with methicillin.

TREATMENT

In regard to therapy two orders of problems arise, firstly the patient who develops a clinical staphylococcal infection in an environment where methicillin-resistance is prevalent and the pathogen must be presumed to be of the resistant variety, and secondly when clinical or bacteriological evidence is consistent with infection with more sensitive staphylococci. Clearly in these two situations a different chemotherapeutic approach is justified; great difficulty may arise in deciding which course to take in individual acute infections.

Methicillin-resistant staphylococci are invariably resistant to a number of other antibiotics and because many patients with methicillin-resistant organisms are seriously ill it has been impossible to get any kind of controlled trial of different chemotherapeutic agents. Combined therapy with at least two drugs is probably the wisest initial therapy; methicillin with kanamycin or cephalothin or possibly fucidin have been tried. Jensen and Lassen (1969) suggest a combination of fucidin with novobiocin, rifamycin, or erythromycin. In any resistant staphylococcal infection vancomycin, despite its toxicity and difficulty in administration should be considered. In these infections good laboratory control is obligatory.

REFERENCES

Barber, M. (1947) Staphylococcal infection due to penicillin-resistant strains. Brit. med. J., **2**, 863

Casman, E. P. (1965) Staphylococcal Enterotoxin. Ann. NY Acad. Sci., **128**, 124

Gould, J. C. (1958) Environmental penicillin and penicillin-resistant *Staphylococcus aureus*. Lancet, **i**, 489

Jensen, K. and Lassen, H. C. A. (1969) Combined treatment with antibacterial chemotherapeutical agents in staphylococcal infections. Quart. J. Med., **38**, 91

Parker, M. T. and Hewitt, J. H. (1970) Methicillin resistance in *Staphylococcus aureus*. Lancet, **i**, 800

Parker, M. T. and Jevons, M. P. (1964) Survey of methicillin resistance in *Staphylococcus aureus*. Postgrad. med. J. Suppl. **40**, 170

15. Antibiotics in Gastro-intestinal Disorders

INTRODUCTION

A nice balance is reached between the very large numbers of bacteria within the intestinal lumen and their immediate environment. Normally these organisms adapt to wide fluctuations in the volume and character of the diet with little noticeable effect on function. Infection with specific micro-organisms such as Salmonella typhi or Entamoeba histolytica can clearly alter bowel function by mechanisms that appear to depend for the most part on the mechanical effects of ulceration. At the other end of the spectrum bacterial products introduced into the gut may be innocuous unless they are absorbed into the blood stream where they are carried to medullary centres, stimulation of which causes vomiting. Staphylococcal enterotoxin acts in this way.

Between these extremes of disorders resulting from pathogenic micro-organisms on one hand and bacterial toxins on the other there falls a group of conditions caused by an increase in bacteria normally present within the bowel. This results when the local anatomy and physiology of segments of the bowel favour multiplication of certain bacterial populations and is found in association with diverticuli and the 'blind loop' syndrome.

In this chapter the use of antibiotics in these various intestinal disorders is considered.

SPECIFIC BOWEL INFECTIONS

Infection with Shigellae, Salmonellae, and the pathogenic strains of Escherichia coli are common causes of diarrhoea and vomiting. These organisms are grouped together because the majority of infections caused by them do not respond to and therefore do not require administration of antibiotics. From this generalisation are excluded infections due to S. typhi and those patients with other salmonella infections with blood stream or tissue invasion.

(i) Bacillary Dysentery

The genus Shigella comprises four groups of organisms responsible for bacillary dysentery; in the United Kingdom the commonest pathogen is

Shigella sonnei. Children are most frequently affected. At the onset there is fever, headache and curiously, meningism. Vomiting may be present. Diarrhoea occurs within a few hours; the stools are watery and frequently contain blood, or blood-streaked mucus. Mild attacks are common with little constitutional upset, and diarrhoea in which the stools may be free of blood. The majority of patients are asymptomatic in two to three days although a high proportion continue to excrete the organism for a variable period and a few become chronic excretors for months or even years.

Treatment of Sonne dysentery with antibiotics has been widely practised, but there are many contradictory claims in the literature. If the criterion of cure is confined to relief of symptoms there is little to choose between treatment with or without antibiotics. Many authors take as evidence of the effectiveness of antibiotics the fact that shigellae cannot be cultured from the patient's stools during the period in which the drug is being taken. The author does not consider this a valid criterion; more relevant is a number of negative stool cultures after the antibiotic has been stopped, preferably with an interval between the termination of therapy and the collection of the first clearance stool sample. Using these criteria the author was unable to demonstrate the superiority of orally administered streptomycin over no treatment in a series of 33 cases of sonne dysentery (Smith & Young, 1966).

Experience of a number of other drugs, including sulphonamides, tetracyclines, colomycin, neomycin, or ampicillin, has not altered the view that chemotherapy is of no avail in obtaining bacteriological clearance in Shigella sonnei infections.

Dysentery resulting from infection with Shigella flexneri, dysenteriae or boydii is much less common in the United Kingdom; these organisms tend to cause a more severe illness, especially in warm climates. If the author encounters a patient with dysentery caused by one of these organisms, it is the practice to prescribe a five day course of oral tetracycline. Cases are not sufficiently common to form an adequate assessment of the efficiency of this therapy and the literature is equally unhelpful (eg Barrett-Connor, 1966).

(ii) Salmonella Infections

There are more than 1,000 salmonellae which are differentiated by their antigenic structure. By a simple **clinical** classification this very large genus can be separated into three sub-groups:

Group I. S. typhi
S. paratyphi A, B and C

Infection with these organisms results in an illness which is often severe, in which blood stream invasion is characteristic and in which diarrhoea may or may not be prominent. The antibiotics which are most useful in this group are chloramphenicol and perhaps sulphamethoxazole-trimethoprim in the acute stage of illness; ampicillin and sulphamethoxazole-trimethoprim may be tried in the chronic carrier stage. Chemotherapy in typhoid and paratyphoid infection is fully discussed in the chapter on chloramphenicol (page 77).

Group II. S. typhi-murium
S. enteritidis
S. cholerae-suis

Infection with organisms in this group usually results in gastro-enteritis, often with severe bloody diarrhoea. Occasionally blood stream invasion occurs. S. typhi-murium is the commonest cause of salmonella infection and has worldwide distribution. S. cholerae-suis has considerable invasive characteristics.

Group III. This includes,
All the remaining salmonellae

Organisms in this group are frequently called after the city in which the isolation of the organism was first made, such as S. dublin, S. brandenburg, S. newport, S. london.

Illness resulting from infection with organisms in Group III is of the gastro-enteritis type and cannot readily be distinguished from that resulting from Group II organisms, except that they are less commonly encountered, unless in local epidemics.

TREATMENT OF GROUPS II AND III INFECTIONS

The treatment of infections resulting from salmonellae in Groups II and III is symptomatic and supportive; intravenous infusions of electrolyte solutions and plasma may be required especially in the very young and old. Antibiotics are contraindicated except when there is evidence of blood stream invasion. The reasons for withholding antibiotics in uncomplicated salmonella enteritis are twofold. First there is good evidence that using antibiotics prolongs the length of time the patient excretes the organism. In a study of children with S. typhi-murium infection Dixon (1965) concluded that antibiotics did not shorten the period of symptomless excretion. Table XVI taken from his paper shows the comparison between the length of time to effect clearance in 67 treated and 64 untreated children, and it is plain that the untreated group fared better.

Rosenstein (1967) investigated 70 contacts of children with salmonella gastro-enteritis who had positive stool cultures. Her conclusion was that the duration of salmonella carriage was shortest in patients who had not initially received antibiotic therapy, intermediate in those treated with ampicillin or neomycin and longest in patients who received chloramphenicol. The failure of oral neomycin in non-invasive salmonella infections was well demonstrated in a prospective trial carried out by the Members of the

Table XVI. Number and percentage of children whose faeces harboured Salm. typhimurium at weekly intervals after infection in two outbreaks

WEEK OF INFECTION

	1	2	3	4	5	6	7	8	9	10	11	12	13	14	15	16	17	18
SUFFOLK, 1964 (TREATED CHILDREN)																		
No. of children with positive faeces	67	66	63	60	50	39	30	25	20	19	10	9	6	2	2	1	1	0
Percentage	100	98.5	94.0	89.6	74.6	58.2	44.8	37.3	29.9	28.4	14.9	13.4	9.0	3.0	3.0	1.5	1.5	0
SOUTH WALES, 1954 (UNTREATED CHILDREN)																		
No. of children with positive faeces	64		55	35	20	8	3	2	2	2	1	1	1	1	1	1	1	0
Percentage	100		85.9	54.7	31.3	12.5	4.7	3.1	3.1	3.1	1.6	1.6	1.6	1.6	1.6	1.6	1.6	0

(Reproduced by permission of the author and the Editor British Medical Journal)

Association for the Study of Infectious Disease (1970). There were 168 patients (78 given neomycin, 90 given placebo) and there was no difference in clearance rate between the neomycin and placebo-treated groups. Those given the antibiotic were more likely to be symptomless excretors for a six week period after treatment than those given the inert substance. Similar views on antibiotic failure have been expressed by Lafleur et al (1966) and Gotoff et al (1966).

The second reason for withholding antibiotics in these groups of patients is the probability that multiple antibiotic resistance will be induced not only in salmonellae, but in other enterobactericeae leading to formidable therapeutic and epidemiological difficulties. The episomal transfer of resistance factors is now well established as a mechanism of rapid acquisition of drug resistance in enteric bacteria (see Chapter 2 Transmission of Drug Resistance).

It must be made plain, however, that full doses of chloramphenicol, or possibly sulphamethoxazole-trimethoprim should be used when there is evidence of septicaemia (Smith, 1967). The only reason for prescribing these drugs is to remove the organism from the blood stream as quickly as possible, so that metastatic focal infection may be avoided.

(iii) Enteropathogenic E. coli

Gastro-enteritis resulting from infection with enteropathogenic strains of E. coli is virtually confined to children under three years. Epidemics in nurseries and institutions are common. Not only diarrhoea, but abdominal distention and vomiting may be troublesome. In this condition it is extremely difficult to assess the efficiency of antibiotic therapy because of the mild nature of many cases and the different criteria selected for assessment. A really large controlled trial does not seem to have been undertaken. Some authors have found neomycin effective in controlling diarrhoea (Wheeler et al, 1954; Rogers et al, 1956), but it is uncertain if the eradication of the organisms from stool samples is expedited by antibiotics. The dose of neomycin recommended is 30 to 50 mg/kg/day in divided doses.

In gastro-intestinal infections two facts should be stressed. Firstly, that in vitro sensitivity is often a poor guide in selecting effective chemotherapy; secondly, that stool samples taken when the patient is receiving an antibiotic, especially a non-absorbable compound, will contain some of the drug and may well inhibit culture of the organism. Clearly this can lead to spurious negative results.

(iv) Amoebic Dysentery

The protozoa Entamoeba histolytica may invade the wall of the large intestine causing ulceration which manifests clinically as diarrhoea. The course of the illness is often relapsing over a period of years and there may be extention of the infection to other organs, especially the liver. Specific therapy involves the use of drugs which are tissue amboebicides, luminal amoebicides, and drugs which act indirectly on the amoebae.

TISSUE AMOEBICIDES

Emetine hydrochloride in intramuscular doses of 1 grain (65 mg) daily for 10 to 12 days is the most effective drug. Emetine is widely distributed in the tissues and may be cardio-toxic; it rarely completely clears the intestinal infection. A synthetic emetine-like compound dehydroemetine may prove equally effective, but has not yet been fully tried.

Chloroquine is an amoebicide which is concentrated in the liver, its action on parasites being confined to that organ.

LUMINAL AMOEBICIDES

For treatment and elimination of intestinal amoebiasis emetine bismuth iodide (EBI) is used. It is administered orally as enteric coated pills in a daily dose of 1 g three times which is continued for ten days.

Many other amoebicides are available, including arsenicals such as acetarsol, carbasone, diphetarsone and iodo-quinoline compounds such as chiniofon, and di-iodohydroxyquinoline. These are usually less effective than EBI.

OTHER DRUGS

Metronidazole (Flagyl) is effective in all forms of amoebiasis. The dose is 800 mg three times daily for ten days. Alcohol should be avoided during administration.

Tetracyclines, 2 g daily may sometimes help in controlling amoebic dysentery.

CLINICAL USE OF COMBINED THERAPY

In treating amoebiasis the combination of drugs used depends on the localisation of the major lesions.

An acute attack of amoebic dysentery will require emetine hydrochloride followed by emetine bismuth iodide. Tetracyclines may also be prescribed.

When there is hepatic involvement emetine is given concurrently with chloroquine.

(v) Diarrhoea from bacterial toxins

Staphylococcal enterotoxin and possibly toxins produced by Clostridium welchii cause acute food poisoning. Antibiotics are not indicated, treatment being directed to relieving symptoms and restoring body fluid and electrolyte losses.

(vi) **Cholera**

The profuse watery diarrhoea of cholera kills when fluid and electrolyte replacement is inadequate or inept; skilful management of fluid balance has markedly reduced the mortality. No antibiotics appear to be active against Vibrio cholerae but the use of tetracycline may reduce stool volume and therefore the duration of infusion of large volumes of fluid.

NON SPECIFIC GASTRO-INTESTINAL DISORDERS

The ecology of the bowel flora is such that alterations in bacterial populations may lead to disordered bowel action, the most conspicuous of which is usually diarrhoea. Weight loss, anaemia and vitamin B_{12} deficiency are long-term effects which may be encountered.

(i) **Diverticulitis and Blind Loop Syndrome**

Diverticulitis of either the small or large bowel may result in diarrhoea, vomiting, and occasionally abscess formation. The latter most frequently presents as 'left sided appendicitis' with tenderness, diarrhoea and a palpable mass in the left lower abdomen. Treatment by conservative regime should include chemotherapy; a non-absorbable sulphonamide, or antibiotic such as neomycin is often helpful. Tetracycline or ampicillin can be used to achieve a combined antibiotic action both within the gut and in the tissues.

Proliferation of bacteria in the small bowel may be the common aetiological basis for steatorrhoea in blind loop syndromes resulting from surgery or fistula formation with demonstrable anatomical abnormality, and physiological disturbances resulting in hypomotility which can occur in conditions like scleroderma and diabetes mellitus. The syndrome includes anaemia, low serum albumen and calcium, and neurological abnormalities, related to malabsorption of vitamin B_{12}. The precise mechanism by which bacteria deprive the body of vitamin B_{12} is far from clear. The most plausible explanation is that the presence of bacteria results in degradation of bile salts to the unconjugated state in which they have a toxic inhibitory action on the intestine (Rosenberg et al, 1967). The organisms which have been shown to cause deconjugation include enterococci, clostrida and bacteroides; treatment with antibiotics such as tetracyclines and erythromycin (Rosenberg et al, 1967) will often reduce steatorrhoea and objective improvement in vitamin B_{12} absorption may be demonstrated.

(ii) Antibiotic induced entero-colitis

The best example of this condition is the enterocolitis seen in surgical patients who have been taking wide spectrum antibiotics orally. Suppression of susceptible flora by a drug which reaches a high concentration in the small bowel leads to an overgrowth of organisms, and staphylococci are the chief offenders. Any wide spectrum drug or combination of drugs will cause this complication;

tetracyclines are frequently implicated. Treatment is directed at correcting fluid and electrolyte losses, withholding the wide spectrum antibiotic and substituting drugs which are effective against the causative organism. When staphylococci are responsible, cloxacillin both orally and parenterally is the best choice.

(iii) Hepatic coma. Portal systemic encephalopathy

Certain amines are produced by intestinal micro-organisms in the breakdown of protein; these metabolites are normally detoxicated by the liver but may reach the brain in toxic concentrations when liver cell function fails. The resulting coma or encephalopathy is therefore rationally treated by dietary restriction of protein combined with a broad spectrum antibiotic to inhibit intestinal flora. The drug most often used is neomycin in doses of 4-8 g daily.

(iv) Gastro-enteritis of obscure aetiology

In the majority of patients who have symptoms of acute vomiting and diarrhoea no aetiological agent is isolated. These symptoms are common in travellers and a variety of factors are held responsible — all of them conjectural. Alteration in bowel flora, viruses, mechanical factors such as different methods of cooking have all been blamed. Treatment of these upsets which can be harassing is symptomatic. Antibiotics are contraindicated.

(v) Prophylaxis in bowel surgery (see Chapter 23)

REFERENCES

Barrett-Connor, E. (1966) Shigellosis in the adult. J. Amer. med. Ass., **198**, 717

Dixon, J. M. S. (1965) Effect of antibiotic treatment on duration of excretion of Salmonella typhimurium. Brit. med. J., **2**, 1343

Gotoff, S. P., Boring, J. R. and Lepper, M. H. (1966) An epidemic of Salmonella St. Paul infection in a convalescent home. Amer. J. med. Sci., **251**, 16

Joint Project by members of the Association for the Study of Infectious Disease (1970) Effect of neomycin in non-invasive salmonella infections of the gastro-intestinal tract. Lancet, **ii**, 1159

Lafleur, L., Lavoie, R. and Chicoine, L. (1966) Salmonellose chez les enfants; etude de 95 cas a l'Hopital Ste-Justine, Montreal en 1963-64. Canad. med. Ass. J., **94**, 1304

Rogers, K. B., Benson, R. P., Foster, W. P., Jones, L. F., Butler, B. B. and Williams, T. C . (1956) Phthalysulphacetamide and neomycin in the treatment of infantile gastro-enteritis. Lancet, **ii**, 599

Rosenberg, I. H., Harrison, W. G. and Bull, D. M. (1967) Abnormal bile salt patterns and intestinal bacterial overgrowth associated with malabsorption. New Engl. J. Med., **276**, 1391

Rosenstein, B. J. (1967) Salmonellosis in infants and children. J. Pediat., **70**, 1

Smith, Hillas, Clinical aspects of Kanamycin. Discussion, page 12. Supplement May 1967. Postgrad. med. J.

Smith, Hillas and Young, S. E. J. (1966) Treatment of Sonne Dysentery (c) Brit. med. J., **1**, 481

Wheeler, W. E. and Wainerman, B. (1954) The treatment and prevention of epidemic infantile diarrhoea due to E. coli 0-111 by the use of chloramphenicol and neomycin. Pediatrics, **14**, 357

16. Septicaemia and Bacterial Endocarditis

INTRODUCTION

In this chapter septicaemia and bacterial endocarditis are taken together because they have several important features in common. In both conditions bacteria are present in the blood stream, multiplying in the case of septicaemia and resulting often in profound prostration, toxaemia and circulatory disorder. It follows from this that blood cultures are of paramount importance in both conditions, providing the means for definitive bacteriological diagnosis. The term bacteraemia requires explanation; it implies the presence in the blood of organisms which are not multiplying, is often transient, and of less serious import to the patient than septicaemia. It should be made clear, however, that the distinction between bacteraemia and septicaemia is something of an academic one and is most convincingly made in retrospect when the course of a particular infection has been observed over a sufficiently long period for the outcome to be clear.

In bacterial endocarditis the reservoir of infection is the heart valves which disseminate emboli into either the systemic or pulmonary circulations. In the common form of endocarditis, when the aortic or mitral valves are involved, there are cardiac signs and evidence of emboli in the systemic circulation; pulmonary lesions may give the first indication of involvement of the right side of the heart in endocarditis. Although bacterial endocarditis still predominantly affects heart valves affected by rheumatic disease or congenital abnormality, a proportion of patients, especially in older age groups, show no abnormalities other than those ascribed to arteriosclerosis (Lerner & Weinstein, 1966). The type of infecting organism modifies markedly the clinical picture in endocarditis – Staphylococcus aureus, for instance, causes a fulminating infection with metastatic foci in bones, brain, lungs and other organs. Endocarditis due to Streptococcus faecalis may be almost a chronic disease with anaemia, mild fever, lethargy, and cardiac murmurs as the major features.

TECHNIQUE: BLOOD CULTURES

It cannot be overemphasised that blood cultures must be taken before therapy is started, that they must be taken in sufficient numbers, and that they should be incubated both aerobically and anaerobically. The patient's life may depend upon the correct identification of the infecting organism, and it is impossible to plan logical or effective antibiotic therapy if full bacteriological studies are not available. To achieve this ideal those in clinical charge of patients must realise the importance of routine blood cultures, for it is in the minority of patients whose illnesses are not cured by the passage of time or the promiscuous use of antibiotics, that blood cultures provide the key to cure. It is not proposed that every patient with pyrexia requires blood cultures; but if pyrexia is due to infection of any degree of severity and especially if a firm diagnosis cannot be made on clinical grounds, then blood cultures are not only indicated but are imperative. It must also be emphasised that the absence of fever in no way precludes a diagnosis of infection and does not constitute a contraindication in any sense to obtaining blood cultures.

Positive results are usually obtained after three cultures; persevering to obtain at least six is often justified and may be rewarding. In very acute cases, multiple cultures at short intervals should be obtained.

METHOD OF OBTAINING BLOOD CULTURES

Select a prominent vein and clean the overlying skin with ether followed by an antiseptic solution such as 2% tincture of iodine. Allow the iodine to dry and do not touch the cleaned area until venepuncture is performed. Enter the vein with a single movement and withdraw at least 10 ml of blood into a dry sterile syringe. Transfer the blood into two bottles containing nutrient media injecting about 5 ml into each. It is useful to have a supply of culture bottles containing penicillinase; this destroys any penicillin which is present in the blood sample and may permit organisms present to grow.

Culture bottles should be taken to the laboratory without delay, where they are incubated both aerobically and anaerobically. This is the basic technique and does not require elaborate equipment. There are many modifications, such as taking larger volumes of blood and using more than two culture bottles. Quantitive cultures may be made by pouring a measured volume of citrated blood on to plates containing melted agar. A combination of nutrient broth and solid agar slope (Castaneda) may be used in the same bottle; colonies appearing on the slope can be easily identified and transfer to other media facilitated.

INTERPRETATION OF RESULTS

There are two chief difficulties, false positive cultures, and failure to isolate organisms which may be present in the patient's blood stream.

(i) **False positive cultures**

This implies an error in technique, either in taking the culture or in the laboratory. Contaminants are usually scanty and may be present only in a single bottle. A contaminant which is known to be aerobic may produce some colonies in the bottle cultured anaerobically, but fail to grow in the sample cultured aerobically. Diphtheroids and Staph. albus are common contaminants.

In some circumstances it is impossible to be sure if the organisms cultured are in fact derived from the patient's blood. Many pathogenic organisms have been dismissed as contaminants. The situation calls for repeated cultures.

(ii) **Failure to isolate organisms**

The first and most obvious reason for failure is that the diagnosis is incorrect, the patient is not suffering from septicaemia or endocarditis. Occasionally endocarditis is due to Rickettsiae and diagnosis depends on serology not blood cultures.

Failure may result from poor technique, such as allowing the cultures to remain too long outside the incubator, use of unsuitable media or conditions of growth. The presence of organisms which require prolonged incubation such as bacteroides may be unsuspected if cultures are discarded too soon. Blood cultures should be kept for at least three weeks. Some of the reasons for negative blood cultures are given in Table XVII.

Table XVII. Reasons for negative blood cultures

1. Incorrect diagnosis
2. Infection due to organisms which cannot be cultured, eg Rickettsiae
3. Too few cultures taken
4. Recent antibiotic therapy
5. Failure in technique:
   - (i) Incorrect Media
   - (ii) Incorrect conditions of growth, eg no anerobic culture
   - (iii) Discarding cultures too early
6. Right-sided endocarditis
7. Infection with bacterial L forms

LABORATORY AID TO TREATMENT

In treating endocarditis one attempts to do what is rarely possible in the majority of infections, namely, to kill all the invading organisms. This requires prolonged and effective chemotherapy with a bactericidal drug or combination of drugs. It is therefore important that bactericidal as well as bacteriostatic concentrations of the drugs used should be known to the clinician. A useful method is for various dilutions of the patient's serum to be incubated with the organism isolated from the patient; a bactericidal effect should be obtained with dilutions of at least 1:4.

CLINICAL DIAGNOSIS OF BACTERIAL PATHOGEN

In most cases of bacterial endocarditis when the infection is not acute it is possible to obtain bacteriological confirmation of the diagnosis before starting therapy. On the other hand septicaemia often presents acutely and may be life-threatening and it is in this situation that the clinician must act, making a diagnosis on the evidence available which is always incomplete, his guide to 'best guess' chemotherapy being his own clinical judgement. Certain features suggest infection with particular bacteria and so dictate antibiotic therapy; occasionally several features conflict and the diagnosis is uncertain while in some the clinical features provide no clues to the bacterial pathogen. It is, however, always worth attempting to make a bacteriological diagnosis and in the following section some of the points indicating appropriate therapy will be examined.

(i) Streptococci

Although streptococci of various types may be occasionally cultured from the blood stream and, with the exception of Str. pyogenes, their presence does not often cause an acute illness. Septicaemia due to the latter, now a rarity, is sometimes encountered in the post-partum period and results in a fulminating infection which can end fatally within a few days. Fortunately penicillin G is highly effective. The presence of a punctate erythema occurring in this context may suggest the bacteriological aetiology. Str. faecalis septicaemia is found in women with genital tract sepsis, and in older men who have had genito-urinary manipulations. Although these infections may be severe they do not frequently cause a fatal illness unless endocarditis develops.

About 90% of cases of endocarditis are due to streptococci. Infection with Str. viridans usually results in what might be called the classical form of subacute bacterial endocarditis. There is fever, malaise, anaemia, cardiac murmurs and plenomegaly. A variety of minor and major embolic phenomena is encountered. The evolution of this condition is such that the usual time from onset of symptoms to diagnosis is five to six weeks. A few cases run a moderately acute course. Conversely Staph. aureus usually responsible for an acute illness may cause a protracted subacute infection. Assessment of the bacterial pathogen in cases of endocarditis which are based solely on the acuteness of the illness and the length of the history are therefore frequently erroneous. It is, however, worth preserving a clinical distinction between acute and subacute endocarditis whatever the bacterial aetiology, for in the former therapy must be undertaken without delay.

Septicaemia and endocarditis due to Str. pneumoniae is usually associated with infection in sites where the bacterial cause can be suspected on clinical grounds and confirmed bacteriologically. These include acute pneumonia especially of the lobar variety, meningitis often associated with chronic sinusitis or otitis, and the pneumococcus is probably one of the commonest pathogens responsible for septicaemia in children after splenectomy. This is a highly invasive organism and the presence of either septicaemia or endocarditis in pneumococcal infections alters the prognosis adversely.

(ii) Staphylococci

Staphylococcus aureus is usually responsible for an acute blood stream infection with a marked tendency to localisation in tissues. Thus, when the possibility of septicaemia is considered in the presence of symptoms and signs suggestive of infection of bones, perirenal tissues or lungs the organism likely to be responsible is the staphylococcus. The presence of staphylococcal skin lesions, boils, abscesses and carbuncles, indicates the bacterial pathogen. In the majority of cases, the total leucocyte count is normal or only slightly raised, though there may be an increase in the proportion of polymorphonuclear cells; a marked leucocytosis often develops within 48 hours of starting therapy. In a number of patients an erythematous skin eruption, usually of short duration, is found. Two other features, inconstant though they are, should be sought, namely a history of some looseness of the bowels in the very early stages of the illness, and a relative bradycardia. The latter appears to be quite rare.

Endocarditis resulting from Staph. aureus is frequently fatal; heart valves are rapidly destroyed. A fact which should not be forgetten is that a high proportion of cases of staphylococcal endocarditis are diagnosed only at post-mortem and that in any patient with staphylococcal septicaemia cardiac involvement must be suspected and therapy continued for a prolonged period even in the absence of overt cardiac signs.

Staph. albus is frequently responsible for a low-grade infection in valves and prostheses inserted surgically. This occurs in two situations – the Spitz-Holter valve implanted in infants with hydrocephalus to drain cerebrospinal fluid from the dilated cerebral verticules into a systemic vein, and after implantation of cardiac valves. Infection of these inserted valves gives a high yield of positive blood cultures; in the case of the Spitz-Holter valve the cerebrospinal fluid is usually sterile. It is thought that the valves are infected at the time of insertion and cure usually demands replacement.

(iii) Anaerobic Organisms

These include non-spore forming anaerobic streptococci, spore forming clostridia, and bacteroides. Mixed infections are common. In this group the most clear-cut clinical picture is seen in septicaemia due to Clostridium welchii (perfringens). It occurs in relation to gastro-intestinal haemorrhage, cholecystitis or peritonitis, but is particularly related to post-abortum infection. It causes an acute illness with marked intravascular haemolysis, producing in severe cases a mahogany brown colour of the skin and sclerae; profound hypotension, often irreversible, is accompanied by a strange degree of mental clarity. Those who survive frequently develop oliguric renal failure. Not all cases of Cl. welchii septicaemia present such well marked features: for instance, intravascular haemolysis is not always seen, but it is characteristically noted in post-abortum cases. A marked polymorphonuclear leucocytosis accompanied by thrombocytopoenia is frequently present.

The genus Bacteroides includes Gram-negative non-spore forming, rod shaped bacteria which require anaerobic conditions for growth. They are present in large numbers in the bowel. While there are some 30 species, only two are of clinical importance, Bacteroides funduliformis, and Bacteroides fragilis which appears to be less virulent and less common than the former. Infection may take origin in the oro-pharynx, gastro-intestinal tract, female pelvic organs, surgical wounds or decubitus ulcers. The clinical features of septicaemia resulting from bacteroides, include hectic swinging temperature, marked polymorphonuclear leucocytosis and thrombophlebitis at the initial focus or in metastatic lesions. When pus forms it has a particularly foul odour and gas formation may be demonstrated. Young adults are often affected.

Although patients with acute bacteroides septicaemia are clearly ill, the diagnosis is frequently not confirmed even though suspected. This results from the fact that bacteroides require anaerobic conditions for growth, and that it may be difficult to sustain growth even after initial isolation.

(iv) Gram-negative organisms

The incidence of infections with Gram-negative bacilli is increasing. This is seen in hospital units as diverse as general medical wards and premature infant units where streptococcal and pneumococcal infections have been largely replaced by, first, a great increase in staphylococcal infection, and, in recent years, by infection with Gram-negative organisms. The classical study by Finland and colleagues (1959) at the Boston City Hospital showed that while in 1935 there was a 60% mortality in 286 cases of septicaemia in 1957 there was a total of 588 cases with a mortality of 40%. The mortality of 42% for the 36 cases of Gram-negative infection in 1935 had increased to 54% for 182 cases treated in 1957. At the Mayo Clinic for the period 1940-1954 there were 137 cases of bacteraemia due to Gram-negative bacilli, but from 1955 to 1959 there were 113 cases (Apittel et al, 1956). Between 1953 and 1964 in the New York Hospital McCracken and Shinefield (1966) reported an increase in the incidence of meningitis and septicaemia due to Gram-negative infection in the neonatal period and also recorded an increased mortality.

The reasons for this increased incidence in Gram-negative infection relate to alterations in bacterial populations resulting from treatment with antibacterial drugs, to the intensive use of mechanical equipment predisposing particularly to pseudomonas infection, and especially to host factors which have been altered by the increasing age of the population, frequent use of radiotherapy, corticosteroid and immuno-suppressive drugs. The outcome in infections of this nature bears a close relation to the severity and prognosis of the underlying disease.

When septicaemia or endocarditis results from infection with Gram-negative species certain general features may indicate that this group of organisms is involved; occasionally some special features point to a specific organism. In general severe Gram-negative infections are prevalent in the neonatal period, in genital tract sepsis and in patients over 50 years suffering from peritonitis, hepato-biliary disease, urinary tract infection. Particularly vulnerable are those suffering from diseases such as diabetes mellitus, leukaemia or myelomatosis or in situations where immune host responses are altered by drugs such as corticosteroids or antimetabolites. Frequent antibiotic therapy may favour the multiplication of Gram-negative organisms.

Shock occurs in some patients with Gram-negative septicaemia; it is often not clearly realted to fluid and electrolyte loss and may be difficult to treat. The various syndromes are discussed in the section on the chemotherapy of septicaemia.

In many patients with Gram-negative septicaemia the leucocyte count is not conspicuously raised; indeed, leucopoenia and an accompanying thrombocytopoenia are expected, but these haematological findings are inconstant and require caution in interpretation.

SPECIFIC GRAM-NEGATIVE INFECTIONS

Escherichia coli is important because it is the commonest organism encountered; statistically it is most likely to be responsible for septicaemia in the absence of special distinguishing features. There are usually no special features to indicate a diagnosis due to proteus or to the Klebsiella-Aerobacter group of organisms.

Pseudomonas septicaemia may present with shock accompanied by leucopoenia; debilitated patients with leukaemia and other haematological disorders or those suffering severe burns are particularly susceptible. Jaundice, arthritis, and neurological abnormalities such as disorientation, tremors and convulsions are not uncommon. The diagnosis may be suspected when typical skin lesions occur. Four different types have been described (Barker, 1897; Forkner, 1958). The most striking are round indurated ulcerated areas with black necrotic centres commonly situated in the ano-genital area. Inflammatory reaction and pus formation are not conspicuous. These lesions are termed ecthyma gangrenosa.

Vesicular lesions occur in small clusters with an erythematous base; these are inflamed and painful and Ps. aeruginosa may be cultured from the opalescent fluid contained in these blebs. A third type of lesion is a flat sharply demarcated cellulitis which enlarges rapidly, becoming haemorrhagic and necrotic. The fourth category of lesion includes oval maculopapular nodules on the trunk. These may occur early, cause no symptoms, and usually measure less than 2.0 cm in the greatest diameter.

Haematological abnormalities, especially agranulocytosis, perhaps accompanied by thrombocytopoenia are often present in pseudomonas septicaemia; this has been referred to as 'the paradox of pseudomonas bacteraemia' as these haematological disorders predispose to pseudomonas septicaemia, and in acute pseudomonas infections in patients without underlying disease secondary haematological abnormalities occur. Hypotension, and cardiac arrhythmias are common.

Meningococcal septicaemia usually presents acutely; there is a petechial or purpuric skin eruption which may be very marked, hypotension is characteristic and many patients die so quickly that the meningeal reaction which is nearly always present does not develop into clinically recognisable meningitis. Less acute cases show evidence of both meningitis and septicaemia.

A much rarer form of septicaemia due to N. meningitidis presents a subacute or chronic course lasting weeks or months. Recurrent fever, malaise and especially arthritis are dominant features. Skin eruptions, sometimes resembling erythema nodosum may occur, and of course petechiae may be present. The course of this subacute form may be altered at any time by manifestations of florid meningococcal septicaemia or meningitis.

Septicaemia due to salmonellae is not common except with S. typhi and S. paratyphi when it is characteristic. Patients with acute gastro-intestinal symptoms due to salmonellae, especially if these symptoms are severe, and if pyrexia persists for more than a few days, will sometimes produce an organism on blood culture. S. cholerase-suis has marked invasive properties, and S. typhi-murium because of its ubiquity are the two most likely to be encountered, but any salmonella will give a similar picture.

In typhoid and paratyphoid fevers, leucopoenia, relative bradycardia, splenomegaly, and the presence of 'rose' spots are clinical indications of the bacteriological pathogen. In septicaemia accompanying uncomplicated salmone

Table XVIII

PATHOGEN	SPECIAL FEATURES OF SEPTICAEMIA
1. Streptococcus	
(i) Group A	Punctate erythema: appearance of tongue; circumoral pallor
(ii) Group D (enterococci)	Suspect in young women or older men after genito-urinary manipulation
(iii) Pneumoniae	Presence of lobar pneumonia; occasionally jaundice; post splenectomy
2. Staphylococcus	
(i) aureus	Skin lesion, eg boils or carbuncles; erythematous rash; mild diarrhoea
(ii) albus	Inserted cardiac or Spitz-Holter valves
3. Escherichia coli	Underlying infection – urinary tract, biliary tract, peritoneum. Shock, leucopoenia, thrombocytopoenia
4. Pseudomonas aeruginosa	Presence of severe burns or haematological disorder. Much steroid and antibiotic therapy. Typical necrotic skin lesions – ecthyma gangrenosa
5. Bacteroides	Hectic temperature with rigors; recent pregnancy or abdominal surgery. Foul pus. Emboli especially pulmonary
6. Clostridium welchii	Severe intravascular haemolysis; shock oliguria, leucotytosis. Common in septic abortion
7. Neisseria meningitidis	Petechial skin eruption; shock; meningitis
8. Salmonella typhi, paratyphi	Fever, leucopoenia, bradycardia, 'Rose' spots. Diarrhoea

enteritis leucopoenia is usually present, but there are no other constant distinguishing features.

Table XVIII gives a list of features which may be found helpful in distinguishing on clinical evidence septicaemia resulting from certain bacterial pathogens.

TREATMENT OF BACTERIAL ENDOCARDITIS AND SEPTICAEMIA

Patients with blood stream infection fall into two categories, those requiring urgent treatment before full bacteriological results are available, and included in this category are nearly all patients with septicaemia and a proportion of those with endocarditis. A deliberate approach, assessing both clinical and bacteriological findings can usually be made in the majority of patients with endocarditis, though acute cases, notably those due to infection with Staphylococcus aureus, must be treated urgently. In both categories, as stressed previously, blood cultures must be obtained before starting treatment.

TREATMENT OF ACUTE CASES

These patients constitute one of the greatest medical emergencies; treatment must be decided upon quickly, administered vigorously, and modified as the situation demands. Large doses of antibiotics parenterally are the rule. It is in this group of patients, where diagnosis is necessarily clinical, that the foregoing section may provide a basis for selecting immediate treatment.

(i) Gram-positive cocci

The most fulminating infections in this group are commonly due to staphylococci, much less frequently to Group A streptococci or pneumococci which respond to penicillin G. For staphylococcal infection a combination of penicillin G and cloxacillin is recommended. An adult should receive at least 12 mega penicillin G per 24 hours; this dose can be administered as 2 mega 4 hourly by the intramuscular route. Most patients will not tolerate these injections for more than 24 to 48 hours and a good solution is to give the drug intravenously when at least 24 mega should be administered, provided renal function is not severely disturbed. Cloxacillin, in doses not less than 1 g four hourly, either intramuscularly or intravenously, should also be administered. These large doses, suitable for the initial period of treatment may be modified if the response is satisfactory. The combination of these two penicillins is highly effective and used in the way described even the most acute cases will come under control within 48 hours. Improvement may not occur and may be impossible in late cases where focal damage to vital organs is advanced; inadequate doses may also cause failure.

Methicillin can be used instead of cloxacillin, but as it is rather more toxic and probably less active, it is not recommended. Cephaloridine is not as effective as cloxacillin against penicillinase-producing staphylococci but has a wider antibacterial spectrum. Fucidic acid and lincomycin are useful antistaphylococcal drugs, especially for penetration into tissue such as bone. Vancomycin may prove useful in methicillin-resistant cases.

Enterococcal septicaemia or endocarditis is probably best treated by a combination of penicillin G and streptomycin; some will respond to penicillin alone if the dose is high enough, but a few will require addition of a third drug such as bacitracin. Before abandoning penicillin-streptomycin therapy the dose of penicillin may have to be raised to very high levels (eg 100 mega per 24 hours).

(ii) Gram-negative septicaemia

In many cases the presence of Gram-negative organisms in the blood stream does not cause major circulatory disorder, but when shock does occur the prognosis is poor with a mortality of upwards of 50%. The main features influencing the outcome are the prognosis of the underlying condition and the severity of the shock.

In some cases of Gram-negative septicaemia so-called low resistance or 'warm' shock is present. Clinically there is hypotension with normal or low venous pressure and relatively warm limbs. This picture is a result of vasodilation of arterioles caused by endotoxin; electrolyte imbalance, various toxins or drugs and adrenal insufficiency can cause similar abnormalities.

A second type of circulatory disorder may be observed in which the most conspicuous feature is depression of cardiac function with low cardiac output. This can result in the apparently anomalous situation characterised by severe hypotension and markedly elevated central venous pressure. Clearly the precise haemodynamic upset is very complex, being a result of interaction of many features which modify venous and arteriolar tone, cardiac output and the capacity of the various sub-divisions of the vascular compartment. The marked differences in haemodynamic and metabolic disorders associated with Gram-negative shock have been emphasised by Udhoji and Weil (1965) who stressed that while most patients had reduced cardiac output, increased peripheral resistance and metabolic acidosis, those patients with cirrhosis had an alkalosis, which was sometimes metabolic and sometimes of the uncompensated respiratory type.

Treatment of Gram-negative septicaemia is therefore twofold – correcting any underlying circulatory disorder, and controlling the infection with appropriate chemotherapy. In the initial stages methods designed to improve perfusion of vital organs are imperative; the blood stream infection may be eradicated but the patient may die of shock. A combination of some of the following measures may be used:

Treatment of Shock

(i) Adequate fluid replacement with blood, plasma, electrolyte and mannitol solutions. Monitoring of central venous pressure is desirable.

(ii) Corticosteroids; controversy continues about their use; if administered, large doses such as 1000 mg several times per day should be tried.

(iii) Vasoactive drugs; blockade of alpha receptors to prevent sympathetic constrictor activity, eg phenoxybenzamine (Dibenzyline); stimulation of beta receptors causing peripheral vasodilation and increased cardiac contractility, eg isoprenaline; vasoconstrictors such as metaraminal are best avoided; theophylline — ethylenediamine and digitalis may be useful in selected circumstances; heparin may be used if there is a clotting defect resulting from disseminated intravascular coagulation.

(iv) Hyperbaric oxygen: toxin production by anaerobic organisms (eg Cl. welchii) may be inhibited leading to improved clinical state.

(v) Exchange transfusion; some evidence suggests that this may be effective in shock due to both aerobes and anaerobes.

Chemotherapy in Gram-negative septicaemia

1. In 'blind' therapy where infection with Pseudomonas aeruginosa is considered unlikely, a useful combination is high doses of intravenous penicillin (eg 20-60 mega/24 hours), combined with kanamycin 1 g daily intravenously in divided doses.
   Alternatives include chloramphenicol (2-4 g IV daily); ampicillin (2-4 g IV daily); cephaloridine (2-6 g IV or IM daily).
2. If pseudomonas septicaemia is suspected then one of the following may be used: colomycin, polymyxin B, or gentamicin. These drugs even though their effective and toxic doses are close are often successful.
   Carbenicillin — a recently introduced penicillin, active against Gram-negative bacilli, especially pseudomonas — may prove to be the drug of choice because of its apparent lack of toxicity. Doses of at least 20 to 30 g daily intravenously will be required. Carbenicillin and gentamicin may be used together.
3. The response of bacteroides septicaemia to antibiotics is variable; if the diagnosis is considered likely and therapy urgently required, large doses of penicillin G intravenously combined with streptomycin should be started.
4. Neisseria meningitidis infections should be treated with penicillin and sulphonamides as described in the section on meningococcal meningitis (Chapter 17).
5. Acute typhoid and paratyphoid infection are treated with chloramphenicol (Chapter 6).

In septicaemia, the treatment may demand modification if the clinical response is not satisfactory and further therapy can be planned on the basis of antibiotic sensitivity tests. Length of treatment will depend on the severity of the infection and its response to therapy; few serious infections will be treated for less than one month.

Septicaemia due to Cl. welchii should be treated with large intravenous doses of penicillin G; tetracycline and cephaloridine may also be used.

Treatment of less acute septicaemia and endocarditis

In this situation treatment can usually be delayed 24 or 48 hours until the results of at least the initial blood cultures and the sensitivity pattern of any organisms isolated are available. Thus therapy can be planned.

Subacute endocarditis is most often due to Str. viridans – a heterogenous collection of streptococci which vary in their sensitivity to penicillin G. The majority will respond to penicillin in doses of 4 mega per day; the addition of streptomycin is probably not necessary, but in those patients infected with enterococci or any streptococcus resistant to 0.5u/ml penicillin G the combination of streptomycin and penicillin G is likely to be the most effective therapy.

In subjects hypersensitive to penicillin, alternative drugs are cephalosporin derivatives and lincomycin. Experience with these antibiotics is limited and their use in this situation should be approached with caution.

Although bacteristatic drugs and oral penicillin have sometimes been successful in the treatment of bacterial endocarditis their use is not recommended.

For endocarditis due to staphylococci and Gram-negative organisms the principle of therapy described in the foregoing section on septicaemia should be followed. Salmonella endocarditis, most commonly due to S. cholerae-suis, has been treated effectively using kanamycin (Geraci & Dearing, 1962); ampicillin and chloramphenicol are likely to be most useful alternatives.

Endocarditis with persistently negative cultures

The reasons for negative blood-cultures have been mentioned at the beginning of this chapter (page 187). Patients with persistently negative cultures after Rickettsial infection has been excluded should be treated with high doses of intravenous penicillin (40-100 mega) combined with streptomycin (1 g) daily and therapy should usually continue for six weeks.

REFERENCES

Barker, L. F. (1897) The clinical symptoms, bacteriologic findings and post-mortem appearances in cases of infection of human beings with Bacillus pyocyaneous. J. Amer. med. Ass., **29**, 213

Finland, M., Jones, W. E. Jr. and Barnes, M. W. (1959) Occurrence of serious bacterial infections since introduction of antibacterial agents. J. Amer. med. Ass., **170**, 2188

Forkner, C.E., Frei, E., Edgcomb, J.H. and Utz, J.P. (1958) Pseudomonas septicaemia. Observations on 23 cases. Amer. J. Med., **25**, 877

Geraci, J. E. and Dearing, W. H. (1962) Salmonella panama endocarditis cured with kanamycin therapy. Mayo Clin. Proc., **37**, 552

Lerner, P. I. and Weinstein, L. (1966) Infective endocarditis in the antibiotic era. New Engl. J. Med., **274**, 259

McCracken, G. H. Jr. and Shinefield, H. R. (1966) Changes in the pattern of neonatal septicaemia and meningitis. Amer. J. Dis. Child., **112**, 33

Spittel, J. A. Jr., Martin, W. J. and Nichols, D. R. (1956) Bacteraemia owing to Gram-negative bacilli: experiences in the treatment of 137 patients in a 15 year period. Ann. intern. Med., **44**, 302

Udhoji, V.N. and Weil, M.H. (1965) Haemodynamic and metabolic studies on shock associated with bacteraemia; observations on 16 patients. Ann. intern. Med., **62**, 966

17. Bacterial Meningitis

INTRODUCTION

A reduction in mortality from more than 80% to probably less than 20% has been achieved in meningitis of bacterial origin excluding tuberculous meningitis. This markedly improved prognosis is in large measure due to chemotherapy; it has been observed, not only in parts of the world where improvements in living standards have been noticeable during this period, but also in those countries where advances in public health, housing and nutrition have not been conspicuous.

Nevertheless an overall mortality in the region of 20% is formidable; it must not be forgotten that however sophisticated modern therapy the mortality from late cases and fulminating cases of meningitis is probably just as high today as it ever was.

Another factor which emerges as a result of different mortality in relation to rapidity of diagnosis is the difficulty in comparing results of treatment by various authors and different methods. Good results in a small series of cases may reflect not only good treatment but perhaps the absence of late and fulminating cases.

ANATOMICAL AND PHYSIOLOGICAL CONSIDERATIONS

The brain is enclosed in the cranium and the spinal cord lies in the spinal canal of the vertebral column. The dura mater is a thick fibrous membrane lining the interior of the skull and forms a loose sheath around the spinal cord. The dura forms fibrous septa, most obvious of which are the falx and the tentorium which partially divide the contents of the cranial cavity. Venous sinuses draining blood from the brain are formed along certain lines when the two layers of the dura are separated. The dura mater is known as the pachymenix; pachymeningitis is unusual except in syphilis, but may occur as an extention of infection originating in the bones of the skull.

Interior to the dura mater is the arachnoid beneath which lies the pia mater, a delicate membrane which dips into the sulci and intimately follows the contours of the brain surface. Between the arachnoid and the pia mater is the sub-arachnoid space which contains cerebrospinal fluid. As the spinal cord descends to the level of the first or second lumbar vertebra and the meninges to the level of second sacral vertebra samples of cerebrospinal fluid may be obtained with safety and convenience between these two levels. The pia arachnoid membranes are referred to as the leptomeninges and infection in this area is known as leptomeningitis or simply meningitis.

CEREBROSPINAL FLUID

Cerebrospinal fluid is found in the lateral cerebral ventricles and the third ventricle which are in communication by the foramina of Munro; the third ventricle communicates by the aqueduct of Sylvius with the fourth ventricle and thence to the central canal of the spinal cord. The fluid leaves the fourth ventricle by way of the medial foramen of Magendie and the paired foramina of Luschka to escape into the subarachnoid space. This space has several expansions which constitute the basal cisterns, the largest being the cisterna magna beneath the cerebellum.

Cerebrospinal fluid is formed, circulates and is absorbed; despite modern methods of investigation the precise way in which these functions occur is not agreed. The fluid is produced from the blood, predominantly but probably not exclusively, by the choroid plexuses of the cerebral ventricles. It is likely that the perivascular spaces and possibly the lymphatics of the cranial nerves contribute to the formation of the fluid.

The volume of the cerebrospinal fluid in an adult is usually between 120 and 150 ml; its rate of formation varies and will be an equilibrium derived from rate of absorption and pressure within the system. In the normal state probably 100 ml to 200 ml are formed daily; disease states can markedly alter this rate of production.

The fluid is removed from the subarachnoid space by absorption by the arachnoid villi and pacchionian bodies and then into the venous sinuses and directly through the arachnoid into the cortical vessels. Some is absorbed into the venous plexuses around the foramen magnum and a small amount escapes along the perineural sheath of the cranial nerves into extra-cranial lymphatics.

It should be remembered that there are virtually two separate pools of circulating cerebrospinal fluid — the fluid in the ventricular system and that in the subarachnoid space. It may take a very long time for a substance injected into the lumbar subarachnoid space to be carried to the cortex of the brain, and it is unlikely that it can enter into the ventricular system at all

BARRIERS: BLOOD/BRAIN; BLOOD/CEREBROSPINAL FLUID

Blood/Brain

Early workers demonstrated that dyes injected intravenously reached equilibrium in tissue like muscle within minutes of injection, whereas the same process in the brain took hours. This restricted entry into the brain led to the concept of a blood-brain barrier. Despite the difficulties and errors inherent in these early experiments modern workers using more sophisticated techniques, especially radioactive isotopes, have confirmed the basic concept of a barrier between certain substances in the blood and their entry into brain. This barrier can be interpreted as having a protective effect, preventing blood-born foreign substances such as sucrose and penicillin or naturally occurring humoral agents like acetylcholine and serotonin from acting on sensitive brain and spinal cord centres. Certain substances pass rapidly from the blood into the brain, notably ethyl alcohol and highly fat soluble anaesthetics like ether or thiobarbitone.

Blood/Cerebrospinal Fluid

It is well established that substances present in high concentration in blood plasma may be virtually excluded from the cerebrospinal fluid. Penicillin G, for instance, even in plasma concentrations of several hundred units per ml, crosses the normal meningeal membrane in only very small amounts.

The fact that certain antibiotics can be demonstrated in cerebrospinal fluid in concentrations of 50% or more of the simultaneous plasma level has led to the view that high cerebrospinal fluid levels augur good therapeutic response. In this context it is of particular interest to note the concept of brain extracellular fluid as proposed by Davson (1958, 1963, 1967). This suggests that glial tissue and neurones present closely packed cellular elements which offer only a very limited 'extracellular' space in which substances present in plasma may be distributed. Penicillin, when present in plasma is almost absent in brain tissue for the simple reason that there is so little extracellular fluid into which the drug can penetrate. Inflammation in this anatomical region may be expected to expand the space and could permit relatively high concentrations of antibiotic at the point where they are most required. Increased entry into the extracellular space may or may not be accompanied by an increased cerebrospinal fluid/plasma ratio. This concept of a small extracellular space, expanded in meningitis, permitting increased entry of antibiotic without necessarily increased cerebrospinal fluid concentration is consistent with the findings of various authors that cerebrospinal fluid concentrations of, for instance, ampicillin are not necessarily related to the clinical outcome of the infection (Thrupp et al, 1964; Pickup & McWilliam, 1966).

PATHOGENESIS

With the advent of modern chemotherapy interest has been deflected away from experimental studies in the pathogenesis of meningitis. A continued mortality rate of 20% must in part reflect our inadequate understanding of the manner in which meningeal infection occurs, its mode of dissemination and its precise influence on the physiology and metabolism of the brain, cerebrospinal fluid and cerebral vasculature. The mode of death, for instance, has never been adequately explained in patients with meningitis in whom the cerebrospinal fluid is sterile.

METHOD OF INVASION

Micro-organisms may reach the meninges via the blood stream or by extension from neighbouring infected tissue. Despite the failure of animal studies to produce a consistent model of experimental meningitis by intravenous injection of bacteria, bacteraemia is a common clinical finding in primary meningitis and often associated with bad prognosis. Focal infection at a site distant from the meninges will frequently explain the origin and even the nature of the infecting organism. It is less easy to explain why an apparently harmless colonisation of the pharynx with Neisseria meningitidis may result in meningococcal meningitis, usually with an intervening phase of septicaemia.

Microscopically in early cases of purulent meningitis there is oedema of the pia arachnoid, congestion of vessels and frequent ecchymosis. Polymorphonuclear cells appear in a few hours and fibrin strands are laid down. Bacteria are usually demonstrated in large numbers; after several days lymphocytes predominate. Later, detached arachnoid lining cells and reticulin fibres contribute to diffuse fibrosis. In some cases, even from the earliest stages the meningeal reaction is accompanied by suppurative encephalitis, the inflammation being especially marked along the perivascular spaces spreading down into the cerebral cortex. In endocarditis and septicaemia there may be formation of what amounts to multiple micro-abscesses. In fatal cases the meningeal surface is covered by a thick layer of purulent exudate, abundant in the basal cisterns with flattening of the cerebral convolutions and obliteration of sulci.

Chronic infection of the middle ear or accessory nasal sinuses, fractures of the skull, defects of the cribriform plate, are frequently associated with meningitis and inexplicably this is often pneumococcal meningitis. Osteomyelitis of the bones of the skull or extention of soft tissue infection of the face and scalp usually along venous channels can also result in purulent meningitis.

RELATION OF SYMPTOMS TO MORPHOLOGICAL CHANGES

Post-mortem studies suggest that symptoms of confusion, impaired consciousness and fits are usually related to damage to the cerebral cortex from vascular occlusion, or cortical necrosis of obscure though possibly vascular origin. Cerebral hypoxia or reaction of cerebral tissues to infection without evidence of bacterial invasion, may also be responsible for so-called 'toxic encephalopathy'. Internal hydrocephalus may be responsible for coma, fits or deterioration in condition.

CLINICAL MANIFESTATIONS

Patients suffering from acute meningitis of whatever bacteriological origin may present certain common manifestations, those due to infection and those due to an increase in intracranial pressure. Certain signs may distinguish meningitis of particular bacteriological aetiology.

Fever, tachycardia, chills, leucocytosis suggest infection. Headache, neck and back stiffness, tense fontanelle, vomiting, back pain, drowsiness or coma may be caused by raised intracranial pressure and meningeal inflammation.

These features combined with a petechial or purpuric eruption suggest a meningococcal infection; occasionally pneumococci cause a similar picture; rashes in viral meningitis tend to be either maculo-papular or finely petechial.

Focal infection, especially in the lungs, middle ear and sinuses, is suggestive of a pneumococcal origin.

In children under three years of age, although there may be no particular distinguishing features, meningitis is frequently due to H. influenzae.

Staphylococcal meningitis is usually a late manifestation of generalised staphylococcal infection.

REACTIONS MIMICKING MENINGITIS

While the differential diagnosis of purulent meningitis including other central nervous system infections due to spirochaetes, viruses, fungi and neoplasms or abscesses is well understood, some less well known conditions may cause difficulty. The commonest clinical problem is meningism.

MOLLARET'S MENINGITIS

This curious condition described by Mollaret in 1944 is characterised by recurrent episodes of fever, malaise, headaches and signs of meningeal irritation. Fits sometimes occur. Between attacks the patients are asymptomatic. The cerebrospinal fluid is remarkable in that it contains several thousand polymorphonuclear leucocytes, lymphocytes, and during the first twelve hours large fragile poorly staining cells. The protein content rarely exceeds 80 mg/100 ml and the sugar content is normal. It is clearly only a diagnosis to be made in retrospect after several episodes have been well documented and serious underlying disease excluded.

BEHCET'S SYNDROME

Nervous system involvement in this condition may occur in at least 10% of cases and is frequently accompanied by evidence of meningeal irritation. The cerebrospinal fluid shows a pleocytosis, in the majority of cases either polymorphs or lymphocytes predominate, numbering less than 100 cells/c.mm. The protein content may be slightly raised and the sugar content is within the normal range.

MENINGEAL IRRITATION FOLLOWING LUMBAR PUNCTURE

After lumbar puncture meningeal reaction may be due to trauma, chemical irritation, or the introduction of micro-organisms.

HYPERSENSITIVITY MENINGITIS

Rarely meningeal reaction may be a manifestation of hypersensitivity to drugs or serum sickness, and may occur in collagen disease.

BACTERIOLOGICAL AETIOLOGY

Very many micro-organisms can cause purulent meningitis, but three pathogens predominate. They are Neisseria meningitidis, Streptococcus pneumoniae and Haemophilus influenzae. Neonatal meningitis is usually caused by Gram-negative coliform organisms. An indication of the incidence in England and Wales of various forms of meningitis is shown in Figure 5.

MENINGOCOCCAL MENINGITIS

INCIDENCE

Meningococcal meningitis occurs in most parts of the world as an endemic disease, at times becoming epidemic. In central Africa large epidemics are

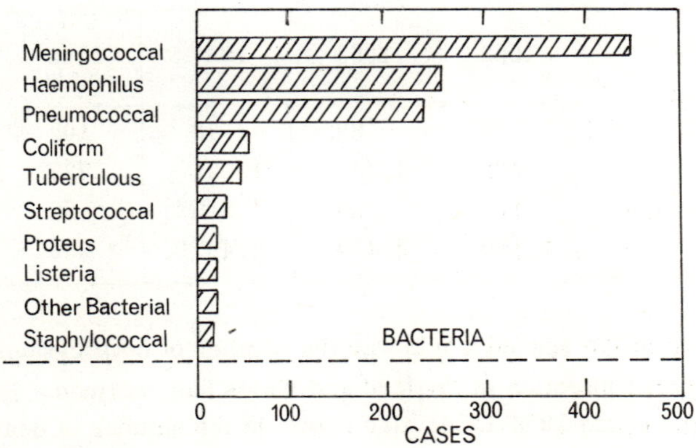

Figure 5. Infectious Diseases in England & Wales, 1963. Meningitis, Encephalitis and other Neurological Disease. From Public Health Laboratory Service (1964) Monthly Bulletin of the Ministry of Health & the Public Health Laboratory Service, 23, 59 (Crown copyright: reproduced by permission of H.M. Stationery Office)

Table XIX. The incidence of cerebrospinal meningitis (1954-1963) in the five 'leading' countries of the Meningitis Belt

NUMBER OF CASES

	1954	1955	1956	1957	1958	1959	1960	1961	1962	1963
Upper Volta	2,968	3,796	7,114	16,617	3,660	2,834	3,344	2,762	1,904	1,046
Nigeria	1,864	1,002	999	1,031	842	2,555	29,848	13,479	23,754	3,246
Sudan	3,470	3,371	9,933	4,214	1,033	797	1,138	7,775	5,326	1,032
Niger	176	114	234	406	211	94	1,434	3,349	15,564	2,585
Chad	1,624	207	270	1,268	1,105	171	430	4,721	996	384
Total	10,102	8,490	18,550	23,536	6,851	6,451	36,194	32,086	47,544	8,293

(Reproduced from Meeting on Neisseria Research First Report. WHO/BED/Men/1.65)

common. Table XIX shows the great variation in the number of cases in the so-called 'meningitis belt' of Africa.

In Europe and the United States much less variation in notifications is apparent; Table XX shows this for the period 1962-1965. The disease is common where there are many carriers of the organism and where living conditions are crowded, and there is a seasonal incidence.

Table XX. Notifications of meningococcal meningitis (Extracted from WHO Bulletin)

Country	1962	1963	1964	1965
Austria	78	88	78	102
France	583	1,541	1,021	727
Switzerland	114	189	119	58
USA	2,150	2,470	2,487	3,039

Since the end of the second world war the number of notifications of acute meningococcal infection in England and Wales has declined. Figure 6 shows this for the years 1956-1964; also shown is the number of deaths and this has ceased to fall at the same rate. This disparity between the number of notifications and deaths has been noted by others in Africa and in the USA (Lapeyssonnie, 1963; Carpenter & Petersdorf, 1962). Less awareness of

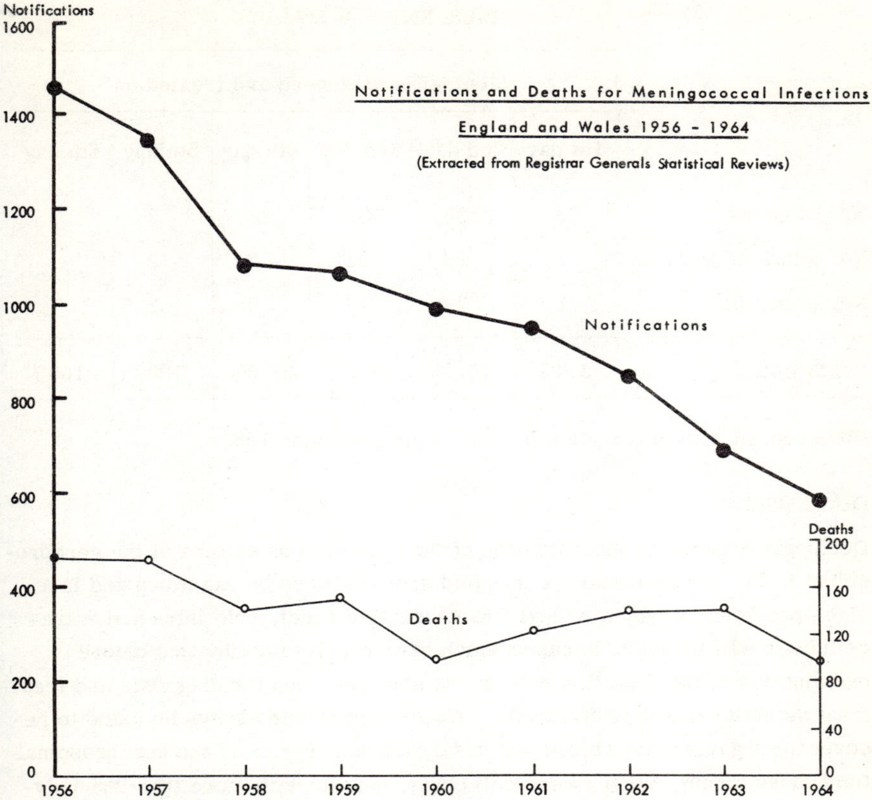

Figure 6. Rate of decline in number of notifications has not been accompanied by a similar rate of decline in number of deaths due to acute meningococcal infection.

the disease in non-epidemic periods and therefore relatively late diagnosis and treatment probably explains this feature.

CLINICAL PRESENTATION

An apparently simple upper respiratory tract infection with pharyngitis, fever and lethargy is the common initial presentation. Some patients then progress to develop signs of meningeal irritation, confusion and purpuric skin eruption. This orderly march of events may take 2-3 days to become fully developed. Unfortunately some patients have an illness which from first symptoms to death lasts only 4-6 hours.

Two groups of patients may be distinguished, fulminating acute cases, which are usually recognised at once, have a bad prognosis, secondly the more slowly evolving cases, with less dramatic signs. In this group survival depends on institution of specific therapy as soon as possible. The influence of early treatment on survival is shown in Table XXI.

Table XXI

	Meningitis diagnosed and treated on					
	1st day	2nd day	3rd day	4th day	5th day	6th day
No. of cases	29	138	35	11	2	1
No. admitted in coma	2	18	21	7	2	1
No. of deaths	1	23	17	7	2	1
Death Rate	3.4%	16.6%	48.5%	63.6%	100%	100%

(Reproduced with permission from L. Lapeyssonnie, 1963)

DIAGNOSIS

Diagnosis depends on identification of the organism on culture of the cerebrospinal fluid. A Gram stain of the fluid should always be examined and in a high proportion of cases typical Gram-negative cocci, both intra and extracellularly will be seen. In cases which have received antibiotics before examination of the fluid this may be the sole criterion for diagnosis and treatment as cultures are often sterile. An attempt should always be made to recover the organism from blood and nasal pharynx. Typically the cerebrospinal fluid looks turbid, has a raised cell count, usually with more than 90% polymorphonuclear cells, a raised protein content and a reduced sugar content. Some cases, clearly septicaemic, may die before localisation of the infection in the meninges, and in these patients the cerebrospinal fluid is normal.

A genuine, though quite rare diagnostic difficulty may arise with the possibility of infection due to Mima polymorpha; this organism usually attacks patients with serious underlying disease. It is a pleomorphic, non-motile, short, Gram-negative bacillus or coccobacillus; diplococcal forms may predominate showing variable staining. Meningitis resulting from infection with M. polymorpha is clinically indistinguishable from that caused by N. meningitidis. Typical cases with the Waterhouse-Friderichsen syndrome have been described (Townsend et al, 1954). The main importance in distinguishing this organism is in therapeutic implications, for usually the response to penicillin and sulphonamides is not consistent. Other antibiotics such as chloramphenicol may be more helpful (Burrows & King, 1966).

TREATMENT

The treatment of meningococcal meningitis can be conveniently discussed under the headings of specific chemotherapy directed against the infecting organism and measures to treat such complications as shock, fits, or the Waterhouse-Friderichsen syndrome.

Specific chemotherapy

Sero-therapy although effective has now been discarded in favour of simpler and more convenient treatment with sulphonamides and antibiotics.

Of the four main serological groups (A, B, C, D) of meningococci, group A is the commonest cause of infection. Some sporadic cases, and small epidemics in the United States and the Sudan have been caused by group B strains. Group C strains cause some sporadic cases and group D infections are very rare.

Sulphonamides

The drugs of choice in treating meningococcal infections will depend to some extent on the prevalence of the various serological groups in the community. In the United Kingdom sulphonamide-resistant strains of meningococci have not been identified and these drugs are considered the specific therapy of choice. In the United States sulphonamide-resistant group B, and to a lesser extent group C strains have been isolated and there have been some treatment failures in sulphonamide-treated patients. The sulphonamide resistance of B strains is not a new feature, but the prevalence of this group has altered the emphasis of specific therapy of these infections in the US from sulphonamides to penicillin G. The subject is reviewed by Feldman (1966 a & b).

Initially the first dose of soluble sulphonamide such as sulphadiazine is best given intravenously; 3-6 g are given to an adult, and if there is no vomiting or shock, treatment can be continued orally, 1-2 g/4 hrly will be required. In shocked or seriously ill patients, treatment by the intravenous route must be continued. In this way water and electrolyte solutions can be administered as well as specific chemotherapy. For an adult the initial 24 hour intravenous dose is 6-12 g at least two of which are given as a priming dose when the infusion is set up. Adequate urine output must be ensured. Table XXII shows the **intravenous dose** of sulphonamide.

Table XXII

Age	Priming IV dose of Sulphonamide	Total Dose/ 24 hours
Adult	3 - 6 g	6 - 12 g
5 years	1.0 g	4 - 5 g
1 - 2 years	0.5 g	3.0 g
0 - 1 years	0.5 g	1.5 - 2.0 g

Intravenous therapy is seldom required for longer than 48 hours; patients who respond to therapy usually do so very quickly. Seven to ten days treatment is sufficient.

When this form of intensive sulphonamide therapy is used penicillin may well be unnecessary but is frequently given in doses of 6 to 12 million units either intravenously or intramuscularly.

In contemplating large intravenous doses of sulphonamides it is of interest to recall that in Africa Lapeyssonnie (1963) used a single intramuscular injection of sulphamethoxypyridazine (45-70 mg/kg) and claimed a cure rate of greater than 90% in over seven thousand patients in whom the diagnosis was confirmed.

Penicillin G

Unlike sulphadimidine, of which perhaps 30% of the plasma concentration reaches the cerebrospinal fluid, penicillin G only crosses into the spinal fluid in very small quantities. However, when meningitis is present appreciable concentrations are reached in the fluid. Table XXIII shows a small series studied by the author in which cerebrospinal fluid penicillin levels

Table XXIII. Penicillin G concentration in blood/cerebrospinal fluid

NORMAL MENINGES

Clinical State	Penicillin Dose. IV	Plasma Pen. Conc. u/ml	Time after dose	CSF Pen. Conc. u/ml	Time after dose
1. Female 75 pyelonephritis	5 mega	122	30 min	0.96	45 min
2. Female 41 lung abscess	50 mega (constant infusion)	61.44	-	0.96	-

MENINGITIS

Clinical State	Penicillin Dose. IV	Plasma Pen. Conc. u/ml	Time after dose	CSF Pen. Conc. u/ml	Time after dose
3. Female 9/12 pneumococcal	0.5 mega	600	1½ hr	3.8	1½ hr
4. Male 6/12 pneumococcal	0.1 mega	-	-	7.78	1½ hr
5. Male 14/12 H. influenzae	0.75 mega	-	-	3.84 (i) 3.84 (ii)	1 hr
6. Male 78 pneumococcal	2.0 mega	28.6	1 hr	1.7	1 hr
7. Male 3/12 no organism	0.75 mega	-	-	7.68 (i) 1.9 (ii)	1 hr

were estimated after intravenous infusion of the antibiotic. Each dose of penicillin was dissolved in 200 ml saline and the infusion time was 20-30 minutes.

As the usual inhibitory concentration of penicillin G for meningococci ranges from 0.01 to 0.6 u/ml it is clear that bactericidal concentrations are obtainable in the cerebrospinal fluid when large doses are given intravenously. However, there are some doubts about the relevance of cerebrospinal fluid antibiotic concentration and these have been expressed in the section on the Blood/Cerebrospinal Fluid Barrier (page 200).

An adult patient, without renal insufficiency, may be given 20-30 mega intravenously in each 24 hour period. For children a 24 hour dose of 0.5-1.0 mega/kg may be sufficient, but higher doses may be warranted. The dangers of fits and electrolyte disturbance must be remembered (see section in Intravenous Penicillin Therapy, page 36). Cerebrospinal penicillin concentrations above 10 u/ml should be avoided (Smith et al, 1967).

A series of adult patients with acute meningococcal infection treated with 12-24 mega units of penicillin G daily without other antibiotics is reported by Levin and Painter (1966). Of their 28 patients 26 returned to duty within one month of the onset of their illness. There was one death, and one patient suffered from neurological sequelae.

Other antibiotics

If for any reason neither sulphonamides nor penicillin G can be used, chloramphenicol, ampicillin or erythromycin can be administered. Chloramphenicol diffuses well into the cerebrospinal fluid and meningococcal infection will usually respond, though less quickly than with either penicillin G or sulphonamide. Ampicillin may be used, but large doses should be given. In one study eight patients were given ampicillin in doses ranging from 150-250 mg/kg per day in six intravenous doses with results that compared favourably with a series of patients treated with penicillin G (Barrett et al, 1966). Using similar methods Mathies also found ampicillin comparable to penicillin G, though more expensive (Mathies et al, 1966). Cephaloridine produces a slower response than conventional therapy (McKenzie et al, 1967).

Intrathecal therapy is not necessary in treating meningococcal meningitis when large doses of penicillin are given intravenously.

MANAGEMENT OF COMPLICATIONS AND SIDE EFFECTS

Waterhouse-Friderichsen syndrome

This syndrome, here defined as a clinical state of profound shock in a patient with fulminating septicaemia, frequently though not exclusively of meningococcal origin, usually, perhaps invariably, proceeds to fatal outcome when adrenal haemorrhages may be demonstrated post-mortem. It is said to occur in about 3% of patients with infection due to Neisseria meningiditis.

The correct method to manage this crisis is not known; it is a rare condition which does not lend itself to controlled trial. The following factors deserve consideration.

(i) The dramatic appearances of the adrenal glands at autopsy led to the conclusion that the condition resulted from failure of secretion of adrenal hormones. Clinical and experimental experience has not substantiated this view. Clinically corticosteroids have been most disappointing (eg Smith, 1967); when levels of circulating steroids have been measured in overwhelming infection they have been high, tending to be higher in fatal cases than in survivors (Melby et al, 1958). Removal of both adrenal glands from normal monkeys, performed with care, does not result in profound circulatory failure, but is followed by a gradual deterioration which may take up to three weeks before death occurs. Hypoglycaemia causes fits and hastens the issue. Saline or glucose solutions, or **small** quantities of corticosteroids can save apparently moribund animals (Greep et al, 1952).

Corticosteroids have been thought to make the clinical condition worse; this is impossible to assess adequately without controlled trial for the most seriously ill patients are those usually given steroid hormones. However, in one series of 166 patients with acute meningococcal infection, not presumed to be in shock at the time of admission to hospital, 43 were given steroids and 123 were not. The steroid-treated group had a mortality of 21% and the non-steroid group only 7% (Margaretten & McAdams, 1958).

(ii) The altered physiological responses of patients in circulatory failure due to infection include increased peripheral arteriolar resistance, but the total blood volume and inferior vena caval pressure are normal. The function of the myocardium is not significantly affected, yet cardiac output is decreased Pooling of blood in peripheral capillaries or veins would seem to be the correct conclusion to draw from these observations. In animal experiments minute amounts of meningococcus endotoxin injected intravenously produces similar circulatory failure to that in humans overwhelmed by meningococcal infection. In these animals venous return to the heart is diminished because of pooling of blood in the liver and mesenteric vessels (Ebert et al, 1955; Weil et al, 1956).

(iii) Endotoxins are found only in Gram-negative organisms; the lipopolysaccharide-complex, irrespective of its bacterial origin, produces the same type of reactions when injected into animals. These consist of immediate and delayed, local and systemic responses. The immediate systemic reaction to a single injection of endotoxin produces shock — the so-called primary lethal effect. The local skin reaction resembles the tuberculin reaction in time and microscopical appearance. The delayed local and systemic reactions to two properly spaced injections of endotoxin are known as the Shwartzman reactions.

The results of injecting endotoxin were noted to be similar to that of large doses of adrenaline. Intradermal injection of small doses of adrenaline into animals previously injected with endotoxin results in marked haemorrhagic necrosis of the skin, the lesions resembling those of fulminating meningococcaemia.

A cortisone-treated animal responds to a single sub-lethal dose of endotoxin as though already prepared for the Shwartzman reaction. That is cortisone appears to act in a way similar to a primary dose of endotoxin. The theoretical implication here is that patients given cortisone, if infected with an endotoxin-producing organism, may be made vulnerable to the accelerated type of Shwartzman reaction, which causes characteristic lesions in the skin and kidneys.

(iv) The role of intravascular coagulation in producing haemorrhages in skin, adrenals, and other organs in patients with Shwartzman-like lesions is far from clear. Where there is clear evidence of defibrination heparin used cautiously would seem to be warranted.

Recommended management

1. Specific chemotherapy as outlined in section on treatment (pages 206-209).
2. General measures such as maintaining adequate airway; oxygen should be administered.
3. Fluid and electrolyte administration. Obvious dehydration should be corrected; care must be taken to avoid overhydration especially if oliguria is present. Blood transfusion appears to have no special advantages unless there has been bleeding or destruction of red cells.
4. Vasopressors. Patients who remain markedly hypotensive when 1, 2 and 3 have been adequately carried out are unlikely to respond to any form of therapy. Vasopressor substances such as metaraminol or noradrenaline are justified until our understanding of the altered physiology indicates better measures. These substances will sometimes provide a recordable blood pressure reading but seldom alter the prognosis.
5. Corticosteroids. Not recommended.
6. Untried methods which may in the future prove useful include hypothermia, adrenergic blocking agents and especially heparin.

Fits

These may occur as a result of:

(i) Cortical irritation from inflammation, vasculitis or haemorrhage.

(ii) Cerebral oedema; acute hydrocephalus.

(iii) Drug toxicity, eg penicillin (see page 38).

(iv) Electrolyte imbalance; overhydration depressing an already low serum sodium value should be avoided.

Recognition of these groups will often indicate the measures required for the prevention and control of fits.

Raised intracranial pressure

Brain compression resulting from raised intracranial pressure can cause death. Dehydration using either mannitol (10%) or urea (1 g/kg in 10% sucrose 8 hourly) intravenously may be useful. Corticosteroids may also be helpful in this situation.

Arthritis

This occurs in about 10% of patients; any joint may be involved, the knee and shoulder joints are those most commonly affected. Arthritis may result from direct invasion of the joint by meningococci, or more usually it is an 'allergic' manifestation. The prognosis is good.

PNEUMOCOCCAL MENINGITIS

INCIDENCE

Although pneumococcal meningitis shows some seasonal variation in incidence it does not show the marked epidemic variation of meningococcal infection. The pneumococcus is therefore usually responsible for less cases than the meningococcus in most reported series. Bevan-Jones and Miller (1967) for instance collected a series of 1,225 cases of meningitis in which an aetiological agent was isolated by the Public Health Laboratory Service during a one-year period ending in July, 1963. There were 521 Neisserian infections and 268 due to Streptococcus pneumoniae. Conversely, however, Carpenter and Petersdorf (1962) reported 209 cases of meningitis, 63 of which had pneumococcal and 53 meningococcal infection. This may reflect the older age group studied by the latter authors.

RELATION TO FOCAL DISORDERS

Pneumococcal meningitis frequently complicates acute or chronic infection in the middle ear, accessory nasal sinuses or lungs; it may follow head injury with or without skull fracture, and is associated with congenital dermal sinuses or when there is a cerebrospinal fluid 'leak' as in the cribriform plate defect. It is probably the commonest cause of meningitis in the post-splenectomy syndrome. Why the pneumococcus should predominate as the cause of meningitis in these circumstances is not known.

RECURRENCE

Recurrent attacks of pneumococcal meningitis are not uncommon and may of course be related to a residual focus of infection. In some cases no focus can be found; Whitecar (1966) reported a patient who suffered eleven episodes of meningitis due to five different serotypes of pneumococci and reviewed 37 other cases reported in the literature.

MORTALITY

Pneumococcal meningitis has a mortality rate of 25-30% highest in those under one month and over 50 years of age, in which groups it is most common. The incidence is higher in males than in females. Fatality rates in meningitis according to the causative organism is shown in Table XXIV,

Table XXIV. Fatality rates according to causative organism

Infecting Organism	Number of cases	Number of deaths	Fatality rate %
Neisseria spp	521	24	5
Streptococcus pneumoniae	268	34	13
Haemophilus spp	243	8	3
Gram-negative enteric organisms	68	10	15
Mycobacterium tuberculosis	58	2	3
Streptococcus spp (other than S. pneumoniae)	24	0	0
Staphylococcus spp	18	5	28
Listeria monocytogenes	13	2	15
Leptospira spp	12	0	0
	1,225	85	7

taken from Bevan-Jones and Miller (1967). These authors comment that the death rate is probably under-estimated because deaths are not normally reported after the causative organism is reported. In their follow-up postal enquiry they found an overall mortality of 36% in 189 cases, shown in Table XXV.

A number of patients showing temporary improvement may be found to have pneumococcal endocarditis. The triad of pneumococcal meningitis, endocarditis and pneumonia is particularly lethal.

Table XXV. Details of 189 cases of Pneumococcal Meningitis by age and sex (Obtained by postal enquiry)

Age	All cases	Male	Female	Deaths	Fatality rate %
0-	38	24	14	12	32
1-	27	18	9	2	7
5-	27	15	12	2	7
15-	7	7	0	1	14
30-	28	15	13	11	39
50 and over	62	35	27	40	65
Total	189	114	75	68	36

(Tables XXIV and XXV are reproduced by kind permission of the authors and the Controller of HM Stationery Office, from Monthly Bulletin MOH and PHLS 1967, **26**, 22)

CLINICAL FEATURES

Meningitis of pneumococcal origin will present evidence of infection and of meningeal irritation; focal infection should be sought when the pneomococcus seems the likely pathogen.

The history is often a little longer, extending perhaps 3, 4 or more days, and the onset less abrupt than is customary with meningococcal infection. A petechial eruption is not usually present.

TREATMENT

There are two common regimes for treating pneumococcal meningitis; one involves administration of penicillin G intramuscularly and intrathecally, frequently accompanied by full doses of sulphonamides, although the latter drug is probably unnecessary; the other, introduced by Dowling (1949) consists of large parenteral injections of penicillin G only. Two million units of penicillin G can be given intramuscularly every two hours, but this is a painful method of administration, and today it is common practice to give 20-30 million units intravenously per 24 hours. Intrathecal injection is not required. Treatment should be continued for two weeks, and even though the clinical response appears satisfactory lumbar puncture should be repeated in the third week. Persistence of cerebrospinal fluid abnormality suggests incomplete resolution and possible abscess formation.

Other Antibiotics

These include ampicillin, erythromycin, cephaloridine and chloramphenicol

(i) **Ampicillin.** Large doses will be required as in treating meningococcal infection: 150-260 mg/kg/day given in 6 intravenous doses.

(ii) **Erythromycin.** This drug has been used with success (Mead, 1963). 1 g every six hours is given intravenously, each dose being dissolved in 50 to 100 ml dextrose or saline solution.

(iii) **Cephaloridine.** This drug has been used to treat pneumococcal meningitis with some success. In their initial series McKenzie and colleagues (1967) used doses up to 200 mg/kg/day given as three intramuscular injections with an initial 2 g intravenous dose combined with intrathecal therapy (50 mg for an adult; 12.5 mg for infants). Of the 15 patients treated all survived and three had residual neurological damage. More recently these same authors (Love et al, 1970) reported on the treatment of 51 attacks of pneumococcal meningitis treated with a similar cephaloridine regimen. They had an overall mortality of 13.7% and they compare this with an expected mortality of 28% for patients treated with penicillin and sulphonamide.

Clearly cephaloridine is effective but whether it is more effective than appropriate penicillin therapy or is less dangerous remains unsettled.

(iv) **Chloramphenicol.** As in many forms of bacterial meningitis chloramphenicol may be useful. There is good diffusion into the cerebrospinal fluid but the clinical response is usually more delayed than that achieved by optimum penicillin therapy.

Antibiotic combinations in pneumococcal meningitis

In 1951 Lepper and Dowling reported that patients with pneumococcal meningitis treated with penicillin alone had a better prognosis than when penicillin was combined with chlortetracycline. Carpenter and Petersdorf (1962) considered that the addition of a second antibiotic to penicillin resulted in much greater mortality; further, Weinstein quoted by Swartz and Dodge (1965) suggests that chloramphenicol and penicillin combined gives inferior results to penicillin alone.

The implications are clear; when the diagnosis of pneumococcal meningitis is established use one antibiotic (preferably penicillin) only.

In patients, however, with purulent meningitis of unknown aetiology, especially in young children, a combination of penicillin and chloramphenicol is recommended as **initial** therapy.

INFLUENZAL MENINGITIS

Meningitis due to Haemophilus influenzae type B affects children, predominantly under 3 years of age; cases in older children and in adults occur rarely.

The clinical presentation may occasionally be acute with an encephalitic picture. More often there is a history of preceding respiratory tract infection followed by vague illness with fever, refusal of feeds, and vomiting. Signs of meningeal irritation on first examination may not be obtrusive, but can usually be found.

In this infection brain injury may occur early and is not always associated with vascular thrombosis, arteritis, or subdural effusion. Effusion occurs during the course of the illness and should be sought as a cause of pyrexia in an infant apparently adequately treated with chemotherapy. Transillumination of the skull can indicate the site of an effusion. It is not clear how the presence of subdural effusion alters prognosis; aspiration will sometimes be necessary and in long-standing cases removal of the effusion and its membrane will have to be undertaken.

TREATMENT

Of the many antibiotic regimes used to treat H. influenzae meningitis, two, possibly three, offer the hope of good results.

(i) Chloramphenicol

H. influenzae meningitis is one of the few unequivocal indications for the administration of chloramphenicol. The organism is sensitive and the drug penetrates into the cerebrospinal fluid in concentrations approaching half that reached in the plasma. This is a simple form of therapy and intrathecal injections are not required.

In the initial stages of therapy it is best to administer chloramphenicol intramuscularly. The sodium succinate is used in doses of 100 mg/kg/day; if intravenous therapy is required the initial dose for a child is calculated on the basis of 5-10 mg/kg. The daily intravenous dose given at 6-hourly intervals is 75 to 150 mg/kg. If capsules can be taken the daily dose is 125 mg/kg; the palminate is less satisfactory as absorption is not predictable. The daily requirement is given in three or four equal doses and treatment is continued for at least 10 days. Premature infants and neonates should not receive more than 25 mg/kg/day.

(ii) Streptomycin, intramuscularly and intrathecally with sulphonamide

There is no doubt that used in the way described by Weinstein (1965) summarised on page 55, good results may be obtained. It is, however, a demanding technique requiring careful intrathecal injection.

(iii) Ampicillin

This could prove to be the drug of choice, but at the time of writing it is an interesting, though not fully proved, alternative to chloramphenicol. If this drug is used it should be remembered that large doses will be required, with at least the initial dose being administered intravenously. If the intravenous route is employed intrathecal injections may not be necessary. The idea that ampicillin in conventional oral doses can be used to treat H. influenzae meningitis should be resisted. Lambert (1967) has voiced a warning on this point. Barrett et al (1966) and Mathies (1965) using doses of ampicillin of at least 150 mg/kg/day (occasionally 250 mg/kg/day) had results comparable to conventional therapy. Recently there have been reports of failure of intravenous therapy.

STREPTOCOCCAL AND STAPHYLOCOCCAL MENINGITIS

These forms of meningitis are now relatively uncommon. Streptococci of various groups are occasional causes of meningitis in the neonatal period, especially in infants with meningoeceles or spinal canal defects.

Staphylococcal meningitis is almost invariably a late manifestation of generalised staphylococcal infection. Septicaemia and endocarditis may be present resulting in multiple metastatic foci especially in bones and lungs and in this context meningitis occurs often accompanied by cerebral abscesses.

In these two forms of purulent meningitis the drugs which are most likely to give good results are penicillin G, sulphonamides and, for penicillinase-producing staphylococci, cloxacillin, methicillin or other penicillinase stable compounds. Large doses should be used, and it must be re-emphasised that successful outcome is largely dependent on early treatment with bactericidal drugs or combinations of drugs. In vitro sensitivity tests are vital.

NEONATAL MENINGITIS

INCIDENCE

Neonatal meningitis is defined as meningitis occurring within the first 30 days of life. It has a close association with perinatal maternal infection, especially uterine and urinary tract infection; obstetric difficulties such as delay in delivery, early rupture of the membranes, prematurity, toxaemia, frequent manipulation and instrumentation are often found in mothers whose children develop neonatal meningitis. Males appear to be affected more frequently than females.

BACTERIAL AETIOLOGY

Gram-negative organisms, always a common cause of meningitis in this age group, have become more prevalent and now account for more than 80% of neonatal meningitis. In most series Escherichia coli is the single most common organism; the so-called 'pathogenic' strains of E. coli associated with diarrhoea in infants do not apparently cause neonatal meningitis. Although agglutinating antibodies to coliform bacteria appear in the 19 s macroglobulin fraction of serum protein (IgM) they are not transferred across the placenta, but the infant has the capacity to produce these globulins within the first week of life. Delay in immunological maturity combined with other unknown factors may result in infection.

Other Gram-negative organisms encountered include Pseudomonas aeruginosa, Aerobacter aerogenes, Proteus spp., Vibrio foetus and various strains of salmonellae. Of Gram-positive organisms staphylococci and streptococci predominate; Listeria monocytogenes is sometimes encountered.

CLINICAL FEATURES

Typical signs of meningitis are often few or absent; if they are conspicuous the diagnosis has almost certainly been made too late for treatment to succeed. Fever, apathy, alteration in feeding habit, diarrhoea, may be the only suggestive features; concurrent neonatal sepsis such as cord stump infection, pneumonia, abscesses, pyoderma and especially septicaemia should be diligently sought. Spina bifida with cord defects frequently predisposes to this type of infection. In some infants there may be no signs, merely failure to thrive, and in these infants lumbar puncture is indicated.

TREATMENT

It must be emphasised that mortality in neonatal meningitis is high; a fatality rate of 60% or more is not uncommon, and that antibiotic therapy is merely one factor important for survival in this condition.

When neonatal meningitis is diagnosed treatment must be instituted immediately before the bacteriological cause is certain. The following antibiotic regimes should be considered, while awaiting the results of bacteriological cultures.

(i) Kanamycin and Penicillins

Kanamycin is an effective drug against many Gram-negative organisms especially E. coli which is the commonest pathogen in neonatal meningitis. In young and premature infants the daily dose is 10-15 mg/kg, which may be given as two equal intramuscular doses. It is wise to give at least one intrathecal injection of not more than 5 mg. Unfortunately, a number of patients will be suffering from pseudomonas infection, and may not respond to kanamycin; likewise salmonellae are usually resistant.

Penicillin G is also given intramuscularly in doses of up to 2 mega units per day. This of course will be effective if streptococci or non-penicillinase-producing staphylococci are the responsible organisms, but cloxacillin or similar semi-synthetic penicillin will be required if penicillinase-producing staphylococci are the pathogens. Massive intravenous penicillin has some attractions in this context for many Gram-negative organisms can be brought under control; pseudomonas and indole producing strains of proteus are likely to be resistant (Weinstein et al, 1964). It is, however, a very demanding technique to employ in new born infants.

(ii) Chloramphenicol

This is an excellent drug for treating Gram-negative infections and is more likely to succeed than any other drug when salmonellae are the responsible pathogens. Unfortunately, premature and neonatal infants cannot safely be given chloramphenicol in doses greater than 25 mg/kg/day. Imperfect conjugation with glycuronic acid in the liver combined with reduced urinary excretion render doses greater than these hazardous.

(iii) Polymyxin B, Colistin

These drugs will be required if Pseudomonas aeruginosa proves to be the pathogen. Doses are as follows:

Colistin (Colistin sulphomethate)	250,000 u/24 hr given as 2-4 intramuscular injections
	500-1,000 units/kg each 24 hours, intrathecally
Polymyxin B (Thiosporin) (Aerosporin)	80,000 u/24 hr given as 2-4 intramuscular injections
	5,000 units/kg each 24 hours, intrathecally

Other Antibiotics

Newer antibiotics which are not yet proved in the treatment of neonatal meningitis include cephaloridine, ampicillin and gentamicin. This latter drug, which is active against staphylococci and Pseudomonas aeruginosa, has good prospects. Newman and Holt (1967) treated three infants with meningitis, two due to Kl. aerogenes and one due to Ps. aeruginosa, with gentamicin. They had good results without toxicity, but found that intramuscular doses of at least 2 mg/kg/day and intraventricular doses of 0.5 to 1 mg/day were required.

Carbenicillin (disodium α-carboxybenzylpenicillin) is a recently introduced semisynthetic penicillin active against Ps. aeruginosa and other Gram-negative species which has been used in the treatment of meningitis. Richardson and colleagues (1968) treated two adult patients with meningitis, one due to Ps. aeruginosa, and one due to the paracolon bacillus with improvement in both cases. Four infants (aged 11 days, 9 months, 1 week, 2 days) with proteus meningitis were treated by Ross and associates (1970) with recovery in every case. Doses ranged from 300 mg to 800 mg/kg/day administered intravenously and intrathecal therapy was used in only one patient.

Tuberculous meningitis is secondary to tuberculosis elsewhere in the body; treatment is therefore that of generalised tuberculosis, combined with specific measures to deal with meningeal invasion.

The onset is insidious; the realisation that the patient, often a child, is unwell comes after a time. Headache, lethargy, fever, suggestive of tuberculous toxaemia will often be present for one or two weeks before vomiting, drowsiness, neck stiffness are apparent. Focal neurological signs, especially cranial nerve involvement, may be present from an early stage. A curious and unexplained finding is the preservation of the ankle jerks while the knee jerks are depressed or absent. There may be clear evidence of previous tuberculous infection; family contacts must be sought. Choroidal tubercules are diagnostic; papilloedema may be present.

The cerebrospinal fluid is under pressure and clear or opalescent. Very early in the disease polymorphonuclear cells predominate, but this is quickly replaced by a lymphocytosis, up to several hundred cells per c.mm. The protein content is raised, sometimes markedly, usually between 100 and 200 mg/100 ml. The sugar content is characteristically reduced, but this may not always be apparent in the early phase of the illness. In doubtful cases, lumbar puncture should be repeated in 24 hours; a further decrease in sugar content is strong presumptive evidence of tuberculous meningitis. It should be emphasised that cerebrospinal fluid glucose readings should always be interpreted in conjunction with simultaneous blood glucose levels. A patient with hyperglycaemia may have normal glucose levels in the cerebrospinal fluid even in the presence of tuberculous meningitis. On standing, in cases of tuberculous meningitis, a fine fibrin web is often observed; this occasionally occurs in poliomyelitis.

Films of the fluid must be studied and searched microscopically for the presence of tubercle bacilli. This may be tedious, but can be most rewarding. Culture and guinea pig innoculation must be performed.

TREATMENT

The most useful drugs in treating tuberculous meningitis are streptomycin, INAH, PAS, ethionamide. There is probably a place for corticosteroids, and possibly intrathecal purified protein derivative (PPD).

Streptomycin and INAH

Given together these two drugs constitute the major attack in this disease; almost all are agreed on this point, but there is some controversy as to whether they need to be given intrathecally. Honor Smith contends that intrathecal therapy is required (Smith, 1964) and administers both drugs by this route. Most others reserve intrathecal streptomycin for very severely ill patients, especially during their initial week or so of therapy, and few use intrathecal INAH. Streptomycin is given intramuscularly, 1 g daily until 60-80 g have been administered. It is important to use streptomycin sulphate, not di-hydrostreptomycin, to avoid damage to the auditory branch of the 8th cranial nerve. When 80 g have been given, the drug may be discontinued for one month and then started in doses of 1 g twice weekly for a further 3 month period.

INAH is given by mouth to a total of 300 to 600 mg daily; pyridoxine is also prescribed.

Para-amino-salicylic acid

This drug, which has little antituberculous activity, has a limited place in the treatment of tuberculous meningitis. Its chief use appears to be potentiation of the action of INAH by competitive inhibition of acetylation. Adults should receive 12-16 g daily. Intestinal upset is common.

Ethionamide

This is a powerful antituberculous agent and crosses easily into the cerebrospinal fluid. Its place is not fully assessed, but, despite the fact that it is unpleasant to take, it may be a useful drug in this context. The daily oral dose for an adult is 1 g; the initial dose should be 250 mg twice daily and this is increased over one week until a daily dose of 1 g is reached.

Corticosteroids

In tuberculous meningitis these compounds may have four effects:

(i) They make the patient feel better and toxicity is lessened. These effects may be temporary.

(ii) As they are powerful anti-inflammatory agents they may reduce tuberculous exudate at the base of the brain. Abnormalities in the cerebrospinal fluid become less marked. If exudate is abundant they do not facilitate its absorption.

(iii) It is doubtful if these drugs prevent the extension of arteritis, but they are worth trial in this respect. It is well to remember that the action of corticosteroids on the blood/cerebrospinal fluid barrier is a tendency to restore permeability towards normal.

(iv) A short course of corticosteroids (dexamethazone may be most effective 4-8 mg IM/day) can lessen cerebral oedema.

PPD

Honor Smith and her associates at Oxford have shown that the brisk meningeal reaction resulting from intrathecal injection of tuberculin may promote resolution of basal exudate. Small doses (0.0075 μg in 1 ml saline) are given by the lumbar route, the dose being increased until a reaction occurs. Severe reactions can be aborted by cortisone.

This treatment is:

(i) Technically demanding

(ii) Useful only in patients who are Mantoux positive

(iii) Potentially dangerous

(iv) Unpleasant for the patient

(v) Best carried out in units where neurosurgical facilities are available

LENGTH OF TREATMENT

Treatment should not be limited by time but by effectiveness. The initial period will seldom be less than six months; the total period of treatment will extend to two or three years.

REFERENCES

Barrett, F. F., Eardley, W. A., Yow, M. D. and Leverett, H. A. (1966) Ampicillin in the treatment of acute suppurative meningitis. J. Pediat., **69**, 343

Bevan-Jones, H. and Miller, D. L. (1967) Bacterial Meningitis 1962-63. Monthly Bulletin of the Ministry of Health and the Public Health Laboratory Service, **26**, 22

Burrows, S. and King, M. J. (1966) Meningitis due to Mima polymorpha. Amer. J. clin. Path., **46**, 234

Carpenter, R. R. and Petersdorf, R. G. (1962) The clinical spectrum of bacterial meningitis. Amer. J. Med., **33**, 262

Davson, H. (1958) Some aspects of the relationship between the cerebrospinal fluid and the central nervous system. 'The Cerebrospinal Fluid'. Ciba Foundation Symposium. J. & A. Churchill, London. Page 189

Davson, H. (1967) 'Physiology of the Cerebrospinal Fluid'. J. & A. Churchill, London

Davson, H., Kleeman, C. F. and Levin, E. (1963) The blood-brain barrier. First International Pharmacological Meeting, Vol.4. Page 71. Pergamon Press, Oxford

Dowling, H. F., Sweet, L. K., Robinson, J. A., Zellers, W. W. and Hirsch, H. L. (1949) The treatment of pneumococcic meningitis with massive doses of systemic penicillin. Amer. J. med. Sci., **217**, 149

Ebert, R. V., Borden, C. W., Hall, W. H. and Gold, D. (1955) A study of hypotension (Shock) produced by meningococcus toxin. Circulation Research, **3**, 378

Feldman, H. A. (1966a) Meningococcal Disease 1965. J. Amer. med. Ass., **196**, 391

Feldman, H. A. (1966b) Meningococcal Infections - the military and the civilians. Ann. intern. Med., **65**, 1148

Greep, R. O., Knobil, E., Hofmann, F. G. and Jones, T. L. (1952) Adrenal cortical insufficiency in the rhesus monkey. Endocrinology, **50**, 664

Lambert, H. P. (1967) Chloramphenicol (c) Brit. med. J., **2**, 243

Lapeyssonie, L. (1963) La Meningite Cerebro-spinale en Afrique. Supplement to Vol.28, Bull. Wld. Hlth. Org.

Lepper, M. H. and Dowling, H. F. (1951) Treatment of pneumococcic meningitis with penicillin compared with penicillin plus Aureomycin: studies including observations on apparent antagonism between penicillin and Aureomycin. Arch. intern. Med., **88**, 489

Levin, S. and Painter, M. B. (1966) The treatment of acute meningococcal infection in adults. Ann. intern. Med., **64**, 1049

Love, W. C., McKenzie, P., Lawson, J. H., Pinkerton, I. W., Jamieson, W. M., Stevenson, J., Roberts, W. and Christie, A. B. (1970) Treatment of pneumococcal meningitis with cephaloridine. Postgrad. med. J. Suppl., **46**, 155

McKenzie, P., Love, W. C., Lawson, J. H., Pinkerton, I. W., Jamieson, W. M. and Stevenson, J. (1967) Cephaloridine in pneumococcal and other forms of pyogenic meningitis. Postgrad. med. J. Supplement Vol. 43 (Cephaloridine), 142

Margaretten, W. and McAdams, A. J. (1958) An appraisal of fulminent meningococcaemia with reference to the Shwartzman Phenomenon. Amer. J. Med., **25**, 868

Mathies, A. W. Jr., Leedom, J. M., Thrupp, L. D., Ivler, D., Portnoy, B. and Wehrle, P. F. (1966) Experience with Ampicillin in bacterial meningitis. Antimicrob. Agents Chemother. 1965. Page 610

Mead, H.R. III (1963) Treatment of meningitis. J. Amer. med. Ass., **185**, 1023

Melby, J. C. and Spink, W .W. (1958) Comparative studies on adrenal cortical function and cortical metabolism in healthy adults and in patients with shock due to infection. J. clin. Invest., **37**, 1791

Mollaret, P. (1945) La meningite endothelioleucocytaire multi-recurrent benigne, syndrome nouveau ou malade nouvelle? Documents humoraux et microbiologiques. Ann. Inst. Pasteur, **71**, 1

Newman, R. L. and Holt, R. J. (1967) Intrathecal Gentamicin in treatment of ventriculitis in children. Brit. med. J., **2**, 539

Pickup, J. D. and McWilliam, P. K. A. (1966) Intrathecal and intramuscular ampicillin in the treatment of Haemophilus influenzae meningitis in infants. Postgrad. med. J., **42**, 312

Richardson, A. E., Spittle, C. R., James, K. W. and Robinson, O. P. W. (1968) Experiences with carbenicillin in the treatment of septicaemia and meningitis. Postgrad. med. J., **44**, 844

Ross, S., Krayhill, E. N. and Khan, W. (1970) Treatment of proteus meningitis with carbenicillin: a report of four cases. J. Infect. Dis. **22**, suppl. 62

Smith, H. (1964) Tuberculous meningitis. International Journal of Neurology, **4**, 134

Smith, Hillas (1967) Treatment of pyogenic meningitis (discussion). Postgrad. med. J. Suppl. **43**, 119

Smith, Hillas, Lerner, P. I. and Weinstein, L. (1967) Neurotoxicity and massive intravenous therapy with penicillin. Arch. intern. Med., **120**, 47

Swartz, M. N. and Dodge, P. R. (1965) Bacterial meningitis - a review of selected aspects. New Engl. J. Med., **272**, 779

Thrupp, L. D., Leedom, J. M., Ivler, D., Wehrle, P. F., Brown, J. F. Mathies, A. W. and Portnoy, B. (1964) H. influenzae meningitis: a controlled study of treatment with Ampicillin. Postgrad. med. J., Suppl. **40**, 119

Townsend, F. M., Hersey, D. F. and Wilson, F.W. (1954) Mima polymorpha as a causative agent in the Waterhouse-Friderichen syndrome. US Armed Forces med. J., **5**, 673

Weil, M. H., MacLean, L. D., Visscher, M. B. and Spink, W. W. (1956) Studies on the circulatory changes in the dog produced by endotoxin from Gram-negative micro-organisms. J. clin. Invest., **35**, 1191

Weinstein, L. (1965) 'The Pharmacological Basis of Therapeutics'. (Ed) L. S. Goodman and A. Gilman. 3rd Edition. Page 1239

Weinstein, L., Lerner, P. I. and Chew, W. H. (1964) Clinical and bacteriological studies on the effect of 'Massive' doses of penicillin G on infections caused by Gram-negative bacilli. New Engl. J. Med., **271**, 525

Whitecar, J. P. Jr., Reddin, J. L. and Spink, W. W. (1966) Recurrent pneumococcal meningitis. New Engl. J. Med., **274**, 1285

18. Chemotherapy of Tuberculosis

INTRODUCTION

Chemotherapy with effective antituberculous drugs has markedly altered the outlook in this disease which has been, and still is, one of the greatest scourges of mankind. In London in 1801, for instance, 30% of all deaths were due to tuberculosis; not only death, but disability, misery and a very great deal of unhappiness and poverty can be directly attributed to this disease. The situation has improved, at least among populations who have access to proper medical care. Even in less evolved societies great advances have been made, but unfortunately there are still many people in the world dying from undetected and untreated tuberculosis. So effective is the best of possible regimens that in new cases, despite the hazards of drug toxicity and hypersensitivity, and the problems of resistant bacilli, effective therapy can nearly always be achieved. In long-standing cases the outlook has been improved and when surgery is required it may be undertaken with a boldness, not to say nonchalance, unknown in the days before chemotherapy. The various techniques of collapse therapy such as artificial pneumothorax, and phrenic nerve paralysis have now been virtually discarded; disfiguring surgery is seldom necessary.

It is proper to state that chemotherapy is the most important single factor in the management of patients with tuberculosis; all other factors are secondary, but the hard lessons learned in the days before specific therapy cannot be too readily discarded. Adequate rest and food, optimistic outlook by medical and nursing attendants and cheerful surroundings have still some part to play in the management of the patient with this chronic disease.

PATHOGENIC MYCOBACTERIA

It has been recognised for many years that mycobacteria other than Mycobacterium tuberculosis can cause disease in man. Infection with M. bovis is a well established entity; M. avium is very rarely pathogenic in man though exposure to this organism may in some areas be a cause of increased tuberculin skin sensitivity. In recent years other groups have become relatively common. First among these are tubercule bacilli that have become modified by chemotherapy; not only does modification occur in staining and morphological characteristics, but also in development of resistance to chemotherapy. Further, tissues resected from patients who have received prolonged therapy may contain acid fast bacilli capable of causing atypical tuberculosis in guinea pigs. Another strain, sometimes called the Asian strain because it is frequently encountered in that continent, seems to cause less severe disease, presumably because of reduced virulence.

An important group are the so-called atypical or unclassified mycobacteria. These have been designated into four groups:

Group I	Photochromogens: so called because they produce yellow pigment on exposure to light.
Group II	Scotochromogens: produce pigment when growth takes place in the dark.
Group III	Nonphotochromogens: there is little or no pigment formation when grown in light or darkness.
Group IV	Rapid Growers: colonies appear in three to four days; most produce no pigment.

The disease caused by atypical mycobacteria cannot be distinguished clinically from that resulting from M. tuberculosis; two factors, however, may suggest that they are responsible for infection. Firstly, atypical mycobacteria may be resistant to the standard antituberculous drugs, and secondly, skin hypersensitivity is usually demonstrated only when high concentrations of mammalian tuberculin are injected. This second feature can be used as a basis for confirming the diagnosis if differential Mantoux tests are performed — that is a greater skin reaction occurs when tuberculin prepared from anonymous mycobacteria is injected compared with the response to mammalian tuberculin.

In Figure 7 the mycobacteria pathogenic for man are shown schematically.

Mycobacterium

(i) tuberculosis	(ii) bovis	(iii) avium	(iv) Atypical (unclassified)
Strains modified by Chemotherapy			Photochromogens (M. kansasii)
Asian Strain			Scotochromogens
			Nonphotochromogens (Battey bacillus)
			Rapid Growers (M. fortuitum; M. balnei)

Figure 7. Pathogenic Mycobacteria

It should therefore be obvious that the only reliable way to proceed in infections due to mycobacteria is to identify the causative organism bacteriologically and to determine its sensitivity to anti-tuberculous drugs. M. kansasii and the Battey bacillus are the commonest atypical organisms responsible for infection and are particularly prevalent in certain areas of the United States.

STANDARD DRUGS

(i) **Streptomycin**

The main facts about streptomycin are in Chapter 4. The discovery of this antibiotic was the result of an extensive search among soil micro-organisms for a compound that was effective without causing excessive toxicity.

Because streptomycin was the first effective anti-tuberculous agent it was used alone; today anti-tuberculous drugs are almost always used in combination. However, as a result of its early use a good deal of information became available. The drug was shown to be effective; clearing of pulmonary lesions was sometimes noted, sputum conversion was commonly attained and tuberculous meningitis, previously so often fatal, could now be treated successfully. These dramatic results left no doubt that streptomycin was an effective antituberculous drug.

However, two of its main disadvantages also became apparent; drug resistance and 8th nerve damage were frequently encountered. When streptomycin was used alone, especially in chronic pulmonary tuberculosis, there was often marked improvement in the patient's condition, fever was reduced, there was an increase in weight and sputum volume decreased. This state persisted for two or three months after which the disease frequently got worse. This was the result of the survival and multiplication of resistant bacilli although sensitive bacilli had been suppressed or killed. It has been shown that about 75% of patients treated for four months with streptomycin alone develop resistant tubercle bacilli. Resistance to streptomycin is permanent and irreversible (Yegian & Vanderlinde, 1950); it is therefore a serious event for the patient, who is henceforth denied the benefit of the antituberculous activity of this drug.

ACTION OF STREPTOMYCIN

The action of streptomycin has been for the most part elucidated using bacteria other than M. tuberculosis but there is no reason to believe that its action on tubercle bacilli differs from its action on other sensitive bacteria. There appear to be two phases of activity initiation, first cell membrane protein is altered, and secondly a lethal process other than an attack on protein synthesis is involved.

Within the cell streptomycin interferes with polyamines in ribosomes and probably prevents the normal attachment to 'messenger' RNA (mRNA).

In cells sensitive to the action of streptomycin protein synthesis is disrupted, in resistant mutants ribosomes are less affected, and in dependant mutants (cells which require the presence of streptomycin for their survival) the presence of streptomycin seems to be necessary for attachment of mRNA to ribosomes.

TOXICITY

Toxic reactions to streptomycin are described in Chapter 4. Only certain aspects, mainly applicable to the use of the drug in tuberculosis, will be discussed here.

Eighth nerve damage is important because it is relatively common, may be permanent and can often be avoided. In its prevention the following factors must be considered:

1. Reduced dosage (ie less than 1 g daily) for patients over 40 years of age.
2. Reduced dosage for patients with glomerular insufficiency. To adjust the dose estimation of streptomycin blood concentrations may be required.
3. Courses consisting of more than 70-90 g in an adult should be avoided.
4. Evidence of acute vestibular disturbance (headache, vertigo, nausea and vomiting aggravated by movement) should be sought, and streptomycin therapy stopped if they are present.

It must be emphasised that these remarks refer to **streptomycin sulphate**; dihydrostreptomycin may cause deafness **without** preceding vestibular upset.

HYPERSENSITIVITY

The commonest hypersensitivity manifestation is a maculo-papular eruption occurring within two weeks of starting streptomycin therapy in a patient not previously exposed to the drug. Other rashes, urticarial, haemorrhagic, and occasionally exfoliative dermatitis have been described. Eosinophilia and fever may be present. In this situation there are four possible courses of action:

1. To withdraw the drug
2. To continue the drug; this may become difficult or dangerous, but is often possible
3. To desensitise the patient to streptomycin
4. To change to dihydrostreptomycin which does not have cross-immune reactions with streptomycin. This is perhaps the only indication for the use of this toxic drug which is painful to inject.

Desensitisation may sometimes be carried out rapidly starting with an initial dose of 1 mg and doubling the dose on alternate days, thus reaching a dose of 1 g in 21 days.

To minimise the danger of drug resistance developing during the period of desensitisation, Lal and Ferguson (1963) introduced a very rapid method

Day	Dosage	Day	Dosage	Day	Dosage
1	10 μg	11	1.0 mg	21	40.0mg
2	20 μg	12	1.5 mg	22	60.0mg
3	40 μg	13	2.0 mg	23	100.0mg
4	75 μg	14	2.5 mg	24	150.0mg
5	100 μg	15	4.0 mg	25	200.0mg
6	200 μg	16	6.0 mg	26	250.0mg
7	300 μg	17	8.0 mg	27	350.0mg
8	450 μg	18	12.0 mg	28	500.0mg
9	600 μg	19	16.0 mg	29	750.0mg
10	750 μg	20	25.0 mg	30	1000.0mg

involving six hourly injections. On the first day the initial dose is 0.5 mg streptomycin and the fourth injection is 2.0 mg; on the fourth day a total daily dose of 850 mg is reached.

Sensitivity reactions to streptomycin are thought to be due to two types of antibody, the one, carried by lymphoid cells and associated with lymphadenopathy and maculo-papular eruptions; the other is presumed to be a circulating antibody. This sort of sensitivity is rarer and causes urticarial rashes and anaphylactic reactions. If desensitisation is attempted in the latter group it should be carried out starting with very low doses as in the schedule recommended by Cohen (1966) above.

(ii) **Isoniazid** (Isonicotinic acid hydrazide)

Isoniazid was first synthesised in 1912, but it was not until 40 years later that its antituberculous activity was announced, for the discovery of its action happened by chance. The occurrence of isoniazid as an intermediate in the synthesis of one of the thiosemicarbazone compounds led to its testing in vitro and subsequently in vivo during the period 1950-1952. The Medical Research Council report of 1952 described a controlled trial and established the value of isoniazid in the treatment of tuberculosis (Medical Research Council Report, 1952).

PHARMACOLOGY

Isoniazid is an odourless white crystalline powder soluble in water. It is thermostable and resists autoclaving at 110°C for fifteen minutes. Alteration in the structure of isoniazid leads to the formation of compounds which have either less effective antituberculous action or greater toxicity than the parent substance.

The drug is well absorbed when administered either orally or parenterally; so effective is oral absorption that parenteral therapy is very rarely used. A single oral dose of 3mg/kg produces blood concentrations of 1.3 μg to 3.4 μg/ml in about an hour, and in some individuals tuberculostatic levels may persist for periods up to 24 hours.

After absorption isoniazid remains either in the free form or is conjugated to acetylisoniazid. Smaller quantities of other metabolites are also produced. The free form has much greater antituberculous activity than the metabolites.

The ability to acetylate isoniazid varies markedly from person to person, but appears to be constant for any individual and this ability may be genetically determined. Patients can thus be divided into 'rapid inactivators' and 'slow inactivators'; unfortunately increasing the dose does not seem to compensate for rapid acetylation. The response of this group of patients is usually not quite so impressive whatever dose of isoniazid is used.

The drug is widely and rapidly distributed in the tissues and body fluids; it appears in saliva and pleural fluid, it passes the placental barrier and is present in foetal blood. The drug penetrates tubercules and diffuses into necrotic centres and is selectively retained in some tissues including caseous masses. In the cerebrospinal fluid a concentration of about one fifth the plasma level is usual, but when meningeal inflammation is present much higher cerebrospinal fluid levels are attained. A dose of 3 mg/kg given to a patient with tuberculous meningitis can give levels of 4 μg/ml in the cerebrospinal fluid, a concentration which may be tuberculostatic. Simultaneous administration of PAS does not affect the distribution of isoniazid.

Excretion of isoniazid is chiefly by the kidney — 50-75% of an ingested dose is excreted within 24 hours. About 1% is excreted in faeces.

MODE OF ACTION

Isoniazid has a useful antibacterial action only on human and bovine tubercle bacilli. The precise mechanism of its action is not understood.

On exposure to isoniazid carbohydrates and phosphates accumulate in the acid-soluble fraction of M. tuberculosis. As the major accumulated material is trehalose, a sugar found in mycobacterial lipids, the presumption is that this drug acts by interference with lipid metabolism. Feingold (1963) has put forward the suggestion that isoniazid may inhibit a lipid fraction of the cell envelope which is essential for its viability.

ANTIBACTERIAL ACTIVITY

Isoniazid is most active against typical human and bovine strains of tubercle bacilli; minimum inhibitory levels of 0.015 μg/ml to 0.25 μg/ml are usual. The saphrophytic mycobacteria are usually inhibited by 10 μg/ml and M. avium may require 100 μg/ml for inhibition. The atypical mycobacteria vary in their sensitivity some being inhibited by 10 μg/ml while others require 100 μg/ml.

RESISTANCE

Tubercle bacilli cultured in increasing concentrations of isoniazid develop resistance to its action. When patients have been treated with isoniazid alone this phenomenon of resistance may be demonstrated in vitro. However, resistance in vivo does not necessarily follow. This curious lack of concinnity between resistance in the test tube and in the patient, quite unlike the situation noted with streptomycin, remains an enigma. In practice it means that in vitro resistance to isoniazid may not always have the unfavourable significance for the patient that follows resistance to streptomycin.

PRESENTATION AND DOSAGE

Isoniazid is available as tablets of 50 or 100 mg. The usual dose is 5 mg/kg daily, but for very extensive severe disease and in tuberculous meningitis the dose is usually 15 mg/kg initially, reducing to 10 mg/kg when improvement is noted. The tablets are given in two or three equal doses after meals. For children a syrup is available (containing 20 mg in 3.6 ml) and the daily dose is from 5 to 10 mg/kg.

There are many preparations, granules, cachets, powders, which combine isoniazid with aminosalicylate and which are most useful, especially for out-patient therapy.

A preparation containing 50 mg in 2 ml is available for parenteral use.

TOXICITY: SIDE EFFECTS

The incidence of untoward effects with isoniazid is related to the dose rising to about 15% when doses of 10 mg/kg are administered daily.

The commonest toxic manifestation is peripheral neuritis which may occur when doses greater than 5 mg/kg/day are prescribed. Slow inactivators of the drug tend to develop peripheral neuritis more frequently than rapid inactivators. Anaesthesia, paraesthesia and burning pain along the distribution of the sensory nerves in the extremities are the usual manifesations. The precise cause of this peripheral neuritis is not known, but it has been found that isoniazid depletes the tissues of pyridoxine by the formation and excretion of isonicotinyl hydrazone of pyridoxal. The peripheral neuritis may be prevented by the simultaneous administration of 100 mg pyridoxine daily. Pyridoxine does not reduce the therapeutic effect of isoniazid.

Convulsions may occur, usually when large doses are employed and their relation to pyridoxine deficiency is not clear. The vitamin may be successful in terminating fits.

Other central nervous system effects which may be encountered include restlessness, insomnia, muscle twitching and increased tendon responses. Optic neuritis and optic atrophy may occur which resolve when isoniazid is withdrawn. Encephalopathy can occur.

Symptoms probably related to vagal activity, and varying from patient to patient, include dryness of the mouth, epigastric discomfort and retention of urine in the male. A rare effect is anaemia in patients susceptible to pyridoxine-deficiency.

Hypersensitivity reactions to isoniazid are rare; fever, hepatitis and various rashes may occur. Patients who are receiving both isoniazid and PAS and in whom hypersensitivity to the latter drug occurs may develop cross-hypersensitivity to isoniazid.

DESENSITISATION

Desensitisation to isoniazid can be carried out (1) rapidly, (2) over a period of 50 days.

In the rapid method, the patient is given 25 mg three times daily on day one; 50 mg three times daily, day two; 75 mg three times daily, day three; and 100 mg three times daily, day four. During this period corticosteroid drugs are also prescribed and tapered off if no untoward effect is noted.

Desensitisation over a longer period is achieved by starting with minute doses. The following is recommended by Cohen (1966):

Day	Oral dose of INAH in mg	Number of doses per day
1	0.01	1
2	0.02	1
3	0.05	1
4	0.1	1
5	0.2	1
6	0.5	1
7	1.0	1
8	2.0	1
9	4.0	1
.	(dose of INAH increased by 2 mg daily)	.
.	.	.
.	.	.
.	.	.
41	68	1
42	70	1
43	75	1
44	80	1
45	85	1
46	90	1
47	95	1
48	100	1
49	100	2
50	100	3

MERITS OF ISONIAZID AS AN ANTITUBERCULOUS AGENT

Isoniazid is a very effective and the cheapest antituberculous drug; it is well absorbed when administered orally, diffuses rapidly into tissues and fluids, including the cerebrospinal fluid, and penetrates tubercles and caseous masses. Resistance is frequently demonstrated when the drug is used alone; hypersensitivity reactions and toxicity are unusual when conventional doses are used. Isoniazid is perhaps the most useful antituberculous drug.

(iii) **Para-aminosalicylic Acid (PAS)**

Benzoic and salicylic acids were found to increase the oxygen consumption of tubercle bacilli (Bernheim, 1940). It was thought that analogues might inhibit the growth of these organisms and Lehmann (1946) showed that the most active compound tested was p-aminosalicylic acid (PAS).

PHARMACOLOGY

PAS is a white crystalline powder, slightly soluble in water; aqueous solutions are unstable and on standing form irritating compounds. The sodium salt is much more stable, freely soluble in water, and does not decompose at room temperature. It is therefore highly acceptable for clinical use; calcium and potassium salts are also available.

Amino-salicylic acid is well absorbed from the gastro-intestinal tract, the sodium salt even more so. After absorption the drug is distributed throughout total body water; it penetrates into caseous material but does not reach the cerebrospinal fluid.

Within seven hours of an oral dose about 80% is excreted in the urine, about half of which is in the acetylated form. Excretion is reduced by kidney dysfunction, or by simultaneous administration of probenecid.

MODE OF ACTION

PAS is a bacteriostatic drug, a concentration of 1 μg/ml inhibiting most strains of M. tuberculosis; this effect does not appear to interfere with the actions of isoniazid or streptomycin.

Amino-salicylate is thought to act on tubercle bacilli in a similar manner to that of sulphonamides on susceptible bacteria. Para-aminobenzoic acid (PABA) is competitively inhibited. It is not yet clear why PAS is much more active against M. tuberculosis than against other micro-organisms, nor why sulphonamides are ineffective against tubercle bacilli.

RESISTANCE

Resistance to aminosalicylate can be induced in vitro and occurs in clinical practice, though less quickly than with streptomycin. It usually takes about four months for resistance to develop, and after one year about 75% of strains are resistant.

PRESENTATION AND DOSAGE

Sodium aminosalicylate BP is available as 0.5 g tablets; powder, granular forms and cachets are also available. There is a large variety of preparations containing PAS and isoniazid in varying doses, and these are useful for out-patient therapy when the patient can conveniently take only a single preparation. A preparation is available for parenteral use.

The daily dose of aminosalicylate administered by the oral route is 12 to 20 g given in four separate doses for the average weight patient. Gastric irritation is common and smaller doses may be necessary, especially in the initial stages of therapy. The drug is best tolerated when taken with food.

TOXICITY: SIDE EFFECTS

The commonest side effects of aminosalicylic acid relate to the gastro-intestinal tract; anorexia, nausea, burning epigastric pain, occasionally vomiting or diarrhoea may result. A few patients may be unable to take therapeutic doses: in the majority this can be overcome by the following measures:

1. Stop the drug and start with low, gradually increasing doses
2. Try an alternative preparation
3. Give the drug during meals; antacids and milk sometimes give relief
4. Use an enteric coated preparation.

These symptoms while unpleasant are not usually harmful, but they may dissuade patients from taking the proper dosage. Patients with peptic ulcers may have exacerbations of symptoms and ulceration may be induced in some individuals.

In some patients taking high doses, for prolonged periods, goitre and hypothyroidism may occur.

Hypersensitivity reactions occur in 2-3% of patients and are commonest in the second month after starting therapy. Fever, malaise, rashes, lymphadenopathy and eosinophilia occur. Sometimes the fever is sudden in onset and sore throat is present – the clinical picture suggesting infectious mononucleosis. The heterophile agglutination reaction is negative. Jaundice and joint pain occur. If PAS therapy is continued severe jaundice with hepatic necrosis can occur; pancreatitis and nephritis occasionally result. Patients on low sodium diets should not receive any form of the drug which contains this ion.

Haematological abnormalities induced by the drug include agranulocytosis, eosinophilia, lymphocytosis and thrombocytopoenia. Acute haemolytic anaemia may occur.

Two curious pulmonary manifestations of hypersensitivity to aminosalicylate are Loeffler's syndrome, and pulmonary radiological opacities, often related to tuberculous foci. These latter lesions, which can be confused with spread of disease, are thought to result from localised tissue reactions to release of tuberculin.

Hypersensitivity phenomena to PAS are often severe; if possible an alternative drug should be substituted. If it is important for the patient to continue PAS therapy desensitisation may be carried out, and if the risk of this is thought considerable, corticosteroids may be administered simultaneously. The desensitisation method of Berte et al quoted by Cohen (1966) is given below:

ORAL PAS DESENSITISATION SCHEDULE
(Days 1-12: an 0.1% solution of sodium PAS is used)

Day	Amount given in CC	Dose of PAS in mg	No. of doses daily
1	0.12	0.12	1
2	0.25	0.25	1
3	0.50	0.50	1
4	1	1	1
5	1	1	3
6	2	2	3
7	4	4	3
8	8	8	3
9	15	15	3
10	30	30	3
11	60	60	3
12	100	100	3

(Days 13-24: a 1.0% solution of sodium PAS is used)

13	5	50	3
14	8	80	3
15	10	100	3
16	20	200	3
17	20	200	3
18	40	400	3
19	40	400	3
20	60	600	3
21	60	600	3
22	100	1000	3
23	100	1000	3
24	100	1000	3

(Days 25-34: Weighed sodium PAS Powder is used)

Day	Dose of PAS in g	No. of doses daily
25	1	3
26	1	3
27	1	3
28	2	3
29	2	3
30	2	3
31	3	3
32	3	3
33	3	3
34	4	3

MERITS AS AN ANTITUBERCULOUS AGENT

Aminosalicylic acid is a weak tuberculostatic agent in comparison with streptomycin and isoniazid. Its main importance lies in its ability to delay the development of resistant strains when either isoniazid or streptomycin are prescribed with it. The view that its main action was to delay acetylation of isoniazid does not seem to have been substantiated by recent work (Peters, 1960).

It is well absorbed when administered orally, but large doses have to be used and gastro-intestinal upsets are common. Hypersensitivity phenomena are relatively common and are often severe; resistance develops more slowly than to either isoniazid and streptomycin.

TREATMENT WITH STANDARD DRUGS

Successful treatment of tuberculosis involves prolonged (2-3 years) continuous therapy with at least two effective drugs. By effective is meant drugs which have been shown to have in vitro activity against the infecting bacilli. In previously untreated patients before sensitivity tests are available the three standard drugs should be administered. Patients in whom treatment fails due to drug resistance or to withdrawal of standard drugs because of toxicity or hypersensitivity can be treated with reserve drugs, nearly all of which are more toxic than the three standard drugs, but some of which have good antituberculous activity.

In the initial treatment of pulmonary tuberculosis in young adults the following is recommended:

(i) Streptomycin sulphate 1 g IM daily
(ii) Isoniazid 300 mg daily in 3 doses
(iii) PAS 16-20 g in 3 or 4 doses per day

In patients over 40 years it is wise to reduce the frequency of streptomycin injections to three times weekly after one month's therapy at the higher dose.

When 80 g of streptomycin have been given the drug is withdrawn — this will mean that the patient has had between three and five months treatment.

At this stage in the treatment of most patients it is usually possible to continue therapy with isoniazid and PAS, provided the infecting organism is sensitive to these two drugs.

In patients with widespread advanced disease, in miliary tuberculosis and tuberculous meningitis the schedule is modified as follows:

(i)	Streptomycin 1 g IM (total 90 g)	during six months
(ii)	Isoniazid 10-15 mg/kg for 8 weeks reducing to 5 mg/kg thereafter	
(iii)	PAS 16-20 g daily	

In moribund patients and in some patients with miliary tuberculosis corticosteroids may be useful. When isoniazid is administered, especially in doses greater than 5 mg/kg, pyridoxine 100 mg should be administered simultaneously.

In treating children the same principles apply, the doses being as follows:

Streptomycin	Age: up to 2 yrs	200 mg daily
	2 - 5 yrs	250 mg daily
	5 - 12 yrs	500 mg daily
	over 12 yrs	1 g daily
Isoniazid	10-15 mg/kg daily in two or three doses	
PAS	0.2 g/kg daily	

RETREATMENT

Here the factors involved which have led to failure must be examined carefully. Of great importance is the possibility of resistant bacilli; not infrequently the patient may have failed to continue taking the prescribed drugs. Adequate therapy will depend on selection of drugs based on the results of sensitivity tests.

TUBERCULOUS PLEURISY WITH EFFUSION

This is a fairly common form of tuberculosis and occurs frequently in young adults. It is probably always secondary to pulmonary lesions, which cannot be demonstrated radiologically. The diagnosis may be suspected when there is a sharply positive tuberculin reaction and confirmed by finding tubercle bacilli in pleural fluid samples or by pleural biopsy. The condition will often settle spontaneously and chemotherapy has little effect on the effusion itself. The importance of chemotherapy lies in the prevention of subsequent pulmonary lesions, which result in a high proportion of untreated cases. Two standard drugs are used; a good regime is isoniazid 100 mg three times daily and PAS 4 g three times daily. This regime should be continued for two years. Corticosteroids may be useful in the early stages to assist absorption of the pleural exudate.

SKELETAL TUBERCULOSIS

Effective treatment of primary tuberculosis and the near eradication of bovine tuberculosis have greatly reduced the incidence of tuberculosis of bones and joints. The treatment of this form of the infection differs in no particular way from that of pulmonary tuberculosis. The aim is to heal the disease with a minimum of anatomical deformity and functional loss. Major surgical procedures are now seldom required. Chemotherapy with two effective drugs, preferably streptomycin and isoniazid begun as soon as possible and continued for at least two years forms the basic approach to this form of the disease.

GENITO-URINARY TUBERCULOSIS

In both sexes the kidneys are a common site for tuberculous infection; in the male the prostate, seminal vesicles and epididymis, and in the female the uterus and the Fallopian tubes may become involved.

In the treatment of renal tuberculosis certain factors should be remembered:

(i) rest is probably more important than in treating pulmonary tuberculosis

(ii) there is some evidence that three drugs give better results than two

(iii) if one of the three standard drugs cannot be used, probably the best alternative is cycloserine, since it is concentrated in the renal tubules.

RESERVE DRUGS

(i) **Ethionamide**

Ethionamide is a yellow crystalline compound almost insoluble in water and has a chemical structure closely related to isoniazid. Concentrations of approximately 2 μg/ml inhibit most strains of M. tuberculosis; 75% of photochromogens are inhibited by 10 μg/ml but scotochromogens are more resistant. Resistance to ethionamide develops rapidly.

Given orally 1 g ethionamide gives peak plasma levels of 20 μg/ml at 3 hours. After absorption the drug is rapidly and widely diffused, tissue and plasma concentrations being approximately equal. Ethionamide enters the cerebrospinal fluid in useful concentrations, even in the absence of meningeal inflammation. The drug is rapidly eliminated, but its fate in the body is not known; it is thought that it may be converted to a metabolite more active than the parent compound.

Ethionamide is available as tablets containing 125 mg and also as powder. The daily dose for an adult is 1 g; initially 250 mg are given twice daily, and then gradually increased until the full dose is reached. If the full dose cannot be tolerated, smaller doses may be prescribed and may be effective.

TOXICITY: SIDE EFFECTS

Side effects are common and often sufficiently severe to warrant withdrawal of the drug; serious toxic effects are rare.

Anorexia, vomiting, diarrhoea, burning epigastric discomfort are common; patients complain of unpleasant taste in the mouth and in the first few weeks of treatment they may lose weight.

Peripheral neuritis and convulsions are rare occurrences; postural hypotension, depression, and confusion occur.

Abnormal liver function tests occur in about 10% of patients who take ethionamide. Toxic hepatitis appears to be common in diabetics.

Severe allergic disturbances and rashes, gynaecomastia, impotence and menorrhagia have been encountered.

CLINICAL APPLICATION

Ethionamide is a useful antituberculous drug, not as effective as streptomycin or isoniazid; because of its toxicity it is not suitable for initial therapy. Cross resistance with thiacetazone may occur. Since it is usually effective against tubercle bacilli which have become resistant to isoniazid or streptomycin its chief use is in treating tuberculosis due to bacilli resistant to these drugs.

Prothionamide, an n-propyl derivative of ethionamide has similar in vitro activity to the parent compound and probably similar antituberculous activity in man. There is complete cross resistance with ethionamide, but probably no cross resistance with thiacetazone.

Gastro-intestinal disturbances are less with prothionamide than with ethionamide when both drugs are given in the same dose; other toxic effects are similar for both compounds.

(ii) **Pyrazinamide**

Pyrazinamide is a white crystalline powder, sparingly soluble in water and is related chemically to the thiosemicarbazones. In vitro tests show that pyrazinamide at acid pH is active against intracellular tubercle bacilli in concentrations of 12.5 μg/ml.

The drug is well absorbed after oral administration; a dose of 1 g gives peak plasma levels up to 45 μg/ml; it diffuses well into tissues and is excreted by the kidney.

Pyrazinamide is available as 0.5 g tablets. The daily dose is 20 to 30 mg/kg divided in four, with a maximum of 3 g daily. Given alone resistance develops quickly, isoniazid and ethionamide are most effective in prevention of resistance to pyrazinamide.

TOXICITY: SIDE EFFECTS

Liver damage is the most important form of toxicity and may occur in about 15% of patients. It is commoner in older patients, but is not limited to those with previous liver disease. It may occur early or late in treatment and does not appear to be dose related. Liver biopsy reveals widely distributed areas of focal necrosis with complete destruction of the normal cell structure; death may occur.

Patients who receive pyrazinamide must have frequent clinical and biochemical assessment of liver function. Serial estimation of serum transaminase levels are imperative; this means that patients should either be in hospital or have close out-patient supervision.

Other untoward effects include increased absorption of urates, plasma uric acid levels of 9 mg/100 ml are common and after prolonged use of the drug episodes of gouty arthritis may develop in some patients. Colchicine is effective in relieving these episodes and pyrizinamide need not necessarily be stopped.

Anorexia, nausea and vomiting, fever and malaise also occur.

CLINICAL APPLICATION

Pyrazinamide is a useful secondary antituberculous drug, almost as effective as isoniazid in human tuberculosis. It is used as a second-line drug and has been recommended in patients who are to be subjected to pulmonary surgery. In preparation for this a short course of pyrazinamide may be given. Liver toxicity is frequent and patients must be constantly watched for evidence of liver dysfunction.

(iii) Cycloserine

Cycloserine is a white crystalline powder freely soluble in water, which loses potency on exposure to heat and light. It is well absorbed when administered orally. It is highly diffusible and cerebrospinal fluid levels are similar to those in blood. Renal insufficiency produces high blood levels of cycloserine which may lead to increased risk of toxic effects.

In concentrations of 5-20 μg/ml cycloserine inhibits the majority of strains of M. tuberculosis; concentrations of about 10 μg/ml can be attained by using a dose of 250 mg twice daily. This antibiotic also inhibits in vitro growth of E. coli, enterococci and staphylococci probably by inhibition of cell wall synthesis. When cycloserine is used singly resistance develops quickly; it is effective against strains that are resistant to streptomycin and isoniazid and there is no evidence of antagonism to other antituberculous drugs.

Cycloserine is available as capsules or tablets containing 250 mg, and pulvules of 125 and 250 mg. The optimum daily dose for an adult is 1 g; a good regime is to start with 250 mg twice daily and increase the dose by 250mg each week until the full dose of 1 g is reached. In patients receiving more than 0.8 g cycloserine per day there is an excessive urinary loss of pyridoxine and as the major toxicity of this antibiotic is neurological, pyridoxine in doses of 300 mg per day should be administered simultaneously.

TOXICITY: SIDE EFFECTS

Toxicity of cycloserine is principally neurological or psychiatric; these disturbances cannot be predicted unless serum levels in excess of 30 μg/ml can be demonstrated and the drug should probably not be given to epileptics or those with a history of psychosis.

Convulsions, excitation, depression and confusion, impulsive behaviour with hallucinations, have been noted; some patients become suspicious and paranoid and a few have committed suicide. The neurological side effects can be reduced by using pyridoxine, anticonvulsants, and tranquillising drugs, but serious psychiatric disturbances demand withdrawal of the drug. Early recognition of depression is clearly important.

CLINICAL APPLICATION

Cycloserine is a reserve drug for dealing with infection due to tubercle bacilli resistant to the standard drugs. It has formidable neuropsychiatric toxicity which limits its usefulness.

(iv) Kanamycin

Kanamycin is described in Chapter 7. It is a relatively weak bacteriostatic antituberculous drug, the usefulness of which is limited by its toxicity, of which permanent deafness and renal irritation are the major expressions. The usual dose is 1 g per day given intramuscularly; doses in excess of 20 mg/kg should not be given.

The chief application of this drug in tuberculosis is during a period when surgery may be carried out; in this way the duration of kanamycin therapy can be limited.

(v) Viomycin

Viomycin is a basic polypeptide; the white or pale yellow crystalline sulphate powder which is freely soluble in water is used. Aqueous solutions are moderately stable at room temperatures, but are inactivated by heat. Viomycin is weakly bacteriostatic, about one fifteenth as active as streptomycin; most strains of M. tuberculosis are inhibited by concentrations of 1-10μg/ml. Resistance develops rapidly and there is cross resistance with streptomycin and kanamycin.

Because viomycin is poorly absorbed from the gastro-intestinal tract it is administered by intramuscular injection. After an injection of 1 g peak plasma levels from 40 to 100 μg/ml occur in one and a half hours; diffusion into tissues is better than with streptomycin and small quantities reach the cerebrospinal fluid. The drug is excreted mainly by the kidneys.

Viomycin sulphate is available in vials containing 1 g; the usual dose is 1 g daily by intramuscular injection two or three times weekly. For short periods doses of 2 g may be used.

TOXICITY: SIDE EFFECTS

Viomycin causes pain at the site of injection and care should be taken to ensure that the injection is intramuscular.

This antibiotic frequently causes toxic upset of 8th nerve function and electrolyte disturbances. Vestibular upset is commoner than with streptomycin; patients complain of vertigo and caloric tests confirm vestibular dysfunction. This dysfunction usually clears when the drug is stopped. Tinnitus and hearing loss may proceed to complete deafness; occasionally deafness occurs without warning. Some degree of hearing loss is common, often undetected by the patient because it is limited to the high frequency range. It may be detected by audiometric examination. Viomycin and streptomycin should never be used together.

Renal toxicity is common but not usually severe, proteinuria and haematuria occur and may not require withdrawal of the drug. Care should be taken if patients with renal insufficiency are given viomycin as toxic blood levels may easily occur. Electrolyte loss in the urine (calcium potassium and chloride) may lead to muscle weakness and tetany. Renal function usually recovers when the drug is stopped and electrolyte losses replaced. Allergic phenomena such as rashes and eosinophilia occur.

CLINICAL APPLICATION

Viomycin is a weak tuberculostatic antibiotic, similar to, though less active, than streptomycin, which it also resembles by being toxic to the 8th cranial nerve and the kidneys. These two drugs should not be used together. As a reserve drug it may be used successfully combined with cycloserine or pyrazinamide. Strains of mycobacteria resistant to viomycin are also resistant to streptomycin and kanamycin (Tsukamura et al, 1962). This is an important reason for delaying the administration of viomycin.

(vi) Ethambutol

This is a new antituberculous agent which has not been fully investigated, but shows considerable promise. It is an odourless, white crystalline compound active against mycobacteria (human, bovine and atypical strains) at concentrations from 0.5 to 2 μg/ml. A concentration of 1 μg/ml inhibits about 75%

of strains of M. tuberculosis. It has no effect on other bacteria. Resistance develops slowly; there is no cross resistance with other antituberculous drugs, and when used with streptomycin or isoniazid, ethambutol retards resistance to these drugs.

Ethambutol is well absorbed after oral administration and maximum plasma levels are reached in under two hours. The drug enters red cells easily, but little accumulation occurs in other tissues; excretion is predominantly by the kidneys. The usual daily dose is 25 to 50 mg/kg.

TOXICITY: SIDE EFFECTS

In monkeys given large doses of ethambutol, toxicity is confined to central nervous system lesions; in dogs myocardial changes occur and death from heart failure may ensue. In man the drug has not been studied for sufficiently long for adequate assessment. Loss of central vision may occur one to seven months after starting treatment. So far recovery has occurred when the drug has been stopped.

CLINICAL APPLICATION

Ethambutol will often produce good response when failures have occurred with the standard and some of the reserve drugs. Combined with pyrazinamide, cycloserine, streptomycin, PAS or ethionamide a good result may be produced. Toxicity limits its use, but a dose as low as 15 mg/kg may be acceptable and when used with other drugs may delay development of resistance.

(vii) **Capreomycin**

This is a relatively new antituberculous peptide which inhibits the growth of M. tuberculosis in a concentration of 6 μg/ml; it has some activity against M. kansasii.

Capreomycin is available in vials of 1 g, the optimum daily dose being 1 g intramuscularly; it is excreted mostly in the urine.

Resistance to capreomycin may develop, but takes a long time and there is no cross resistance with isoniazid, streptomycin, kanamycin or other drugs. Curiously tubercle bacilli resistant to streptomycin and PAS are twice as sensitive to capreomycin as normal strains.

TOXICITY: SIDE EFFECTS

Major toxicity relates to the kidney and the 8th nerve. Damage to renal tubular epithelium may lead to azotaemia and can cause plasma concentrations to reach toxic levels. Hearing loss occurs, it is permanent, may not be complete and does not progress after the drug has been stopped. Capreomycin causes little disturbance of vestibular function.

CLINICAL APPLICATION

The status of capreomycin in treating tuberculosis cannot be accurately assessed at the moment. Its effectiveness is of the same order as streptomycin and it may well prove to be useful in treating patients with infections due to streptomycin-resistant tubercle bacilli. If toxicity to the kidney or 8th nerve occurs the drug should be stopped.

(viii) **Thiacetazone** (conteben; tibione; amithiozone)

Thiosemicarbazones are open chain closely related derivatives of sulphonamides. The most active antituberculous compound studied proved to be aminobenzaldehyde thiosemicarbazone (thiacetazone) and was used in Germany in 1946. Early adverse reports of toxicity were discouraging, but recently there has been renewed interest in the drug, primarily as a result of two trials in East Africa carried out by the Medical Research Council. In the first trial (Report, 1960) a combination of isoniazid 100 mg twice daily with thiacetazone 75 mg twice daily or PAS 5 g twice daily, produced similar therapeutic results. Toxicity in the two groups was of the same order. In the second study (Report, 1963) three different dose combinations of isoniazid and thiacetazone given once daily were compared with isoniazid 200 mg daily plus PAS 5 g twice daily. They concluded that a thiacetazone/isoniazid combination given once daily to in-patients was as effective as PAS/isoniazid provided that the dose of isoniazid exceeded 300 mg/day and that of thiacetazone 150 mg daily. Thiacetazone dosage was critical.

The commonest form of toxicity is anorexia, nausea and vomiting and the most serious have been reports of liver damage and bone marrow depression. These effects usually disappear when the drug is withdrawn.

Although thiacetazone had been virtually discarded, it is not yet completely clear how secure its recent revival has been. It is a tuberculostatic drug that may yet prove most useful in countries where cheapness and oral administration are of paramount importance.

(ix) **Other Drugs**

Thioureas

Thiocarbanidine is one of the more active among the substituted thiourea derivatives. It is poorly absorbed from the gastro-intestinal tract and shows considerable activity in animal tuberculosis, but has been disappointing in human infections. Isoxyl is a more recently introduced compound, but has not been fully evaluated. Generally these compounds produce little toxicity.

Rifampicin

Rifampicin (see page 125) is a most promising antituberculous agent at present mostly used for treating patients with resistant strains of <u>Myco tuberculosis</u>, but it may well prove effective in initial therapy. Used with ethambutol and probably a third drug such as capreomycin rifampicin may offer the combination of choice in patients with highly resistant organisms (Pines et al, 1970; Crofton, 1970).

Tetracyclines and Erythromycin

Used in high doses tetracyclines have some antituberculous activity. Erythromycin may have some useful action in treating infections caused by the anonymous mycobacteria.

CLINICAL APPLICATION OF THE RESERVE DRUGS

The reasons for using the reserve antituberculous drugs relate either to the development of resistance to the standard drugs or to hypersensitivity. Patients can often be desensitised to the standard drugs (during which time they must be covered with two effective drugs) but if desensitisation is impossible one or more of the reserve drugs will have to be used.

RESISTANCE

The incidence of primary drug resistance varies from country to country. An investigation in two socially different groups, 123 students in Paris and 108 adult out-patients in Tangier, showed a primary resistance of 14% and 16.6% respectively (Rist, 1964), but in Great Britain in 1957 primary resistance was as follows: isoniazid 0.7%; streptomycin 2.3%; PAS 2.2% (Fox et al, 1957) and these proportions had not increased in 1960. Strict discipline and the use of a large number of antituberculous drugs are probably two of the major factors in this low incidence of resistance.

Some idea of the frequency of acquired resistance in previously treated patients is given in an investigation carried out by the International Union against Tuberculosis on patients admitted to 72 hospitals in 17 different countries (Rist & Crofton, 1960). Of 100 patients the percentage of in vitro resistance was as follows:

Resistance to at least one drug:	42
" " " " two drugs:	18.5
" " " " three drugs:	5.5
" " " " INAH:	31.5
" " " " Streptomycin:	21.7
" " " " PAS:	12.1

A report from the British Tuberculosis Association (1963) involving single sputum samples from 514 patients known to have had a positive sputum for at least one year gave an acquired drug resistance of 73.7% for isoniazid, 63.2% for streptomycin, and 52.9% for PAS.

These figures give some idea of how vast the problem can be and emphasize the paramount importance of effective initial therapy.

Patients who may have resistant bacilli present two problems in management, those relating to organisms of known resistance, and those relating to tubercle bacilli in which resistance is suspected. When the drugs to which the bacilli are resistant can be identified then the alterations in therapy can usually be undertaken in some sort of logical sequence at least in the initial stages. Where resistance is suspected, but where the sensitivity to individual drugs is conjectural, the problem is more difficult. The following is offered as a guide in these two situations.

Infections caused by bacilli of known resistance

1. Infection resistant to PAS only may be successfully treated with daily isoniazid and streptomycin.
2. Where resistance to streptomycin alone exists, isoniazid and PAS may not be effective and either pyrazinamide or ethionamide should be added.
3. When there is resistance to isoniazid alone, streptomycin and PAS will be effective only if 20 g daily of the latter can be tolerated. Otherwise either pyrazinamide or ethionamide should be added.
4. Where there is resistance to two standard drugs, ethionamide and pyrazinamide should be added to the remaining standard drug.
5. When there is resistance to the three standard drugs the situation is indeed complex. At the present time the combination most likely to be effective in patients whose bacilli are resistant to all three standard drugs is, rifampicin and ethambutol, with or without the addition of either capreomycin or pyrazinamide. The combinations are likely to alter. Rifampicin looks a most promising drug.

Infections due to bacilli suspected of being resistant

This is the common situation when patients present with active disease and who have been previously treated. Whatever the reason, be it inadequate or ill chosen therapy, or failure on the patient's part to take his drugs, it is extremely likely that the tubercle bacilli being excreted are resistant to one or more of the standard drugs. To institute retreatment with the three standard drugs in this context invites the development of resistance to perhaps the one remaining powerful drug.

The most important move is to get samples immediately for sensitivity tests. If the patient is not clinically ill it may be justified to withhold chemotherapy; clearly experienced supervision is required and careful assessment vital. If the patient is seriously ill or deteriorates during observation then some form of chemotherapy must be offered. One such scheme is: viomycin 1 g b.d. intramuscularly on two days each week, with tetracycline 2 g twice daily. This is at best a weak antituberculous combination, but if toxic effects can be tolerated it may prevent deterioration until sensitivity tests are available. An alternative combination of thiacetazone or rifampicin with ethambutol would seem worthy of trial. To date trials of these combinations have not been reported.

INTERMITTENT THERAPY

This implies that drugs are given at intervals greater than one day and these regimens offer two advantages. Firstly, widely spaces doses may be given under supervision ensuring that dosage and timing are accurate and secondly antituberculous agents used in this way may be less toxic and paradoxically perhaps more effective.

The exposure of a patient to a drug given intermittently will be less than that following continuous administration. In theory this should reduce toxicity and side effects. Clearly of paramount importance is the effect of such intermittent therapy on the tubercle bacillus. In vitro studies by Mitchison and colleagues (1970) indicate that if an antituberculous drug is added to cultures of Myco tuberculosis and removed after a given time that there is a lag period between the removal of the drug and the time the organisms start to regrow. Thus, after an exposure of 24 hours to isoniazid (concentration of 1 μg/ml) there was a lag period of six to ten days, and with streptomycin (concentration of 5 μg/ml) the lag period was eight to ten days whether the exposure time was 24 hours or only six hours (Dickinson & Mitchison, 1966; Mitchison, 1970).

If the toxic effects of drugs administered intermittently are less then larger individual doses may be given and this has the advantage of suppressing growth of mutant organisms with low degrees of resistance unaffected by conventional doses. Using isoniazid alone this theory was put to the test in Madras (Tuberculosis Chemotherapy Centre, Madras, 1960, 1963). The result of these trials indicated that as the dose of isoniazid was increased from 100 mg to 400 mg there was an improved response but that no further improvement occurred when the dose was increased to 650 mg.

In a later trial (Tuberculosis Chemotherapy Centre, Madras, 1964) streptomycin was given in a dose of 1 g intramuscularly twice weekly with isoniazid in a dose of 12.5-16.1 mg/kg orally. After nine months therapy 93% of 72 patients had negative sputum cultures.

These trials indicate that under certain conditions of dosage widely spaced administration of certain drug combinations offer some advantages. The success of this form of management has induced scrutiny of the available and forthcoming drugs for clearly the dose of the individual drugs, the combined effect of those selected, the route and timing of administration are crucial and cannot be decided upon arbitrarily. A trial in Morocco was described by Burzoni and Durante (1967) in which 68 patients with pulmonary tuberculosis were treated twice weekly with isoniazid (mean dose 14 mg/kg)

Table XXVI. Reserve Antituberculous Drugs

Drug	Activity	Usual Adult Dose/Day	Main Toxicity	Resistance	Comments
Ethionamide	++	0.5-1.0 g Orally	G.I. upset; hepatitis Peripheral neuritis	Cross resistance with thiosemicarbazones	High tissue and CSF levels
Pyrazinamide	++	1.0-3.0 g (max) orally	Hepatitis; gout G.I. upset	Develops rapidly	
Cycloserine	+	0.5-1.0 g	Neuropsychiatric. Fits, Depression	Probably emerges slowly	High CSF levels
Kanamycin	+	1.0 g I.M.	Ototoxic; nephrotoxic	Develops rapidly	Beware renal insufficiency
Viomycin	+	1.0 g I.M. twice weekly	Ototoxic; nephrotoxic. DO NOT USE with streptomycin	Develops slowly	Low CSF levels
Ethambutol	++	25 mg/kg orally	Temporary blindness	Develops slowly	Not fully evaluated
Capreomycin	++	1.0 g I.M.	Ototoxic; nephrotoxic	Develops slowly	Not fully evaluated
Thiacetazone	++	75 mg twice daily, orally	Bone marrow depression hepatitis, G.I. upset		
Rifampicin	++	600 mg orally	Red coloured urine; jaundice		Not fully evaluated

and streptomycin 1 g (mean dose 18.5 mg/kg) both drugs being administered intramuscularly. Of the 58 patients available for assessment 46% had negative sputum by culture and microscopy. Although several factors may have contributed to this disappointing result two are obvious — the isoniazid was given intramuscularly and the dose of streptomycin rather lower than that used in the Madras (1964) trial.

REFERENCES

Bernheim, F. (1940) Effect of salicylate on oxygen uptake of tubercle bacillus. Science, **92**, 204

Burzoni, F. J. M. and Durante, C. (1967) Treatment of patients with pulmonary tuberculosis by twice weekly intramuscular injections of streptomycin and isoniazid: a preliminary report of experience in Marrakesh. Tubercle, **48**, 187

Cohen, A. C. (1966) 'The Drug Treatment of Tuberculosis'. Pages 28, 39 and 45. Charles C. Thomas, Springfield, Illinois

Crofton, J. (1970) The assessment and treatment of drug resistance problems in tuberculosis. J. Irish. Med. Ass., **63**, 75

Dickinson, J. M. and Mitchison, D. A. (1966) Short term intermittent chemotherapy of experimental tuberculosis in the guinea pig. Tubercle, **47**, 381

Feingold, D. S. (1963) Antimicrobial chemotherapeutic agents; the nature of their action and selective toxicity. New Engl. J. Med., **269**, 900 & 957

Fox, W., Wiener, A., Mitchison, D. A., Selkon, J. B. and Sutherland, I. (1957) The prevalence of drug-resistant tubercle bacilli in untreated patients with pulmonary tuberculosis. Tubercle (Lond.), **38**, 71

Lal, S. and Ferguson, A. D. (1963) A rapid method of desensitisation to streptomycin. Tubercle (Lond.), **44**, 360

Lehmann, J. (1946) Para-aminosalicylic acid in treatment of tuberculosis; preliminary communication. Lancet, **1**, 15

Mitchison, D. A. (1970) Reserve drug combinations. J. Irish. med. Ass., **63**, 86

Peters, J. H. (1960) Studies on the metabolism of isoniazid. Amer. Rev. resp. Dis., **82**, 153

Pines, A., Siddiqui, G. M. and Aafat, H. R. (1970) Rifampicin and Ethambutol in the treatment of drug resistant and far advanced pulmonary tuberculosis. J. Irish Med. Ass., **63**, 82

Report (1952) Medical Research Council. The treatment of pulmonary tuberculosis with Isoniazid. Brit. med. J., **2**, 735

Report (1960) East African/British Medical Research Council. Thiacetazone/Diphenylthiourea Investigation. Tubercle (Lond.), **41**, 399.

Report (1963) British Tuberculosis Association. Acquired drug-resistance in patients with pulmonary tuberculosis in Great Britain — a National Survey 1960-61. Tubercle (Lond.), **44**, 1

Report (1963) East African/British Medical Research Council. Second Thiacetazone Investigation. Tubercle (Lond.), **44**, 301

Rist, N. (1964) Nature and development of resistance of tubercle bacilli to chemotherapeutic agents. In 'Chemotherapy of Tuberculosis'. (Ed) Barry. Butterworth, London

Rist, N. and Crofton, J. (1960) Drug resistance in hospitals and sanitoria. Bull. Un. int. Tuberc., **30**, 1

Tsukamura, M., Yamamoto, M., Hayashi, M., Noda, Y. and Torii, F. (1962) Further studies on cross resistance in Mycobacterium tuberculosis, with special reference to streptomycin, kanamycin and viomycin resistance. Am. Resp. Dis., **85**, 427

Tuberculosis Chemotherapy Centre, Madras (1960) Bull. Wld. Hlth. Org., **23**, 535

Tuberculosis Chemotherapy Centre, Madras (1963) Bull. Wld. Hlth. Org., **29**, 483

Tuberculosis Chemotherapy Centre, Madras (1964) Bull. Wld. Hlth. Org., **31**, 247

Yegian, D. and Vanderlinde, R. J. (1950) The resistance of tubercle bacilli to chemotherapeutic agents. Amer. Rev. Turberc., **61**, 483

19. Chemotherapy in Undiagnosed Fever

INTRODUCTION

Long before the introduction of the clinical thermometer doctors had shown interest in fever almost to the exclusion of other manifestations of disease; indeed at one time fever was virtually synonymous with disease. In the early part of this century the reputations of some of the great clinical observers such as Horder were based largely on their ability to diagnose febrile illnesses; this ability is still a fair test of clinical acumen.

Of the known quantities that can be measured in man temperature shows the smallest variation; an estimation on 276 medical students in class between 8 am and 9 am gave a mean of $98.1^{\circ}F$ and a standard deviation of $\pm 0.4^{\circ}F$ (Ivy, 1944). Much has been written on pyrexia of unknown origin (PUO) and various authors have defined the term in different ways. In this chapter my primary concern is with illness of any duration accompanied by fever and to explore a rational use of antibiotics in these circumstances.

If there are rules to be observed they are empirical and for the most part relate to the customary admonition not to prescribe antibiotics until a diagnosis has been made – an exhortation more honoured in the breach than in the observance.

Two orders of problems arise, those relating to acute infections demanding immediate therapy, and less urgent problems when patients present with fever which may be of infective origin, but in whom a more leisurely approach is possible and who require investigation and diagnosis rather than immediate therapy. This latter group includes those patients with conditions commonly referred to as PUO.

ACUTE BACTERIAL INFECTIONS REQUIRING IMMEDIATE THERAPY

The chief reason for urgent treatment of acute infections is obviously to lessen or remove the danger to life or to a particular organ, or to give the patient relief of symptoms. In some cases, as in acute pyelonephritis or pneumonia for instance, the best way of doing this includes effective chemotherapy.

Those infections which are likely to endanger life acutely are, endocarditis and septicaemia, meningitis, chest infections and peritonitis. Acute local symptoms in conditions such as osteomyelitis or pyelonephritis may be so conspicuous that the presence of septicaemia is overlooked.

An aetiological diagnosis should always be attempted; as this will be based solely on clinical evaluation, an accurate diagnosis can be made only in a limited number of patients, but even if a broad distinction can be made, for instance, dividing the likely pathogens into Gram-positive or Gram-negative organisms some purpose will have been served. This implies that a bacteriological diagnosis can be made at the bedside; clearly this is often impossible, occasionally the demonstration of certain physical signs point to the correct course of action, and in the majority of cases some conclusion can be reached about the likely pathogen or group of pathogens. It is assumed that in these patients bacteriological results are forthcoming. Diagnosis is achieved by three separate steps which are shown schematically in Figure 8. It is not within the scope of this book to list the many investigations and diagnostic ramifications of PUO.

(I) **Infection** Yes or No?

This is the most important and often the most difficult question. Many

Diagnosis I Infection

NO

- (i) Neoplasms, leukaemia, lymphoma
- (ii) Collagen disease, D. L. E., polyarteritis, vasculitis
- (iii) Allergic states, drug fever
- (iv) Ulcerative colitis, Crohn's disease
- (v) Others: Periodic fever, haemolysis, emboli, endocrine disorders etc.
- (vi) Factitious fever, psychogenic fever

YES

Diagnosis II What kind of infection?

- (i) bacteria
- (ii) viruses
- (iii) spirochaetes
- (iv) Rickettsiae
- (v) mycoplasmas
- (vi) fungi
- (vii) protozoa

Diagnosis III What bacteria?

Figure 8. Schematic representation of steps which may lead to microbiological diagnosis in patients presenting with fever.

conditions can simulate infection and cause fever; some of these are listed below:

NEOPLASMS

Common primary neoplasms which may present with fever are, carcinoma of the kidney, stomach, pancreas and bowel; sarcoma, especially in the retroperitoneal space. Carcinoma of the lung does not usually present with fever, but fever may occur when there is secondary bacterial bronchopulmonary infection distal to the tumour.

Diffuse neoplastic lesions commonly cause fever; involvement of the liver seems particularly likely when a high polymorphonuclear leucocytosis is present.

Leukaemia, lymphoma and sometimes myelomatosis may be associated with fever.

COLLAGEN DISEASES

In women, disseminated lupus erythematosus may be suggested when there is leucopoenia; in men a modest leucocytosis perhaps with eosinophilia suggests polyarteritis; in both conditions a markedly raised erythrocyte sedimentation rate is expected. Rheumatic fever should not be forgotten, especially in adults with no previous history of the disease.

DRUG FEVER

This commonly occurs when patients are receiving many drugs. It may be necessary for a time to stop all therapy and observe the effect on the patient's temperature.

ULCERATIVE COLITIS: CROHN'S DISEASE

Ulcerative colitis may present with fever without bowel symptoms. A history of arthritis, or ocular and skin lesions may suggest the diagnosis which can be confirmed by sigmoidoscopy.

OTHER CONDITIONS, MOSTLY RARE

These include periodic fever, episodes of haemolysis, and repeated emboli, especially pulmonary emboli. These may be manifestations of unsuspected infection such as pelvic infection or involvement of the right side of the heart in endocarditis. Aetiocholanolone fever is a rare interesting condition which is a variant of periodic fever in which bouts of pyrexia occur and are associated with raised levels of this steroid in the plasma (Bondy et al, 1958). Occasionally congestive heart failure may cause fever, so also may thryotoxicosis; pyrexia in some individuals can be psychogenic.

FACTITIOUS FEVER

Patients who produce factitious fever often have some relation to the medical profession, and they may be notoriously cunning. When this diagnosis is suspected and before a confrontation or 'locker searching' procedure is undertaken two simple examinations may be helpful. Usually when the temperature is markedly raised there is a simultaneous rise in pulse rate; in factitious fever this may not occur and can easily be observed from examination of the patient's pulse and temperature record. A recently voided urine sample should reflect body temperature; this will not be so in factitious fever.

This rudimentary account of non infective pyrexia-producing conditions will indicate not only the wide variations in disease which may be encountered, but also the difficulties in making the initial decision on the presence or absence of infection. Clearly if any of these conditions are present, or are strongly suspected of being present, chemotherapy should be withheld. In some cases, even with the most competent observers, there will not be sufficient evidence even to make a tentative diagnosis. If the clinician considers that infection is present then he must proceed to the second diagnosis and try to decide what kind of infection.

(II) What kind of infection?

Consider in turn what group of micro-organisms may be responsible; these include bacteria, viruses, spirochaetes, Rickettsiae, mycoplasmas, fungi and protozoa. It is of course little use just being aware of this list unless the clinician has some knowledge of the pattern of infection resulting from these organisms. In a book of this size detailed examination of the various possibilities is not practicable. Instead some aspects of three groups of infections, those due to viruses, fungi and bacteria, will be explored.

VIRAL INFECTIONS

Viral infections seldom cause fever of prolonged duration, but secondary bacterial infection may; occasionally a prodromal period of up to 10 days in which there is high fever without physical signs occurs in measles and infectious mononucleosis sometimes has a prolonged pyrexial phase. It is usually possible to diagnose the common acute respiratory viral infections which present with high fever, muscle aches and faucial injection. Viral infections are often associated with leucopoenia; a benign course with resolution in a few days is to be expected in the majority of upper respiratory tract virus infections. One virus which may cause diagnostic difficulty is cytomegalovirus; it will probably be recognised when it is the cause of a severe congenital or neonatal infection, when there is salivary gland involvement, or when it causes a glandular fever-like illness. It may, however, occur as an opportunist in adults with lymphoma, leukaemia or after renal transplantation; pulmonary involvement is common.

FUNGI

Fungal infection presenting with fever as the sole manifestation is unlikely to be primary; primary pulmonary histoplasmosis is an exception and poses diagnostic difficulties, especially in certain areas of the United States. More often fungal infections occur secondary to other conditions especially when the immunological responses have been altered by disease such as leukaemia or reticulosis, or treatment with corticosteroids and immunosuppressive durgs. Prolonged treatment with antibiotics also encourages fungi to grow and intravenous catheters offer a portal of entry directly into the blood stream. Fungi which are most likely to be opportunists in these circumstances include Candida albicans, Aspergillus fumigatus and Nocardia asteroides.

BACTERIAL INFECTION

Bacterial infection is probably more frequently associated with undiagnosed fever than any other group of micro-organisms. If physical signs are confusing or absent it is well to remember that statistically one is much more likely to be dealing with an unusual presentation of a fairly common disease rather than a truly rare condition. The possibilities are limitless, but reviewing any number of difficult infections which present with fever one is impressed with the frequency of four conditions, tuberculosis, hidden abscesses especially in the abdomen, septicaemia and endocarditis, and urinary tract infections. Of these conditions septicaemia is likely to be the most acute infection, demanding immediate antibiotic therapy. The third step towards selection of chemotherapy is the diagnosis of the bacterial pathogen.

(III) **What bacteria?**

It is understood that a careful history and physical examination is carried out; the history must include details of the patient's pets and hobbies, recent contact with others known to have infections, travel, previous similar infective episodes and a very careful assessment of the patient's movements in the period prior to the onset of symptoms. All this is well enough known to be trite; in retrospect it is often failure to pursue these factors in detail which leads to incorrect diagnosis. It is also important to note the response to antibiotics previously administered; failure may occur not only from use of an inappropriate drug, but in many cases from incorrect (usually too low) dosage of an effective drug. When the various clinical manifestations are assessed and their possible microbiological causes considered, a precise bacteriological diagnosis can sometimes be made; more often one or several organisms can be suggested as the pathogen.

The chapter dealing with endocarditis and septicaemia (Chapter 16) deals with the chemotherapy of these acute infections and should be consulted by those requiring details of diagnosis and therapy; likewise meningitis is discussed in Chapter 17.

CHEMOTHERAPY IN ADVANCE OF DIAGNOSIS

In this group of patients the most important requirement is diagnosis. This is imperative, for if any sort of logical antibiotic therapy is to be followed an attempt must be made not only to separate infections from other illnesses, but also having diagnosed infection, to come to some conclusion about the micro-organisms likely to be responsible. The success or partial success of previously administered antibiotics should be noted for the response may offer a clue to an effective alternative. The choice of antibiotic will depend on a clinical assessment of the bacteriological cause, using the three diagnostic steps outlined in the previous section. The following list is offered as a simple guide which should be used in conjunction with Chapters 16 and 17.

ACUTE INFECTIONS: Chemotherapy without bacteriology

Presumed pathogen	
1. Gram-positive cocci	penicillin G + cloxacillin; cephaloridine
2. E. coli: Proteus: Klebsiella	High doses IV penicillin G + kanamycin; ampicillin; cephaloridine; chloramphenicol; trimethoprim/sulphasoxazole
3. Ps. aeruginosa	carbenicillin; gentamycin; polymyxin
4. H. influenzae	chloramphenicol; ampicillin
5. Cl. welchii	High doses IV penicillin
6. Meningococci	penicillin G + sulphonamide
7. Salmonellae	chloramphenicol; ampicillin; trimethoprim/sulphasoxazole

In some severely ill patients, especially children who present with a clinical picture which could result from infection with bacteria or with other micro-organisms, it is wise to treat the patient on the assumption that bacteria are responsible. This situation commonly arises when acute respiratory symptoms are conspicuous. These patients usually warrant anti-staphylococcal therapy.

CHEMOTHERAPY IN CHILDREN WITH FEVER

In the diagnosis and management of children who present with fever the same general principles apply as to adults, but the approach must be modified to take into account the infant's and child's characteristic responses to infection. Two important facts should be emphasised, firstly that children, especially young children, may suffer acute infections and produce few localising clinical manifestations. The infant has a limited repertoire of responses which includes alteration of feeding habit, especially refusal to feed, diarrhoea, fever, tachycardia; in neonates an increase in physiological jaundice or hypotonia, and in older children convulsions. Occasionally the appearance of the child may be more informative than any group of physical signs. The second point is that acute infections in young children may have a very short course, that is an infant who seems only vaguely ill may die within 24 hours from an undetected and untreated disease such as bronchopneumonia.

Infections which may present with fever without other clinical manifestations include septicaemia, meningitis, pneumonia, and urinary tract infection. The first three of these conditions may be rapidly fatal and special care should be taken to consider each in turn. Meningitis can be excluded by lumbar puncture (some cases of meningitis, especially with meningococcal infection die before typical cerebrospinal fluid abnormalities develop); blood cultures will not give a conclusive result for 24 to 48 hours at the earliest, and when these blood samples have been obtained, chemotherapy should be started immediately if septicaemia is considered probable. In the neonatal period Gram-negative organisms, especially E. coli are likely to be the pathogens; in older children meningococci and Gram-positive cocci are frequently responsible. Pneumonia may cause many diagnostic difficulties; fever may not be conspicuous, signs referable to the respiratory system absent, chest film unremarkable and leucocyte count unhelpful. In this difficult situation, provided the child's condition does not deteriorate it may be not only justified but wise to withhold antibiotic therapy until a clear picture of the likely nature and course of the illness is defined. This implies that frequent careful assessment can be made and that laboratory aids are available. If the child's condition becomes worse and there have been no clinical or laboratory developments on which to base a firm diagnosis a wide-spectrum antibiotic such as cephaloridine should be administered.

UPPER RESPIRATORY INFECTIONS

One of the commonest calls made on general practitioners is to see a child of school age who has been found to be pyrexial. In a previously healthy child the most likely conditions to present in this way are infections especially of the upper respiratory tract. A high proportion of these will be of viral origin, when fever, complaints of sore throat and perhaps minimal faucial injection are the only manifestations. Epidemics of this type of infection are common. Treatment is symptomatic; antibiotics are not indicated. Glandular fever may present in this way, but generally there are other signs such as lymphadenopathy, splenomegaly or jaundice which will indicate the true nature of the disease. Antibiotics are contraindicated.

Two conditions which should be treated with antibiotics are tonsillitis and pharyngitis due to group A streptococci and acute otitis media of bacterial origin. Streptococcal tonsillitis should be treated for 10 days and

and the initial therapy at least should be given parenterally (Chapter 13).

OTITIS MEDIA

Otitis media can cause many problems. First, its presentation may be with fever alone, young children may have no pain or discomfort referable to the ears. Second, there is the problem of aetiology, viruses, mycoplasmas occasionally, and more commonly bacteria are responsible. The usual bacterial pathogens are Str. pyogenes, Staph. aureus, Str. pneumoniae and H. influenzae. The third problem is the selection and administration of suitable chemotherapy.

Little is known about the ability of antibiotics to penetrate the middle ear in acute infections. The work of Silverstein et al (1966) showed that fluid taken from the middle ear space of patients with catarrhal otitis media contained quantities of oxytetracycline too low to measure accurately, while penicillin activity was readily measurable and comparable to levels found in patients with acute suppurative otitis media. In treating otitis media due to Str. pyogenes, Str. pneumoniae and non-penicillinase producing staphylococci penicillin G parenterally is the drug of choice. Tetracyclines are best avoided, except when bullous myringitis is present. For infections due to H. influenzae ampicillin is effective; as there is often doubt as to the pathogen and as ampicillin is likely to be effective against the common Gram-positive cocci it is a most useful drug in this context.

REFERENCES

Bondy, P. K., Cohn, G. L., Herrmann, W. and Crispell, K. R. (1958) The possible relationship of etiocholanolone to periodic fever. Yale J. biol. and Med., **30**, 395

Ivy, A. C. (1944) What is normal or normality? Quart. Bull. Northw. Unio. Med. Sch., **18**, 22

Silverstein, H., Bernstein, J. M. and Lerner, P. I. (1966) Antibiotics in Middle Ear Effusions. Pediatrics, **38**, 33

20. The Use of Antibiotics in Special Circumstances:

1. Renal failure

INTRODUCTION

Because many antibiotics are excreted from the body mainly by renal mechanism, some perhaps exclusively so, reduction in the excretory capacity of the kidney imposes certain modifications in antibiotic usage. The most important aspects of this subject are clearly the metabolism of the drug concerned and its precise handling by the kidney. A complication arises when potentially nephrotoxic drugs are used to treat patients in whom renal insufficiency is already present. It is not unusual for patients with chronic renal disease such as pyelonephritis to develop septicaemia accompanied by vomiting which induces further functional renal disturbance, and for such patients to receive antibiotics which themselves interfere with renal mechanisms. In these circumstances there is a complex relationship between several factors which may result in drug toxicity. In this chapter some of these factors are discussed, and the implication for antibiotic therapy explored.

PHYSIOLOGICAL CONSIDERATIONS

In relation to the kidney antibiotics may be classified in three main ways, those that are cleared chiefly by renal mechanisms, those that are cleared mainly by non-renal mechanisms, and an intermediate group which share several modes of excretion. This simple concept takes no account of the biochemical reactions and metabolism of drugs which in some circumstances are relevant to prolonged plasma levels of both active compounds and inactive metabolites, and which can have important implications for toxicity. Antibacterially active chloramphenicol, for instance, appears to be cleared from the blood equally well in uraemic and normal subjects, whereas the inactive metabolic products of chloramphenicol persist in plasma for long periods in uraemic patients (Kunin et al, 1959).

SERUM HALF-LIFE

The serum half-life, defined as the time required for the serum concentration to fall to one half is a convenient measure of the persistence of a drug in the blood after parenteral injection. After a single injection of drug the serum concentration at two separate times appears to give a valid indication of the decay curve as most curves are linear when plotted as the logarithm of the concentration against time. For certain compounds there is an alteration in metabolism resulting from prolonged plasma retention as may result from repeated doses or in uraemia. The half-life of cephalothin, for instance, after a single injection is 2.9 hours, but after prolonged treatment rises to 18 hours; Kabins and Cohen (1964) showed that in uraemic patients cephalothin was converted to deacetylcephalothin which is responsible for the increased half-life of antibacterial compounds after multiple injections.

ANTIBIOTICS CLEARED MAINLY BY THE KIDNEY

Drugs in this category behave like inulin or mannitol, that is their excretion is a function of glomerular filtration, and included in this category are streptomycin, kanamycin, gentamicin, most tetracyclines (not chlortetracycline), polymyxins, vancomycin and probably amphotericin B.

STREPTOMYCIN

The serum half-life of streptomycin after intramuscular injection is about two and a half hours for normal subjects; clearance is probably entirely by glomerular filtration and has been estimated to vary between 30-70 ml/min (Boxer et al, 1949; Marshall, 1948); the relatively low clearance is due to the fact that more than 30% of the drug is bound to plasma proteins (Boxer et al, 1949).

In uraemic patients streptomycin will accumulate in the blood if injected repeatedly. Kunin and Finland (1959) studied the plasma concentration of streptomycin in six uraemic patients; the serum half-life in two anuric (less than 400 ml urine/24 hours for 3 or more days) patients was 52.1 and 110.7 hours respectively; during the early diuretic phase of acute renal failure the half-life was 51.8 and 75 hours in two patients. Two other patients, one making a recovery with full diuresis, had a serum streptomycin half-life of 27.8 hours, while in another patient, who later died in intractable renal failure, the level in the serum dropped only 50% during a period of 20 days after the last injection of the drug.

Streptomycin is probably not nephrotoxic except when administered in very large amounts.

DOSE IN URAEMIA (ADULT)

Loading dose of 1 g IM; half the loading dose may then be given every two to three days (Kunin & Finland, 1959).

KANAMYCIN

Kanamycin is a drug similar in many ways to streptomycin; it differs in being less bound to serum protein and has pronounced ototoxicity with some nephrotoxicity. Excretion is mainly by glomerular filtration, but there may be a contribution by tubular excretion. In normal subjects the serum half-life of injected kanamycin is about three hours. Renal clearance is about 80% of the simultaneous creatinine clearance; children may have a higher clearance

Table XXVII. Correlation between serum creatinine concentration and serum half-life of Kanamycin, and related dosage schedule of Kanamycin

Serum creatinine mg/100 ml	Expected serum half-life of kanamycin (hours)	1st dose mg/kg	Interval (hours)	2nd dose mg/kg	Interval (hours)	3rd dose mg/kg	Interval (hours)	4th dose mg/kg	Interval (hours)
0.75	3.1	6	6	4	6	→			
		(or 8	8	6	8	→)			
1.0	4	6	8	4	8	→			
				(or 6	12	→)			
1.5	5.9	6	12	5	12	→			
						(or 6	16	→)	
2.0	7.6	6	12	4	12	→			
						(or 5	16	→)	
2.5	9.4	6	12	3	12	→			
						(or 4	16	→)	
3.0	11	6	12	3	12	→			
						(or 4	16	→)	
4.0	14	6	12	3	16	→			
6.0	20.5	6	24	3	24	→			
9.0	30	6	36	3	36	→			
12.0	39	6	36	2	36	→			
15.0	48	6	36	2	48	→			

NOTE: The arrows indicate that the previous dose and interval between doses should be continued for as long as treatment is necessary.
(Reproduced by permission of the authors and the editor of the Postgraduate Medical Journal)

rate. Uraemic patients retain kanamycin, and even the very small quantities absorbed from the gastro-intestinal tract may be retained and can lead to therapeutically useful and potentially toxic levels. By estimating serum creatinine levels and kanamycin concentrations Sorenen and associates (1967) derived half-life values on which to base both size and frequency of doses. Table XXVII, from their paper, is reproduced as a guide to dosage.

GENTAMICIN

This antibiotic, poorly absorbed from the gastro-intestinal tract, is excreted entirely by glomerular filtration, urine concentration of up to 100 times those in the plasma being attained. The drug has ototoxicity, some nephrotoxicity and must be prescribed with great caution to those patients with glomerular insufficiency. Estimations of serum concentrations may be required; levels in excess of 10 $\mu g/ml$ should be avoided.

On the basis of studies in 18 patients with varying degrees of renal insufficiency Gingell and colleagues (1969) who assumed that a peak serum level of 7 μg/ml was present, suggest the following dose regimen for gentamicin:

Blood urea mg/100 ml	Creatinine clearance (GFR) ml/min	Dose and frequency of administration
< 35	> 70	*80 mg 8 hourly
50-100	30-50	80 mg 12 hourly
> 200	5-10	80 mg every 48 hr
Twice weekly intermittent haemodialysis	< 5	80 mg after dialysis

*Use 60 mg if body weight is less than 60 kg

TETRACYCLINES

Although the commonly used tetracycline analogues have similar antibacterial range the individual compounds differ pharmacologically, the degree of protein binding, metabolic inactivation, and excretion showing considerable variation. Glomerular filtration is the prime method of excretion and the rate of filtration is determined by the degree of protein binding. The half-life of tetracycline administered intravenously to normal subjects is 6 - 7 hours; marked prolongation of the half-life occurs when the creatinine clearance falls below 30 ml/min (Kunin et al, 1959); oxytetracycline, demethylchlortetracycline, and methacycline behave in a similar way and have serum half-lives roughly proportional to the degree of protein binding. Methacycline protein-bound to the extent of about 80% has a serum half-life of 14.3 hours. Chlortetracycline behaves differently; it is inactivated quickly in the liver so that in renal insufficiency the serum half-life is not markedly prolonged; in one study this rose from 5.6 hours in normal subjects to between 6.8 and 11.0 hours when oliguria was present (Kunin et al, 1959).

As a result of these considerations it is plain that in patients with uraemia chlortetracycline may be used in doses little different from those with normal renal function. Use of any other tetracycline analogue requires major modification to dosage. Chlortetracycline, the simplest compound to use in uraemia has recently not been recommended by Kunin (1967) because there is some evidence that metabolic effects appear despite rapid inactivation in vivo.

There is no doubt that all tetracyclines that have been investigated can produce a catabolic effect which in patients with renal insufficiency may result in progressive azotaemia, nausea, vomiting and weight loss, and that some functional renal disturbances can occur when these drugs are given even to those with normal renal function (see page 70).

Tetracycline may be administered in the following doses: an oral or intravenous loading dose of 0.5 to 1.0 g is followed by 0.5 g every six to eight hours in patients with either normal renal function or when there is a reduction of 75%. Patients in whom glomerular filtration rates are found to be between 10 and 30 ml/min should receive a maintenance dose every 1-2 days: for severely uraemic patients the length between doses should be extended to 3-4 days.

POLYMYXIN B AND COLOMYCIN

These closely related polypeptide antibiotics are used to treat urinary infections due to Pseudomonas species; both are nephrotoxic which effect is increased with pre-existing renal disease. There is thus something of a paradox in that they are often most indicated in patients in whom they are likely to cause severest toxicity. Price and Graham (1970) treated 14 severely ill patients with extremely high doses of colistin sulphomethate (26 mega units/ 24 hours). Acute renal failure developed in all and contributed to death in some of their patients. It seems probable that in future they will be largely replaced by less toxic compounds such as carbenicillin.

There is little data on which to judge doses of these agents in the presence of renal insufficiency. As they are cleared by glomerular filtration doses will have to be markedly reduced; after initial administration maintenance doses may be given every three to four days (Kunin, 1967).

VANCOMYCIN

This drug has a serum half-life in normal subjects of about 6 hours and in glomerular insufficiency this is markedly prolonged. Kunin (1967) suggests a period of nine days between injections. It is plain that if possible an alternative drug should be used in uraemic subjects.

AMPHOTERICIN B

Little is known about the renal handling of this drug; it has a wide range of toxicity and there is often conspicuous deterioration in renal function when the drug is administered with evidence of reduction in glomerular and tubule function, and progressive fatal renal disease can occur. It is impossible to recommend a satisfactory dose in patients with existing renal disease. A cautious trial and error approach seems unavoidable.

ANTIBIOTICS MAINLY CLEARED BY NON-RENAL MECHANISMS

Included in this category of drugs are chlortetracycline, erythromycin, chloramphenicol, novobiocin, isoniazid. As the major route of excretion involves mechanisms that are predominately non-renal little modification to dose schedule is required when uraemic patients are treated.

CHLORTETRACYCLINE

This tetracycline analogue has been discussed in the previous pages; although it can be used in normal doses in uraemic patients toxic metabolites may be formed and it should be used cautiously, if at all.

ERYTHROMYCIN

The serum half-life for intravenously injected erythromycin glucoheptonate is about 1.4 hours in normal subjects, rising to about 5 hours in anuric patients (Kunin & Finland, 1959). This drug is not nephrotoxic and no modifications to dosage are required in treating uraemic patients.

NOVOBIOCIN

This antibiotic is highly bound to serum proteins, but because the bond is readily reversible very variable results have been reported for its renal clearance which is of a low order. As the drug is not nephrotoxic conventional doses may be used in treating uraemic patients.

CHLORAMPHENICOL

Chloramphenicol is inactivated by conjugation with glucuronic acid in the liver. Antibacterially active chloramphenicol is excreted mainly by glomerular filtration at a rate of about 24 ml/min and the inactive glucuronide is cleared more rapidly by renal tubular excretion at a rate of approximately 340 ml/min (Glazko et al, 1949). Active chloramphenicol has a serum half-life of about three hours and is unchanged in the presence of uraemia; in contrast there is marked prolongation of the half-life of chloramphenicol conjugates in the presence of uraemia.

In treating uraemic patients with chloramphenicol similar doses should be used as in patients with normal renal function. It should be remembered that these patients will retain inactive metabolic products the toxicity of which is unknown.

In some patients with liver disease and in the neonatal period glucuronide forming mechanisms are deficient which may lead to prolonged plasma levels of active chloramphenicol. As the neonate has reduced tubular and glomerular functional capacity, retention of chloramphenicol and its metabolites may be expected; the relationship of these metabolites to the circulatory collapse of the 'grey syndrome' is unclear.

DRUGS EXCRETED BY A COMBINATION OF RENAL AND NON-RENAL MECHANISMS

This group of drugs includes the penicillins, lincomycin and the cephalosporin derivatives cephalothin and cephaloridine.

PENICILLIN G

Penicillin G is rapidly cleared by glomerular filtration and tubular excretion; the half-life of a single intravenous injection in normal subjects is about half an hour and after intramuscular injection about one hour. Renal clearance is similar to renal plasma flow which increases with fever, and clearance of penicillin during pyrexia may be augmented by as much as 50% (Rantz et al, 1944). In uraemia, the neonatal period and in patients over 60 years, penicillin is excreted less quickly because of the reduction of functional renal tubular capacity.

Secretion into bile, and possibly inactivation in the liver are other mechanisms of excretion of penicillin. Kunin and Finland (1959) have pointed out that the half-life of penicillin in anuric patients did not exceed 10 hours unless severe liver disease was also present.

In treating the majority of infections in uraemic patients who may be expected to respond to conventional doses of penicillin G, injection every four to twelve hours may be used, depending on the severity of renal impairment. Large doses administered intravenously should be avoided in uraemic patients unless plasma and possibly cerebrospinal fluid penicillin concentrations can be measured.

AMPICILLIN

Ampicillin is handled by the kidneys similarly, if not identically, to penicillin G. Excretion in bile is important, for on reaching the jejunum reabsorption occurs resulting in prolonged high levels in the biliary tract.

Marked impairment of renal function (creatinine clearance less than 30 ml/min) causes prolonged high levels of ampicillin. Hoftler and associates (1966) reported that twelve hours after an intravenous injection of 1 g ampicillin in patients with creatinine clearances of 20 ml/min the serum level was still 25 μg/ml; a level of this order is maintained in normal subjects for only two hours. These authors suggest that in renal insufficiency ampicillin may be used in the following daily doses: patients with creatinine clearances greater than 30 ml/min or serum creatinine concentrations less than 2.0 mg% three intravenous injections of 0.5 g each; when the creatinine clearance is between 20 and 30 ml/min or the serum creatinine lies between 2.0 and 4.0 mg%, two thirds of the normal dose, ie two intramuscular or intravenous injections each of 0.5 g; when the creatinine clearance is below 20 ml/min or the serum creatinine is greater than 4.0 mg%, one intramuscular or intravenous injection of 0.5 g.

METHICILLIN: CLOXACILLIN: OXACILLIN

Methicillin may very occasionally cause renal damage when used in large doses: restriction of dosage in the presence of renal insufficiency is not usually necessary.

Cloxacillin and oxacillin, very similar penicillinase-stable penicillins, are excreted by the kidney and also take part in other extra-renal metabolism. No alteration in dosage is required when treating uraemic patients.

CARBENICILLIN

This recently introduced semi-synthetic penicillin active against Gram-negative organisms and Pseudomonas aeruginosa in particular is excreted like other penicillins both by glomerular filtration and tubular secretion. At present there is only one investigation on which to base doses of this antibiotic in patients with renal failure. Eastwood and Curtis (1968) showed that in order to maintain plasma carbenicillin levels around 100 μg/ml in patients with creatinine clearances of less than 5 ml/min doses of 2 g intravenously every eight hours are required. If haemodialysis is performed (these authors used a Kiil dialyser with a cuprophane membrane PT 150) the dose should be increased to 2 g every four hours. Clearance of carbenicillin is less marked when peritoneal dialysis is carried out and the suggested dose is 2 g intravenously every six hours.

LINCOMYCIN

Lincomycin has a serum half-life of about four and a half hours in normal subjects given a single intramuscular injection; in oliguric patients the half-life may be almost three times that in normal subjects. The antibiotic is not nephrotoxic, is excreted only to a limited extent by renal mechanisms and is metabolised in the liver. It penetrates tissues and may become bound to them.

There is not a great deal of data on which to recommend dose schedules in uraemic patients. It seems that little modification to doses is required; Kunin (1967) suggests that the interval between doses should be twelve hours.

CEPHALOSPORIN DERIVATIVES

Although cephaloridine and cephalothin have many similarities they differ somewhat in excretion and metabolism. Cephaloridine is excreted predominantly by glomerular filtration with little contribution from tubular mechanisms while tubule transport is very active for cephalothin resulting in a renal clearance figure about double that of the creatinine clearance. Administration of probenecid reduces renal clearance of both antibiotics, but the effect is much more marked in the case of cephalothin (Tuano et al, 1966).

Degradation or excretion by non-renal mechanisms are responsible for differences in plasma levels after comparable doses of these two antibiotics. Enzymatic desacetylation in the liver is invoked to explain the relatively short persistence in plasma concentration of cephalothin as opposed to cephaloridin in patients with reduced renal function (Kabins & Cohen, 1964). Kunin (1966) showed that cephaloridine is much more resistant to destruction in the liver than cephaloridine as opposed to 3 hours with cephalothin.

The implications for the use of these drugs in patients with impaired renal function are becoming clearer. When cephaloridine is used the dose must be appropriately reduced (see page 44); cephalothin while probably not completely free from renal toxicity may be used in conventional doses given every 24 hours. Both drugs are removed by peritoneal dialysis (Perkins et al, 1969).

USAGE OF ANTIBIOTICS IN RENAL INSUFFICIENCY

The foregoing sections indicate the renal handling, metabolism and suggested doses of antibiotics with different excretory mechanisms. The object of these dose modifications is to provide plasma and tissue levels in uraemic patients comparable to those known to be therapeutically effective in subjects with normal renal function. This, of course, presupposes that the volume distribution of these drugs is similar in uraemic and non-uraemic subjects — a supposition which is almost certainly incorrect. Further, the alterations in host response resulting from uraemia probably alters the course of infections in uraemic patients. Despite these somewhat theoretical considerations the only guide which can be offered for treatment of infections in the presence of renal insufficiency is to attempt to achieve plasma levels comparable to those expected in subjects with normal renal function. The doses suggested here are taken from several sources in the literature and are only a guide; clearly plasma concentrations of the drug in question may offer better information for dose adjustments.

NEPHROTOXIC ANTIBIOTICS

It should be remembered that patients receiving several antibiotics one of which may be nephrotoxic, can produce side effects due to the accumulation of the alternative drug whose renal excretion has been decreased. Lerner and associates (1967) have pointed out the potentially dangerous effect which the simultaneous administration of kanamycin or polymyxin B may produce in patients receiving large intravenous doses of penicillin G. Renal function should be assessed before and during the administration of such antibiotics and the dose of penicillin reduced if there is deterioration in renal function.

ANTIBIOTICS IN CHRONIC HAEMODIALYSIS

The development and simplification of technique in haemodialysis has led to an increasing number of patients whose lives depend upon frequent dialyses often carried out in the patients' own homes. These patients have permanent access to their circulation by means of various arterio-venous shunts which can be a portal of entry for organisms leading to bacteraemia. It is useful and convenient to treat these patients by intravenous injections (via the shunt mechanism or during dialysis), administering single large initial doses of various antibiotics; care must be taken in the judgement of size and frequency of doses when potentially toxic agents such as kanamycin, gentamicin or even cephaloridine are administered. Long term antibiotic therapy in these patients presents many problems, doses, plasma levels and amount removed by dialysis are dependent on many factors, not least of which are the properties of the membrane used.

Table XXVIII. Behaviour of antibiotics in renal failure (compiled from various reported data chiefly: Kunin, C.M. 1967)

Drug	% Protein bound	% recovered in urine	Serum half-life NORMAL (hrs)	Serum half-life URAEMIA (hrs)	Suggested initial dose in uraemia	Interval between doses in uraemia	Removal by haemodialysis	Removal by peritoneal dialysis
Penicillin G	about 50	58-85	0.5	7.2-10.5	no modification	8-10 hrs	appreciable	
Methicillin	37	71	0.5	4	no modification	no modification	appreciable	
Oxacillin	94	40	0.5	2	no modification	no modification	appreciable	
Cloxacillin	80	30	-	-	no modification	no modification		
Ampicillin	20	60	-	-	0.5 g IM	8-12 hrs		
Carbenicillin	47	80	-	-	2.0 g IV	6-8 hrs	appreciable	little
Cephalothin	56	60-90	0.5-0.85	2.9-18	no modification	24 hrs		
Cephaloridine	slight	70	1.5	20-23	no modification	24 hrs	little	
Erythromycin	18	15	1.4	4.8-5.8	no modification	no modification		
Lincomycin	80-90	10-15	4.4-4.7	10-13	no modification	12 hrs	little	
Tetracycline	24	60	8.5	57-108	no modification	3-4 days	v. little	v. little
Chlor-tetracycline	47	18	5.6	6.8-11.0	not recommended			
Demethylchlor-tetracycline	41	60	14.3		no modification	3-4 days	v. little	
Chlor-amphenicol	24.6		1.6-3.3	3.2-4.3	no modification (except in neonates & severe liver disease)	no modification (except in neonates & severe liver disease)		none
Kanamycin	slight	52-90	3	72-96	see Table XXVII		little	appreciable
Streptomycin	34	30-80	2.4-2.7	52-100	no modification	3-4 days	little	
Colistin	slight	40-80	1.6-2.7	48-72	no modification	3-4 days		little
Gentamicin	25-30	86-100	2.3	2-3	serum levels desirable			

2. Jaundice related to antibacterial chemotherapy

INTRODUCTION

The continued introduction of large numbers of new drugs has been matched by an increasing number of toxic reactions, and antibiotics have been responsible for some of these untoward effects. In many cases the conspicuous manifestations of toxicity are confined to one organ or system, such as the kidney, the central nervous system, or bone marrow, but these overt signs are probably almost always accompanied by a generalised upset which includes hepatic dysfunction. Some drugs produce clear evidence of hepatotoxicity, and the more important reactions are described in the chapters dealing with individual antibiotics. In this section the hepatotoxic actions of chemotherapeutic agents are briefly discussed from the point of view of disordered liver function rather than by discussing each drug individually. The therapeutic implications of the various toxic reactions are also discussed.

MECHANISMS OF HEPATIC TOXICITY OF ANTIBIOTICS

Although it is possible in many cases to indicate specific pathways which have been predominantly deranged, drug toxicity frequently produces combined effects with many complex disturbances so that classification is difficult and arbitrary. The following mechanisms may be considered in the production of jaundice as a result of toxicity by chemotherapeutic agents.

(i) **Haemolytic reactions**

This is a rare cause of jaundice resulting from antibiotic administration; it has been described with penicillin G, novobiocin, para-amino-salicylic acid.

PENICILLIN G

There are at least six cases due to penicillin described in the literature, most recently by Petz et al (1966) and Swanson et al (1966). Haemolytic reactions may occur with or without other evidence of penicillin hypersensitivity and usually only follow prolonged intravenous administration of high doses

(20,000,000 units/day for several weeks in one case). The Coombs antiglobulin test becomes positive in high titre; this is presumed to be due to the presence of anti-penicillin antibodies which may belong either to the 7 S or 19 S fraction of the serum proteins. Haemolysis ceases when the drug is stopped, but in at least one case returned when the patient was re-challenged with penicillin several months after the first haemolytic episode.

NOVOBIOCIN

Haemolytic anaemia, presenting as jaundice has been described in a number of patients treated with novobiocin, a good example being reported by Montgomery (1963). The patient was a six year old girl treated with novobiocin (39 mg/kg/24 hrs) for 5 days because of sore throat and fever. On the fifth day of treatment the patient was noted to be jaundiced and passed dark urine. Laboratory investigations revealed a normal white cell count, with haemoglobin of 7.0 g/100 ml and a reticulocyte count of 1.1%. The direct and indirect Coombs test were positive. Treated with corticosteroids and blood transfusion the patient improved, there was a good reticulocyte response and later the haemoglobin level reached 13.0 g/100 ml. The mechanism of the haemolysis in such cases does not seem to have been fully elucidated, but the presence of a positive Coombs test suggests that this is an acquired haemolytic process similar to that described for penicillin G.

PARA-AMINO-SALICYLIC ACID (PAS)

Although PAS usually causes liver disorder as a part of a generalised hypersensitivity response, there is one case on record of a brisk haemolytic episode apparently as an isolated phenomenon (Rowland, 1958). A 24-year old woman was treated for pulmonary tuberculosis with streptomycin and isoniazid; during five months of treatment the sputum remained positive and the patient was given one dose of 6 g PAS solution. Within two hours the patient felt weak, complained of epigastric pain and vomited. Later she became hypotensive and the urine was reddish-brown. The haemoglobin dropped from the previous level of 14.6 g to 3.7 g/100 ml and the white blood count was 22,000/c.mm. Marked jaundice developed. Treatment with transfusion and later intramuscular iron was successful in restoring the haemoglobin level. Because the patient's sputum remained positive for Mycobacterium tuberculosis desensitisation to PAS was carried out and this was accomplished without further haemolysis.

SULPHONAMIDES

Haemolytic reactions occurring during sulphonamide administration usually present in patients with glucose-6-phosphate dehydrogenase deficiency; occasionally haemolytic anaemia may be associated with the presence of Heinz bodies in the erythrocytes (Gardner & Bargen, 1964).

NITROFURANTOIN

Haemolytic anaemia may occur as a result of nitrofurantoin therapy and is a result of glucose-6-phosphate dehydrogenase deficiency, the process being similar to haemolytic reactions due to sulphonamides (Kimbro et al, 1957).

CHLORAMPHENICOL

Using this drug in the treatment of typhoid fever Robertson and associates (1968) noted three patients in whom haemolysis occurred in association with glucose-6-phosphate dehydrogenase deficiency.

(ii) **Disturbance of conjugation and protein binding**

NOVOBIOCIN

Novobiocin may be associated with a yellow discolouration of skin and plasma which is due to a lipochrome metabolite of the antibiotic. This should not be confused with jaundice which results from an increase in unconjugated bilirubin in the plasma caused by inhibition of glucuronyltransferase, the enzyme that catalyses bilirubin conjugation (Lokietz et al, 1963). The drug has been held responsible for a threefold increase in the incidence of hyperbilirubinaemia in infants treated during a nursery outbreak of staphylococcal infection. A 13-year old girl became jaundiced with no evidence of haemolysis, and normal liver function after long term treatment with novobiocin 2 g daily. She had markedly raised free bilirubin and very low conjugated bilirubin levels (McKay & Lucey, 1964).

CHLORAMPHENICOL

Jaundice due to chloramphenicol therapy is rare. Occasionally in patients with known liver disease, usually severe, jaundice occurs suddenly in association with chloramphenicol administration. This is thought to be due to competition by the drug with the glucuronal transfer mechanism. In severe renal insufficiency the serum half-life of active chloramphenicol is little altered unless there is accompanying liver disease (Kunin et al, 1959). This appears to be due to a slower rate of glucuronide conjugation and a similar process probably contributes to the vascular collapse in the 'grey syndrome' which occurs in newborn infants, whose immature conjugation mechanism is overloaded when chloramphenicol is administered in large doses.

SULPHONAMIDES

Unconjugated bilirubin enters the cerebrospinal fluid more easily than the conjugated form. Sulphonamides compete for binding sites in plasma proteins and so leave a greater proportion of bilirubin free to cross the blood-brain barrier. This may be important in the neonatal period when sulphonamides administered either to the parturiant woman or the newborn infant can induce kernicterus.

(iii) Direct liver cell injury

TETRACYCLINES

Tetracyclines have a direct toxic action on the liver; these drugs are concentrated in the liver and kidneys more than in other organs. Renal insufficiency contributes to high plasma levels of most tetracycline analogues (see previous section) and pre-existing liver disease could be expected to result in increased incidence of hepatic toxicity, but this does not seem to have been proved.

Liver histology, in samples obtained either by biopsy or at post-mortem, has usually shown a fine-droplet fatty change in the liver with involvement in all parts of the lobule. There is little evidence of liver cell necrosis or an inflammatory reaction. Tests of liver function indicate combination of hepatocellular and obstructive features.

The occurrence of hepatic toxicity in pregnancy has been indicated by Schultz and his associates (1963) who described six pregnant women treated with intravenous tetracycline who became jaundiced and died. Dowling and Lepper (1964) reviewing the subject remark on the similarity between the fatty liver syndrome of pregnancy and the hepatic changes found in tetracycline toxicity.

Survey of the reported cases, and relevant literature, allows the following conclusions:

1. Hepatic toxicity due to tetracycline does not seem to occur when conventional doses (2 g/day) are given orally even for prolonged periods. Post-mortem liver samples taken from patients who died of chronic bronchitis who had received tetracycline continuously for 13 to 86 months did not show fatty liver infiltration (Dowling & Lepper, 1964).
2. Toxicity occurs after high doses, usually administered intravenously.
3. Renal insufficiency, resulting in prolonged high plasma levels, is often present in patients with hepatic toxicity.
4. Use of tetracyclines during the last trimester of pregnancy appears to be associated with an added risk.

THIACETAZONE

Thiacetazone is an antituberculous thiosemicarbazone compound synthesised and used in Germany after the second world war. There has been much doubt about its place in therapy, but recently two trials in East Africa (see Chapter 18) have confirmed its usefulness and its hepatotoxicity has been better defined.

The drug has very little toxicity if the daily dose is between 100 and 150 mg; liver dysfunction may be encountered if doses greater than 150 mg daily are used. The duration of administration and the size of dose (if greater than

200 mg/day) appear to be directly related to the degree of liver disorder. Further, those with pre-existing liver disease appear more likely to develop hepatic toxicity to the drug.

Falk and associates (1951) described fatty changes on liver biopsy which regressed when thiacetazone therapy was discontinued. The degree of fatty metamorphosis was closely related to changes in bromsulphalein retention. There is one report of acute necrosis of the liver during therapy in a malnourished East African (Lancet, 1963).

SULPHONAMIDES

Sulphonamides can cause toxicity in many systems; in a review of the world literature Dujovne and colleagues (1967) collected 57 reports of sulphonamide hepatotoxicity and added another well studied case. Their patient was a 38-year old man who received sulphamethoxazole for one week in 1964, and for several weeks in 1966 during preparation for cystoscopy. The drug was stopped but restarted three days later; because of complaints of nausea and the presence of jaundice it was then discontinued. The liver was enlarged, there was marked elevation of the serum alkaline phosphatase, and moderately raised serum bilirubin and transaminase levels. A liver biopsy, one week after the onset of jaundice showed numerous bile casts in the canaliculi, scattered small areas of hepato-cellular necrosis, extracellular hyaline bodies and infiltration with mononuclear cells and eosinophil leucocytes. The patient improved spontaneously, but when later challenged with a test dose complained of nausea and showed a similar biochemical abnormality within twenty-four hours of the first dose of sulphamethoxazole.

This case demonstrates well the combined injurious effects which drugs may produce in liver function; there was direct hepatic cellular injury, cholestasis, and cellular dysfunction. The authors classified this patient's jaundice as 'mixed hepato-cellular'.

PYRAZINAMIDE

The most important adverse effect of this antituberculous drug is hepatoxicity. It is not clear by what mechanism toxicity occurs, but the increasing severity of altered serum transaminase values and jaundice in patients prescribed increasing doses suggests a direct liver cell injury. Hepatic necrosis and death may occur.

(iv) **Hepatitis-like reactions**

Isoniazid and ethionamide, two antibiotics used in the treatment of tuberculosis may produce jaundice suggestive of acute hepatitis (Sherlock, 1965).

Jaundice due to isoniazid is rare; it usually occurs in the first four weeks of therapy, but may be delayed to the seventh week. There is fever in some cases, liver function tests and histology of biopsy material suggest hepato-cellular damage compatible with virus hepatitis.

Ethionamide, a reserve antituberculous drug, may produce raised serum transaminase levels, with or without signs of liver cell damage and manifest jaundice (Conn & Binder, 1964). There may be an increased incidence of this complication in diabetics (Moulding & Goldstein, 1962; Phillips & Tashman, 1963).

(v) Sensitivity-type cholestasis

Jaundice of the cholestatic type has been described after the administration of erythromycin, but it is the esters of both erythromycin and oleandomycin that are particularly associated with hepatic toxicity. The clinical picture is similar to that observed in chlorpromazine toxicity. Jaundice due to erythromycin estolate usually occurs after prolonged administration (ie between the 10th and 20th day) it may be prolonged, but is usually reversible. In some patients who develop this complication there is a strong history of allergy. The clinical presentation is often similar to infective hepatitis, starting with epigastric discomfort, anorexia, vomiting, and followed by jaundice. Liver enlargement occurs and biopsy specimens show changes of intrahepatic cholestasis. The reaction caused by triacetyl oleandomycin is less clearly cholestatic, being a combination of bile stasis and hepatocellular dysfunction.

NITROFURANTOIN

This drug is widely used in the treatment of urinary tract infections and disturbance of liver function appears to be a very rare complication of therapy. Two of twelve patients with varying degrees of liver disorder who received intravenous nitrofurantoin (total dose 3.6 - 6.5 g in from 7-9 days) showed abnormalities of liver function tests suggestive of hepato-cellular damage (Strauss & Jawetz, 1963). There is one well documented case of cholestatic response in a patient treated with nitrofurantoin (Ernaelsteen & Williams, 1961). This patient was a 55-year old woman with recurrent episodes of cystitis who during the third course of nitrofurantoin developed a high fever, maculopapular rash, and later jaundice. The liver was enlarged and tender, but the spleen was not palpable. Liver function tests showed a marked rise in the alkaline phosphatase, increase in serum bilirubin (maximum 6.1 mg/ 100 ml), with little rise in the transaminase values. During the acute phase of the reaction there was marked eosinophilia in the peripheral blood. Liver biopsy (8 days after jaundice was first noted) showed a severe degree of bile stasis with bile thrombi lying in dilated canaliculi; focal areas of liver cell necrosis and inflammatory cell infiltration were present. A second biopsy, six weeks later, showed that bile stasis was still present, absence of liver cell necrosis and considerable regenerative activity.

(vi) Generalised hypersensitivity reactions

Included in this category are drug reactions with marked allergic features accompanied by jaundice. The jaundice may be of various types and may show 'mixed features', and it will be clear that some reactions ascribed to other categories (eg PAS, nitrofurantoin) could equally well be included in generalised hypersensitivity phenomena.

This type of reaction has been described in a patient given penicillin G (streptomycin was also prescribed) and can occur with sulphonamides and PAS. Patients in this group often have histories of allergic responses to other agents including antibiotics and it may be difficult or impossible to decide which drug is responsible for a particular reaction.

THERAPEUTIC IMPLICATIONS OF HEPATOTOXICITY

In general, antibiotics which have caused jaundice or other toxic reactions in individual patients should be avoided. Related compounds should be used with caution. Patients giving a history of allergy should be watched carefully for adverse drug responses; alterations in liver function tests may suggest toxicity at an early stage.

Patients suspected of having glucose-6-phosphate dehydrogenase deficiency which is common in African or Negro populations should probably not be treated with sulphonamides or nitrofurantoin, but this recommendation is not likely to be practicable. Sulphonamides and possibly novobiocin should not be administered to newborn infants.

Tetracyclines should not be used in high doses intravenously for prolonged periods. The presence of severe renal insufficiency is an indication for reduced dosage (except chlortetracycline) and these drugs are better avoided in the last trimester of pregnancy.

USE OF ANTIBIOTICS IN PATIENTS WITH ESTABLISHED LIVER DISEASE

There is no absolute contraindications, but modifications in prescribing are desirable in addition to those implied in the above general suggestions when patients with known liver disease are being treated. The two main variables are the degree of liver disorder, and the metabolism of the prescribed drug. The latter is often so complex that worthwhile conclusions are very difficult.

Patients with established liver disease should be given drugs with known direct liver toxicity such as tetracyclines, pyrizinamide and thiacetazone cautiously. Repeated courses of antibiotics known to cause hypersensitivity-type cholestasis such as the esters of erythromycin are better avoided. Chloramphenicol, if used at all, should be administered in reduced dosage. It may often be possible to use toxic drugs, albeit in reduced doses, by careful and frequent clinical assessment combined with serial biochemical estimations of liver function.

Two points should be emphasised. Firstly, in this section although liver disorders in relation to antibiotic therapy have been stressed, it is imperative that each patient be considered individually and the effects of disease on all systems, including the liver, are fully assessed. Secondly, that in treating any individual patient suffering from liver disease with potentially hepatotoxic drugs the clinician must try and weigh the advantages for and against the use of such drugs. The risks inherent in the use of a particular drug in an individual are very difficult and indeed usually impossible to assess. In this section I have aimed at providing a basis on which a useful therapeutic judgement may be attempted.

3. Treatment of infections in patients with altered immune responses

INTRODUCTION

Patients with altered immunological responses present several difficulties in regard to infections. Firstly, in this group as a whole infections are common, and as many patients in this category now have an improved lifespan due to various effective measures, the treatment of infections must be expected to play an increasing role in their management. Secondly, the diagnosis of infection may be extremely difficult; patients with leukaemia, for instance, who have gross abnormalities of the leucocyte count may develop fever, the true cause of which is elusive. The nature of the underlying disease and the drugs used in treatment may so alter the manifestations of infection and the inflammatory reaction that they remain unrecognised.

Further, this group of patients are particularly susceptible to invasion by opportunist organisms which often produce intractable tissue responses, rather than acute infections and the agents available for the treatment of many of these conditions are far from ideal. In the following section the problems of some of the altered immunity states are briefly discussed, and some general therapeutic principles evolved.

CLASSIFICATION OF IMMUNITY DEFICIENCY STATES

Immunity is a complex phenomenon; the subtlety of interactions between many variables results in a range of body responses disorder of which can result in infection or alternatively in altered reaction to infecting agents. It is convenient for classification, but frequently impossible in practice to divide immunity deficiency states into antibody deficiency, deficiency of cellular immunity and combination of these. Neutropoenia may complicate any of these abnormalities

ANTIBODY DEFICIENCY

Of the common immunoglobulins (IgG, IgM, IgA) deficiency of IgG is most closely related to infections. This occurs in several well defined syndromes such as the sex-linked hypogammaglobulinaemia of boys, and in congenital rubella; it may also occur in myelomatosis and other dysproteinaemias. Deficiency of IgG is frequently present in the lymphoproliferative disorders, and may well be responsible, in part at any rate, for the increased incidence of infection in protein deficiency states. Pneumonia, septicaemia, meningitis and skin infections, due to the common pyogenic cocci or Gram-negative organisms are usual. Infection with Listeria monocytogenes and Pneumocystis carinii also occurs.

DEFICIENCY OF CELLULAR IMMUNITY

Lymphopoenia and altered thymic function are usually linked with deficiency of cellular immunity, also called delayed hypersensitivity. In its purest form this has been found by Fulginiti and associates (1966) to result in frequent infections due to viruses and Pseudomonas aeruginosa. This form of immunity deficiency is common in Hodgkin's disease when it is associated with granulomatous tissue reactions and the usual bacterial infections encountered are tuberculosis, cyptococcosis, and to a lesser extent brucellosis; zoster-varicella virus infections are common.

NEUTROPOENIA

Profound neutropoenia, from whatever cause, is associated with a high incidence of infection. It may occur as an isolated cyclicial phenomenon of unknown aetiology, and abnormal leucocyte function is part of the syndrome of fatal granulomatosis in children. Morphological changes in the leucocytes form the basis for frequent episodes of infection which occur in the Chediak-Higashi anomaly. Reduction in the leucocyte count may be found when disease, drugs or toxins interfere with marrow function. As many of the drugs used in the treatment of malignancy, leukaemia and reticuloses result in a reduction in the number of circulating granulocytes, it is clear that complications of neutropoenic origin may accompany many lympho-reticular disorders. Bodey and associates (1966) were able to relate the prevalence of infection in patients with acute leukaemia to the level of granulocytes and lymphocytes. Infection of bacterial and fungal origin was most common when both types of cell were reduced, and persistently reduced levels had a bad prognosis; patients who were able to increase the granulocyte count even though the initial level was low had a more favourable prognosis.

CORTICOSTEROIDS

It is impossible to be certain how corticosteroid drugs will modify a particular infection. Very often in the acute phase of bacterial infection they are beneficial, reducing fever and increasing well-being apparently in a non-specific and not well understood manner. There is considerable support for the concept that corticosteroids may cause stabilisation of lysosomal mem-

Table XXIX. Types of infection related to various immunity deficiency states

Condition	Disorder of	Common micro-organisms	Type of infection
Myeloproliferative Acute leukaemia Chronic myeloid lcukaemia Polycythaemia vera Myelofibrosis Myelosclerosis Fatal granulomatous disease of children Chediak-Higashi anomaly	Granulocytes	Pyogenic cocci Gram-negative organisms Fungi	Septicaemia Pneumonia
Lymphoproliferative Acute leukaemia Chronic lymphatic leukaemia Reticulosis Myeloma ? Post-splenectomy Hypogammaglobulinaemia	Immunoglobulins	Pyogenic cocci Gram-negative organisms *Listeria monocytogenes* *Pneumocystis carinii*	Pneumonia Septicaemia Meningitis Skin infections
Hodgkins Disease Isolated defect of cellular immunity (Fulginiti et al, 1966)	Cellular immunity	*Candida albicans* *Pseudomonas aeruginosa*	Tuberculosis Cryptococcosis Brucellosis Herpes virus and cytomegalovirus

branes, thus preventing the escape of enzymes capable of digesting phagocytosed parasites (Hirsch, 1962; Iwata et al, 1961). Patients receiving these drugs may develop infections due to micro-organisms, such as brucella or listeria, that prefer an intracellular environment, but infections in these patients are by no means confined to intracellular parasites. If high doses of these drugs are continued for prolonged periods, bacterial, viral or fungal infections are frequent. It is difficult to distinguish the relative roles in the causation of these opportunist infections between the drugs and the diseases for which they are prescribed.

TRANSPLANTATION OF ORGANS

Transplantation of organs from one human being to another is a recent introduction into medicine, and many problems remain unsolved. The phenomenon of rejection of foreign protein underlies all these difficulties. To overcome the rejection process immunosuppressive therapy, combined with corticosteroid drugs, is employed and this has led to a high incidence of infection. Of 42 patients treated by means of renal transplantation from normal donors there were 17 deaths in 14 of which infection was a contributory factor. Pneumonia of bacterial or fungal aetiology occurred in six of the 42 patients, and was fatal in five (Rifkind et al, 1964). The same group of workers have also shown that cytomegalovirus was the commonest organism demonstrated in post-mortem lung cultures; candida species and pseudomonas species were also present in a proportion of cases. Inclusion bodies in lung, as well as other tissues, suggest that cytomegalovirus was pathogenic and not merely a saphrophytic agent (Hill et al, 1964).

Slapak and associates (1968) described four patients who developed a pulmonary disorder after renal homo-transplantation. This syndrome, termed 'transplant lung', occurred during a rejection crisis or when the dose of corticosteroids was reduced. Cyanosis, fever, and pulmonary function studies indicative of alveolar capillary block were noted. These authors suggest that this syndrome is the result of an autoimmune reaction in which antibodies directed against the transplanted kidney cross-react and damage the patient's own alveolar-capillary wall. This reaction may permit opportunist organisms to multiply and dominate the post-mortem findings.

These reports and others of similar nature indicate that after surgical transplantation of organs a number of tissue alterations occur in which micro-organisms, often of unusual nature, play either an aetiological or aggravating role, both of which may have grave consequences for the patient.

THERAPEUTIC SUGGESTIONS

The importance of the host response is emphasised by the high failure rate in treating infections in patients with immunological deficiency. Required are compounds capable of effectively modifying selected facets of the host responses to invasion by parasitic micro-organisms. As these compounds are lacking (but the use of anti-lymphocyte serum may be an important advance) and as drugs directed against the invading parasites are often ineffective, the therapeutic approach has to be indirect. Prevention and prophylaxis become more important than chemotherapy.

PREVENTION

(i) Microbiological investigation

Before any patient receives immunosuppressive therapy not only careful physical examination, but also a full microbiological assessment is advisable. This should include bacteriological cultures taken from nose and throat, skin, and in females, vaginal swabs. Urine and stool samples and also sputum, if available, should be cultured. In this way some idea of the patient's own flora will be known and antibiotic sensitivities will be available. This may be important later if blind therapy has to be instituted for severe infections. Similarly changes in bacterial populations during therapy can be documented.

(ii) Corticosteroids

Where possible doses should be reduced and total courses not unduly prolonged. In a general way this is safe management, but in some circumstances when opportunist infection occurs the steroid dose should be increased. This is best exemplified in the 'transplant' lung syndrome.

(iii) Antimetabolites and radiation

The use of antimetabolites, cytotoxic drugs and radiotherapy should be controlled so that marrow function is not markedly depressed. The granulocyte count is the best single guide. Occasionally there is a striking time relationship between starting treatment with antimetabolites and the onset of opportunist infections.

(iv) Isolation

Patients with reduced immune responses should be treated preferably in single rooms or cubicles and in some patients special precautions will be necessary. This may not always be possible, but leaving such patients in a large general ward exposes them to unjustified hazards.

The use of a protected environment was demonstrated by Levitan and associates (1967) who used a patient isolator system in which the patient's bed was covered with a plastic canopy into which filtered air was ducted. They attempted to provide a sterile environment using tinned food and removing the patient's own micro-organisms by washing the skin with antiseptic solutions and the use of antibacterial and fungicidal drugs. This method of protection and isolation enabled patients to be treated with large doses of antimetabolites in the presence of marked neutropoenia (often with counts less than 500/cm) without an excessive incidence of infective complications. Interestingly, cultures of the patients' stools, nose and skin were sterile for more than 50% of the time in the isolator, but throat swabs were sterile only 1% of the time. Infections were mainly due to Gram-negative organisms which had previously been isolated from the patients' stools or skin.

PROPHYLAXIS

Passive immunity for protection against bacterial infections has limited use. In exceptional circumstances immune human plasma may be helpful in tiding a patient over a severe infective episode, but Feingold and Oski (1965) showed that this was effective in pseudomonas infection. A case could be made for routine administration of pooled gamma globulin to patients at special risk due to virus infections. Kefalides and associates (1964) had some success with this method in protecting patients with burns from infection with pseudomonas infection. Certainly hyperimmune sera should be given to patients who develop varicella-zoster virus infections, who are particularly vulnerable because of chronic lymphatic leukaemia. If hyperimmune gamma globulin can be provided this technique might be a useful measure in protection against cytomegalovirus infection.

Active immunity has not been as widely practiced as would seem warranted. Pneumococcal vaccines are highly effective, but since the introduction of penicillin and other effective antibiotics they have been virtually discarded. In the group of patients under discussion, particularly those underoing transplantation, active immunisation with pneumococcal vaccines should be seriously considered. The same applies to vaccines prepared against Pseudomonas aeruginosa but the results with this organism present many difficulties despite the promising work of Feller and Kamei (1964). An extension of this method of protection is the use of vaccines produced from bacteria which are constantly present in the patient's environment or which have caused infections in other patients treated in the same unit.

ANTIBIOTICS

Prophylactic antibiotics should be avoided. Inevitably they encourage the overgrowth of organisms resistant to the drugs used and this invites disaster in these patients at special risk. Although this did not seem to occur when Levitan and Perry (see above) used their isolation technique, this should be considered an unusual and complex situation requiring much further work and confirmation.

SPECIFIC ANTIMICROBIAL THERAPY

When infections occur in this group of patients with immunity deficiency it is important that they be recognised early and treated efficiently with specific agents if such are available.

BACTERIAL

Very effective antibiotics are available for the treatment of infections due to the common Gram-positive cocci; similarly Neisseria meningitidis and Haemophilus influenzae should present few therapeutic problems. Unfortunately this does not hold for bowel-derived Gram-negative bacteria which may give rise to septicaemia or pneumonia and although the drugs available for treating this type of infection are often effective antibacterial agents, they have disadvantages because of toxicity (eg kanamycin, colistin, gentamicin) or because their wide-spectrum of activity encourages superinfection (eg chloramphenicol, tetracycline, ampicillin). A most useful recent addition for treatment of serious Gram-negative infections, especially those due to Pseudomonas aeruginosa is carbenicillin. This appears to be as non-toxic as other penicillins and is an effective drug with great promise. Salmonella infections may be treated with chloramphenicol or ampicillin. Infections due to L. monocytogenes will often respond to a number of antibiotics; most consistently effective are penicillin G, chloramphenicol and probably ampicillin.

CRYPTOCOCCAL

Systemic cryptococcal infection which usually manifests as meningitis can be effectively treated with only one drug — amphotericin B (see Chapter 11).

FUNGAL

The conditions likely to be encountered are candidiasis and aspergillosis. Local candida infections respond to applications of nystatin or amphotericin B. For generalised candidiasis or aspergillosis only amphotericin B administered intravenously can be expected to produce a good therapeutic result. Nocardiosis may respond to large doses of sulphonamide. No effective chemotherapy is available for the treatment of mucormycosis.

PNEUMOCYSTIS CARINII

Pneumocystis carinii infection was first related to plasma cell or interstitial pneumonia in debilitated infants; in recent years it has been recognised as an opportunist organism in adults with immunity deficiency syndromes and especially following renal transplantation. Prolonged treatment with high doses of corticosteroid drugs appears to be an important predisposing factor. Clinically the pneumonia is characterised by an insidious onset of cough, fever, cyanosis and bilateral alveolar exudate. Simultaneous infection with other opportunist organisms is common. Although the diagnosis may be suspected confirmation is difficult; tracheal aspirate or lung biopsy may be required. Treatment is with pentamidine isothionate and the dose is 4 mg/kg body weight given as a single daily intramuscular injection for 10 to 14 days. Hypotension and gastro-intestinal upsets may occur.

VIRAL

In this category of patient infection with viruses of the herpes group, with the notable exception of herpes simplex, is common. Cytomegalovirus is probably the commonest, but varicella-zoster infection also occurs. There are no drugs effective against these agents.

4 Chemotherapy in the newborn

INTRODUCTION

The newborn infant is in many respects an unusual host possessing opportunity of acquiring infection from unique sources, often with responses which are inadequate to deal with infection, and an immature metabolism which may produce inappropriate clinical manifestations of infection, and which demands special considerations and modifications in the use of chemotherapeutic drugs.

The neonatal period is here defined as the first month of life and it is during this period that major problems of diagnosis, pharmacology and therapy arise. From the point of view of therapy, and dosage related to body weight, the infant over one month old approximates to a miniature adult, whereas in the neonatal period the use of some drugs in doses related to body weight comparable to those used in adults, may result in serious side effects or even disaster. Examples of these untoward responses are, the use of chloramphenicol in the newborn, resulting in vascular collapse or 'grey syndrome', or the administration of sulphonamide which competes for albumin binding sites and thus displaces bilirubin, enhancing the probability of kernicterus.

PHYSIOLOGICAL AND PATHOLOGICAL CONSIDERATIONS

MODES OF INFECTION

(i) **Acquired transplacentally** During the period of gestation the foetus, placenta and mother can be regarded in some respects as a single unit. The developing foetus may show periods of increased vulnerability to certain infectious agents exemplified by the damaging response to invasion by the rubella virus during early pregnancy. This contrasts with vaccinia virus which may affect the foetus at any stage of gestation. In the past syphilis and tuberculosis were noted to be transmitted transplacentally and infection with Listeria monocytogenes, Toxoplasma gondii or cytomegalovirus can occur by this portal unique to the foetus.

(ii) **In the birth canal** In its passage through the birth canal the foetus may be exposed to various micro-organisms particularly due to faecal contamination of the perineum. Herpes simplex virus may be inhaled or it may possibly enter the foetus via the skin or conjunctivae. Pneumocystis carinii may be inhaled at this time but may not cause symptoms until several months after birth. Gonococci or staphylococci acquired in the birth canal may cause ophthalmia. The aspiration of infected amniotic fluid may give rise to various respiratory disorders particularly bacterial pneumonia due to various Gram-negative species, staphylococci and streptococci. This situation is particularly likely to arise when there is premature rupture of membranes with subsequent ascending infection. The skin, notably the area of the umbilicus may be invaded by pathogens and any congenital defects such as dermal sinuses offer obvious portals of entry for bacterial pathogens.

(iii) **Immediately after birth** After birth the newborn infant is exposed to all the hazards of its environment, particularly viral bacterial and fungal pathogens which may be inhaled, ingested or gain entry through the skin or mucus membranes. To a large extent the pattern of infection will reflect the environment — the staphylococcal infection of the umbilical stump is likely to be caused by the particular 'nursery' strain; if instrumentation or mechanical ventilation has been used infection with Pseudomonas aeruginosa may be expected. The antibiotic sensitivity of these pathogens will reflect the prescribing habits current in the obstetric and neonatal departments.

SUSCEPTIBILITY TO INFECTION

In the previous section of this chapter (page 276) the various defence mechanisms are discussed in relation to immunity and resistance to infection. In the neonatal period all these mechanisms are important; the factors most readily assessed are the immunoglobulin concentration and the leucocyte activity.

IMMUNOGLOBULINS

Four major classes of immunoglobulins have been characterised on the basis of their electrophoretic mobility, ultracentrifugal properties and immunochemical characteristics. These are:

1. IgG (gamma G or 7^S-γ_2 globulin), which carries antibodies against diphtheria, tetanus, typhoid H, toxoplasmosis, streptolysin O, Herpes simplex, influenza, vaccinia, measles, mumps, pertussis, incomplete Rh antibodies.
2. IgM (gamma$_1$ M, B_2 M, or 19^S-γ_1 M-globulin), the antibodies carried include: isohaemoglutinins (anti A and anti B), complete Rh agglutinins, heterophile antibodies, rheumatoid factors, reagins against syphilis, antityphoid O.

3. IgA (gamma$_1$ A or B_2A), antibodies against insulin and thyroglobulin as well as skin sensitising allergens are carried by this class of immunoglobulin.

4. IgD

Immunoglobulins

Immunoglobulin	% of total	Molecular weight	Placental transfer
IgG	75%	150,000	Readily
IgM	7%	1,000,000	Very little
IgA	20%		Probably little

NORMAL INFANTS

The healthy newborn infant should have IgG concentrations as high as that of the mother; this transferred immunoglobulin is catabolised with a half-life somewhat lower than in adults reaching its lowest levels between the third and tenth week of life. Synthesis of IgG by the infant starts at about three months and normal adult levels are reached at one to four years of age. Premature infants may have reduced IgG levels and this can be associated with recurrent infection (Hobbs, 1966).

IgM concentrations are necessarily low in the newborn — the levels begin to rise during the second and third month, especially in the presence of infection, during a period of reduced levels of IgG and at a time before IgA has appeared. This account is true in general but it should not be interpreted too literally, for recent work has indicated that the foetus is capable of synthesising IgA and IgM in small quantities (Brasher & Hartley, 1969).

DEFICIENCY STATES

(i) The best defined and most easily recognised of these is the infantile sex-linked agammaglobulinaemia which occurs in boys (Bruton's disease). Recurrent pyogenic infection predominately with extracellular pathogens is expected usually beginning about the time maternal antibody is cleared from the circulation (6-12 months).

(ii) Agammaglobulinaemia with lymphopoenia (Swiss Type) is the most severe form of immunological incompetence and is associated with atrophy of the thymus. This condition is inherited as an autosomal recessive characteristic. The infants have retarded growth and suffer serious infections from the first few weeks of life. The outcome is usually fatal by the second year of life and the end is sometimes hastened by injection of a live organism vaccine.

(iii) Transient hypogammaglobulinaemia probably represents the lower extremes of 'physiological' hypogammaglobulinaemia, is not sex-linked but repeated bacterial infections similar to those occurring in Bruton's disease are found. In some cases IgM and IgG levels remain low.

(iv) There are a large number of miscellaneous disorders probably of the order of twenty different syndromes of immunoglobulin deficiency. Many of these are genetically determined, some result from nutritional disorders or associated disease and are not suitable for discussion here.

(v) Non-specific humoral factors may also be deficient in early life. Serum complement is not produced until late in gestation and at full term is about half the maternal concentration (Dancis & Kunz, 1954). Properdin is a naturally occurring euglobulin which functions in concert with complement to kill protozoa, Gram-negative bacteria and to neutralise some viruses. In the newborn reduced activity of these non-specific humoral factors may contribute to an increased incidence of infection.

GRANULOCYTOPOENIA

Neutropoenia is discussed on page 277; in the newborn severe neutropoenia may be a manifestation of hereditary agranulocytosis transmitted as an autosomal recessive trait, or can occur from drugs administered either to mother or infant, and it should not be forgotten that infection, particularly with Gram-negative species, may result in neutropoenia.

IMMATURE METABOLISM

The newborn infant with immature enzyme systems and tissue differentiation behaves differently from older children and adults in the metabolism and excretion of drugs and these differences must be taken into account when antibacterial agents are used in the neonatal period. Penicillin G, for instance, is cleared almost entirely by the kidney, but in the neonate the immature renal tubule does not excrete penicillin at a rate comparable to the adult kidney and this can lead to excessive blood levels. Novobiocin has been held responsible for an increase in jaundice due it is thought to non-competitive inhibition of bilirubin glucuronide formation, while chloramphenicol in high doses may lead to the 'grey syndrome' which exemplifies two aspects of the neonate's inability to metabolise this drug — namely deficient glucuronide formation in the liver and reduced renal excretion of chloramphenicol metabolites.

We have very limited information on the pharmacology of antibacterial agents in the neonate and even less in the premature infant and this lack of knowledge makes chemotherapy in this age group difficult not to say hazardous. In the section (page 289) dealing with individual drugs these difficulties are further defined in relation to the practicality of therapy.

THE VULNERABLE INFANT

Whilst all newborn infants have reduced levels of IgM and are susceptible to infection with Gram-negative bacteria, those with inherited immunoglobulin disorders will show increased vulnerability to infection with a wide range of micro-organisms. The premature infant deficient not only in IgM but also IgG, is a subject particularly susceptible to infection.

The hazards of the birth canal and the environment together with intra-uterine infection, or disadvantageous antibodies (neonatal thyrotoxicosis, myasthenia gravis, hypoparathyroidism, thrombocytopoenia) together with neutropoenia from any cause and inadequate cellular response are some of the great disadvantages which may threaten survival of the newborn.

MANIFESTATIONS OF INFECTION IN THE NEONATE

The neonate has a limited repertoire of responses so that any untoward stimuli such as anoxia or infection may produce similar manifestations. It is important to realise that the newborn infant may present no specific features indicating infection and yet may succumb within a short period to undetected pneumonia or septicaemia.

Failure to suck accompanied by listlessness is a common finding and in late stages of infection there may be progressive hypotonia and what amounts to stupor. Convulsions may occur. Regurgitation of feeds with loose stools is expected. There is often an increase in jaundice usually of mixed type with some degree of haemolysis. This probably indicates blood stream infection combined with liver cell dysfunction. Alterations in body temperature are important indications in this age group and hypothermia is probably as likely as pyrexia. The classical features of pyrexia and leucocytosis do occur but are much less constant and less helpful than in older children and adults. Signs of meningeal irritation with neck and back stiffness are seldom florid; if they become conspicuous it usually indicates a well advanced meningitis. Fullness of the fontanelle is very important evidence of increasing intracranial tension and if this occurs in an infant whose other manifestations suggest under rather than over hydration then meningitis must be suspected.

It is an important fact that in the newborn septicaemia and meningitis are common. It seems that almost any local infection may be accompanied by blood stream invasion and subsequent dissemination of pathogens particularly to the meninges. The practical implications in this are that in any infant who is suspected of having an infection, blood cultures are obligatory and lumbar puncture may well be desirable.

SELECTED DRUGS: METABOLISM IN THE NEONATE

Knowledge in this field is limited but relevant information of some antibacterial agents commonly used in the neonatal period is discussed on the following pages.

PENICILLIN G

The basic facts on the excretion of penicillin G are given on page 263; modifications of dosage in the neonate are required primarily because of reduced functional excretion by the kidney. Using doses of 20,000 u/kg body weight Barnett and colleagues (1949) showed that peak serum concentrations of approximately 50 u/ml occurred after a single intramuscular injection and 12 hours after injection the mean level was 4 u/ml. With doses of 10,000 u/ml peak levels were slightly lower but no penicillin was detected in the serum 12 hours after administration. With doses of 333,000 u/kg body weight Grossman and Ticknor (1965) reported peak levels of over 200 u/ml and 12 hour levels of approximately 12 u/ml. In the neonate neurotoxicity in the form of generalised or myotonic convulsions may result from excessive penicillin dosage. It is of interest that penicillin G is very much more lethal to the newborn rat than to the adult rat (Michael & Sutherland, 1960).

AMPICILLIN

After a single intramuscular injection of ampicillin in a dose of 10 mg/kg Yaffe and Simon (1970) showed that the mean serum half-life was four hours in nine infants two to seven days old, 2.8 hours in six who were eight to fourteen days old, 1.7 hours in eleven who were fifteen to thirty days and 1.6 hours in nine who were thirty-one to sixty-eight days old. The maximum plasma level recorded in these studies in the youngest infants was 30 μg/ml. The serum half-life in adults is about 1.5 hours and it is of great interest that figures approaching this were obtained at about one month after birth. The clearance of ampicillin increased during the first month after birth and was independant of gestational age.

METHICILLIN

Yaffe and Simon (1970) also found that the clearance of methicillin behaved similarly to ampicillin, that is, it increased up to one month of age. The mean serum half-life was 2.4 hours in ten infants four to seven days old, 1.8 hours in five infants eleven to fourteen days old and 1.4 hours in nine infants seventeen to thirty-three days old. Mean peak serum concentrations of 36.2 to 41.6 μg/ml were reached one hour after injection. In these studies the dose was 20 mg/kg.

OXACILLIN : CLOXACILLIN

Studies with oxacillin showed peak concentrations varying from 47.0 to 51.5 μg/ml one hour after an intramuscular injection (dose 20 mg/kg) of oxacillin. Studies with cloxacillin do not seem to be available but the behaviour of these two compounds is likely to be similar.

CARBENICILLIN

This penicillin derivative has been used in infants but to date the published reports give only clinical details and limited experience with different dosages; no data are available on blood levels in neonates. It must be remembered that this drug will be required in high doses and may have to be administered intravenously. Schulkind and Adler (1970) treated five infants (aged birth to four weeks) with carbenicillin in doses ranging from 200 to 500 mg/kg/day; Ross and associates (1970) in treating neonatal meningitis used doses of 300 to 800 mg/kg/day for periods ranging from 22 to 42 days. The drug was usually given intravenously in four divided doses in 24 hours.

KANAMYCIN

This antibiotic, either alone or in combination, is frequently used in the neonatal period because its antibacterial range includes many Gram-negative pathogens. Davies and associates (1970) reported on blood levels in 34 infants after intramuscular kanamycin. This drug was given in a dose of 5 mg/kg rising to 7.5 mg/kg after the first 48 hours of life in mature, and after the first week in immature infants. The mean serum level one hour after administration on the first day of therapy was 12.8 μg/ml and estimation of blood samples taken on the third and fifth days did not suggest a tendency to accumulate. Yaffe and Simon (1970) showed that in eleven premature infants (weight 0.8-2.5 kg) the mean peak serum concentration was 17.5 μg/ml and occurred one hour after injection of a dose of 7.5 mg/kg body weight. These authors also showed that infants less than 48 hours old excreted only 20% of the administered dose in 12 hours whereas infants aged five to twenty-two days excreted 60% — a value comparable to that found in normal adults.

STREPTOMYCIN

In five premature infants (weight 2-3 kg) peak serum concentrations ranged from 17.2 to 42 μg/ml (mean 29.2 μg/ml) and occurred two hours after an intramuscular injection of a dose of 10 mg/kg body weight. The mean serum half-life was 7.0 hours as compared to 2.7 hours in normal adults (Yaffe & Simon, 1970).

GENTAMICIN

Experience of this drug in neonates is limited and there are few studies which include plasma levels. It is important that the neonatal pharmacology of gentamicin is fully studied for it has bactericidal activity against many pathogens commonly encountered in this age group. Klein (1969) gave details of two newborn infants: a two day old (2.3 kg) infant with myelomeningocoele received a dose of gentamicin of 2 mg/kg and at one hour the plasma concentration was 3.0 μg/ml and at 20-24 hours the level was 0.4 μg/ml. In another anencephalic infant (6 days old, weight 3 kg) a similar dose gave levels of 4.6 μg/ml at one hour and 0.4 μg/ml at 24 hours. In the second infant when the dose was increased to 5.3 mg/kg the one hour plasma concentration was 15.5 μg/ml. When the serum level of this anencephalic infant was 2.3 μg/ml gentamicin two hours after a dose of 2 mg/kg the level of the drug in the cerebrospinal fluid was 0.9 μg/ml.

In neonatal meningitis Newman and Holt (1969) used daily doses of 2mg/kg gentamicin together with intraventricular injections of 1 to 2 mg and stress the importance of repeated plasma and cerebrospinal fluid estimations of gentamicin levels in the control of this type of infection.

CEPHALOTHIN

In full term newborn infants cephalothin (dose 12.5 mg/kg) gave peak serum levels of 25 μg/ml; premature infants given the same dose produced lower peak levels and a steeper fall off at two hours (Sherg et al, 1964). The immature infant therefore metabolised cephalothin at a faster rate than full term infants.

COLISTIN

This drug in adults is excreted predominately by glomerular filtration and renal insufficiency (page 261) demands reduced dosage and it is rather surprising that in premature infants the serum half-life of colistin did not decline with increasing postnatal age, being unchanged in infants aged four to fifty-one days (Yaffe & Simon, 1970). These authors found that after a single intramuscular dose (5 mg/kg) of colistin methanesulphonate mean serum concentrations of approximately 14 to 16 μg/ml were reached two hours after administration and at six hours the level was 6 μg/ml.

CHLORAMPHENICOL

The neonate is unable to metabolise chloramphenicol in a manner similar to adults (see page 262). Conjugation in the liver is impaired and excretion of chloramphenicol metabolites by the kidney is delayed. Toxic effects are common and in the few instances when this drug is required in the neonatal period the dose is 25 mg/kg/day.

PROPHYLAXIS AND THERAPY

To be successful in the neonatal period treatment must be started early; there is very considerable controversy on the usefulness of routine chemotherapy in the neonate and as the manifestations of infection are often vague or ill-defined there seems little reason in many instances to distinguish between prophylactic and therapeutic administration of antibiotic drugs. The essential requirement from the physician is to decide if therapy is required; the

Table XXX. Plasma levels and doses in neonates

Drug	Subject	Dose	Plasma level	Half-life (hours)	Recommended Dose	Reference
Penicillin G	Mature	15,000 u/kg	11.5 μg/ml (mean)		15,000 u/kg 12 hourly increasing to 6 hourly over 2 weeks old	Davies et al (1970)
" "	Premature	15,000 u/kg	11.5 μg/ml (mean)		15,000 u/kg 12 hrly, 1st week 8 hrly, 1-4 weeks 6 hrly, over 4 wks	Davies et al (1970)
" "	Mature	20,000 u/kg	40.0 u/ml (approx) (peak)		50,000 to 100,000 u/kg 12 hourly	Grossman (1970)
" "	Mature	50,000 u/kg	100.0 u/ml (peak)			
Ampicillin	Premature	10 mg/kg	13-19 μg/ml	4 hours (age 2-7 days) 1.7 (15-30 days)		Yaffe & Simon (1970)
"	Mature				100 mg/kg/24 hours day 1-52 12 hourly injections 5 days 8 hourly injections	Grossman (1970)
Carbenicillin	Mature	600-800 mg/kg	200-400 μg/ml (unpublished data Kahn & Ross)		400-800 mg/kg/day I.V.	Ross et al (1970)
Kanamycin	Premature	7.5 mg/kg	17.5 μg/ml (peak)	18 hours (under 2 days) 6 hrs (5-22 days)		Yaffe & Simon (1970)
"	Mature				7.5 mg/kg 12 hourly	Grossman (1970)

Drug	Subject	Dose	Plasma level	Half-life (hours)	Recommended Dose	Reference
Streptomycin	Premature	10 mg/kg	17-42 μg/ml (peak)	7 hours		Grossman (1970)
"	Mature				10-20 mg/kg/day two 12 hourly injections	Yaffe (1965)
Gentamicin	Mature	2 mg/kg	4.6 μg/ml (peak)			Klein (1969)
"	Mature	5.3 mg/kg	15.5 μg/ml (peak)			
"	Mature				2 mg/kg/day	Leedom et al (1969)
Colistin methane-sulphonate	Premature	5 mg/kg	14-16 μg/ml	2.6 (4 days) 2.3 (12-51 days)	2-4 mg/kg every 12 hours	Grossman (1970) Grossman (1968)
Chloram-phenicol	Mature				25 mg/kg/day	Yaffe (1965)
Cephalothin	Premature	12.5 mg/kg	12.5 μg/ml		12.5 mg/kg 6 hourly	Benner (1970)
Cephalori-dine	Mature				30 mg/kg/day	Keay & Fleming (1970)
"	Mature				15 mg/kg/day	Burland et al (1970)

evidence for this decision should be examined carefully and if the conclusion is in favour of therapy then the next step is to decide which drugs to administer.

There are few situations when the choice of drug can be made on the firm basis of bacteriological evidence; in the majority of cases, certainly in the initial stage, 'blind' therapy must be instituted, sometimes the results of culture of amniotic fluid will indicate a particular pathogen and in the infant special attention may be directed against this organism; similarly cultures taken from the infant's umbilicus or skin lesion before the recognition of systemic infection may point to a particular course of action. The pathogens likely to be encountered are Gram-negative species arising in the gastro-intestinal tract, particularly Escherichia coli, Klebsiella species and Pseudomonas aeruginosa. Staphylococcus aureus is still frequently encountered though probably less so than in the past decade. Salmonella species and various streptococci are also encountered.

It is common practice to use drug combinations such as penicillin and kanamycin, gentamicin and cephalothin, or ampicillin and cloxacillin; this merely reflects an attempt to cover a wide range of potential pathogens and there is no good evidence that combinations have any particular merit. In infants with suspected Gram-negative sepsis and especially if Gram-negative rods are seen on stained smears of cerebrospinal fluid then gentamicin and ampicillin may be administered together with gentamicin either intraventricularly or intrathecally. If there is high suspicion that Pseudomonas aeruginosa is the pathogen then gentamicin combined with carbenicillin should be used. Penicillin, cloxacillin and the cephalosporin derivatives can be used when Gram-positive organisms are the likely pathogens. When infection, particularly meningitis, is due to these organisms it is usually possible to sterilise the cerebrospinal fluid quickly, but as Leedom and associates (1969) point out the mortality and the degree of neurological damage is just as high when neonatal meningitis results from these relatively susceptible Gram-positive organisms as when the cause is Gram-negative species.

Whatever drug or combination of drugs is used it should be remembered that therapy policy will require constant scrutiny and revision. This is due not only to the introduction of new antibacterial agents but to the changing antibiotic sensitivity which occurs in any environment when these drugs are in constant use.

Finally even though the chemotherapy is considered appropriate, nutrition must be maintained and the detection, prevention and treatment of acidosis, dehydration and anoxia are crucial considerations in this vulnerable group of patients.

In Table XXX I have summarised some data on blood levels related to dosage in neonates and also provided suggestions for doses. This table may give some basis for selecting drugs and doses in particular infections.

REFERENCES

SECTION I

Boxer, G. E., Jelinek, V. C. and Edison, A. O. (1949) Streptomycin: Clearance and binding to protein. J. Pharmacol. exp. Ther., **97**, 93

Eastwood, J. B. and Curtis, J. R. (1968) Carbenicillin. Administration in patients with severe renal failure. Brit. med. J., **1**, 486

Gingell, J. C., Chisholm, G. D., Calnan, J. S. and Waterworth, P. M. (1969) The dose distribution and excretion of gentamicin with special reference to renal failure. J. infect. Dis. Suppl.1969, 396

Glazko, A. J., Wolf, L. M., Dill, W. A. and Bratton, A. C. (1949) Biochemical studies on chloramphenicol. II Tissue distribution and excretion studies. J. Pharmacol. exp. Ther., **96**, 445

Hoffler, D., Stegemann, I. and Scheler, F. (1966) Ampicillin levels in the serum and urine of patients with impaired renal function. Germ. med. Monthly, **2**, 138

Kabins, S. A. and Cohen, S. (1964) Cephalothin serum levels in the azotaemic patient. Antimicrob. Agents Chemother., **4**, 207

Kunin, C. M. (1967) A guide to use of antibiotics in patients with renal disease. Ann. intern. Med., **67**, 151

Kunin, C. M., Dornbush, A. C. and Finland, Maxwell (1959) Distribution and excretion of four tetracycline analogues in young men. J. clin. Invest., **38**, 1950

Kunin, C. M. and Finland, Maxwell (1959) Persistence of antibiotics in blood of patients with acute renal failure. III. J. clin. Invest., **38**, 1509

Kunin, C. M., Glazko, A. J. and Finland, Maxwell (1959) Persistence of antibiotics in blood of patients with acute renal failure. II. J. clin. Invest., **38**, 1498

Kunin, C. M., Rees, S. B., Merrill, J. P. and Finland, Maxwell (1959) Persistence of antibiotics in blood of patients with acute renal failure. I. J. clin. Invest., **38**, 1487

Lerner, P. I., Smith, Hillas and Weinstein, L. (1967) Penicillin neurotoxicity. Ann. NY Acad. Sci., **145**, 310

Marshall, E. K. Jr. (1948) The absorption, distribution and excretion of streptomycin. J. Pharmacol. exp. Ther., **92**, 43

Price, D. J. E. and Graham, D. I. (1970) Effects of large doses of colistin sulphamethate sodium on renal function. Brit. med. J., **4**, 525

Rantz, L. A., Kirby, W. M. M. and Randall, E. (1944) The absorption and excretion of penicillin following continuous intravenous and subcutaneous administration. J. clin. Invest., **23**, 789

Sorenen, A. W. S., Szabo, L., Pedersen, A. and Scharff, A. (1967) Correlation between renal function and serum half-life of kanamycin and its application to dosage adjustment. Postgrad. med. J. Supplement May, 37

SECTION II

Conn, H. O. and Binder, J. (1964) Ethionamide-induced hepatitis: a review with a report of an additional case. Amer. Rev. resp. Dis., **90**, 542

Dowling, H. F. and Lepper, M. H. (1964) Hepatic reactions to tetracycline. J. Amer. med. Ass., **188**, 307

Dujovne, C. A., Chan, C. H. and Zimmerman, H. J. (1967) Sulphonamide hepatic injury. New Engl. J. Med., **277**, 785

Ernaelsteen, D. and Williams, R. (1961) Jaundice due to nitrofurantoin. Gastroenterology, **41**, 590

Falk, A., Zieve, L., Tucker, W. B. and Hanson, M. (1951) The hepatic toxicity of amithiozone. American Review of Tuberculosis, **64**, 159

Gardner, M. D. and Bargen, J. A. (1964) Haemolytic anaemia secondary to salicylazosulphapyridine. J. Amer. med. Ass., **190**, 71

Kimbro, E. L. Jr., Sacks, M. V. and Torbert, J. V. (1957) Mechanism of the haemolytic anaemia induced by nitrofurantoin. Bull. Johns Hopk. Hosp., **101**, 245

Kunin, C. M., Glazko, A. J. and Finland, Maxwell (1959) Persistence of antibiotics in blood of patients with acute renal failure. II. Chloramphenicol and its metabolic products in the blood of patients with severe renal disease or hepatic cirrhosis. J. clin. Invest., **38**, 1498
Lancet (1963) Leading article. Thiacetazone in tuberculosis, **ii**, 817
Lokietz, H., Dowben, R. M. and Hsia, D. Y. Y. (1963) Studies on the effect of novobiocin on glucuronyl transferase. Pediatrics, **32**, 47
McKay, R. J. and Lucey, J. F. (1964) Neonatology. New Engl. J. Med., **270**, 1231
Montgomery, J. R. (1963) Haemolytic reaction after novobiocin therapy. New Engl. J. Med., **269**, 966
Moulding, T. S. Jr. and Goldstein, S. (1962) Hepatotoxicity due to ethionamide. Amer. Rev. resp. Dis., **86**, 252
Petz, L. D. and Fudenberg, H. H. (1966) Coombs-Positive Haemolytic anaemia caused by penicillin administration. New Engl. J. Med., **274**, 171
Phillips, S. and Tashman, H. (1963) Ethionamide jaundice. Amer. Rev. resp. Dis., **87**, 896
Robertson, R. P., Wahab, M. F. A. and Raasch, F. O. (1968) Evaluation of chloramphenicol and ampicillin in salmonella enteric fever. New Engl. J. Med., **278**, 171
Rowland, H. A. K. (1958) Acute haemolysis following PAS. Brit. med. J., **2**, 92
Schultz, J. C., Adamson, J. S., Workman, W. W. and Norman, T. D. (1963) Fatal liver disease after intravenous administration of tetracycline in high dosage. New Engl. J. Med., **269**, 999
Sherlock, S. (1965) Hepatic reactions to therapeutic agents. Ann. Rev. of Pharm., **5**, 429
Strauss, W. and Jawetz, E. (1963) Nitrofurantoin in patients with hepatic dysfunction. Clin. Pharmacol. Ther., **4**, 297
Swanson, M. A., Chanmougan, D. and Schwartz, R. S. (1966) Immunohaemolytic anaemia due to antipenicillin antibodies. New Engl. J. Med., **274**, 178

SECTION III

Bodey, G. P., Buckley, M., Sathe, Y. S. and Freireich, E. J. (1966) Quantitive relationships between circulating leucocytes and infection in patients with acute leukaemia. Ann. intern. Med., **64**, 328
Feingold, D. S. and Oski, F. (1965) Pseudomonas infection. Treatment with immune human plasma. Arch. intern. Med., **116**, 326
Feller, I. and Kamei, I. (1964) Pseudomonas vaccine and hyper-immune plasma in the treatment of burned patients. Surg. Forum, **15**, 46
Fulginiti, V. A., Hathaway, W. E., Pearlman, D. S., Blackburn, W. R., Reiquam, C. W., Githens, J. H., Claman, N. H. and Kempe, C. H. (1966) Dissociation of delayed-hypersensitivity and antibody-synthesizing capacities in man, Lancet, **ii**, 5
Hill, R. B. Jr., Rowlands, D. T. and Rifkind, D. (1964) Infectious pulmonary disease in patients receiving immunosuppressive therapy for organ transplantation. New Engl. J. Med., **271**, 1021
Hirsch, J. G. (1962) Cinemicrophotographic observations on granule lysis in polymorphonuclear leucocytes during phagocytosis. J. exp. Med., **116**, 827
Iwata, K., Awadaguchi, S. and Yonekura, Y. (1961) Influence of adrenal cortex hormones on phagocytosis, I and II. Jap. J. Bact., **16**, 21, 210
Kefalides, N. A., Arana, J. A., Bazan, A., Velarde, N. and Rosenthal, S. M. (1964) Evaluation of antibiotic prophylaxis and gamma-globulin, plasma, albumin and saline-solution therapy in severe burns. Ann. Surg., **159**, 496
Levitan, A. A. and Perry, S. (1967) Infectious complications in a protected environment. New Engl. J. Med., **276**, 881

Rifkind, D., Starzl, T. E., Marchioro, T. L., Waddell, W. R., Rowlands, D. T. Jr. and Hill, R. B. Jr. (1964) Transplantation pneumonia. J. Amer. med. Ass., **189**, 808

Slapak, M., Lee, H. M. and Hume, D. M. (1968) Transplant lung - a new syndrome. Brit. med. J., **1**, 80

SECTION IV

Barnett, H. L., McNamara, H., Schultz, S. and Tompsett, R. (1949) Renal clearances of sodium penicillin G, procaine penicillin G and inulin in infants and children. Pediatrics, **3**, 418

Benner, E. J. (1970) The cephalosporin antibiotics in antimicrobial therapy. (Ed) Kagan. Page 31. W. B. Saunders, Philadelphia

Brasher, G. W. and Hartley, T. F. (1969) Quantification of IgA and IgM in umbilical cord serum of normal newborn infants. J. Pediat., **74**, 784

Burland, W. L., Simpsom, K. and Samuel, P. D. (1970) Combining cephaloridine and streptomycin for the treatment and prophylaxis of neonatal infections. Postgrad. med. J. Suppl., **46**, 85

Dancis, J. and Kunz, H. W. (1954) Studies of the immunology of the newborn infant. IV. Bacteriostatic and complement activity of the serum. Pediatrics, **13**, 339

Davies, P. A., Darrell, J. H., Chandran, K. R., Waterworth, P. M. (1970) The efficacy of antibiotics in the neonatal period. 'The Control of Chemotherapy'. (Ed) Watt. Page 49. E. & S. Livingstone, Edinburgh

Grossman, M. (1968) Antimicrobial therapy in the newborn infant. Pediat. Clin. N. Amer., **15** (No.1), 157

Grossman, M. (1970) Antimicrobial therapy in the newborn infant. in 'Antimicrobial Therapy'. (Ed) Kagan. Page 189. W. B. Saunders, Philadelphia

Grossman, M. and Ticknor, W. (1966) High doses of penicillin G in the neonate. Antimicrob. Agents Chemother., page 59

Hobbs, J. R. (1966) Disturbances of the immunoglobulins. Sci. Basis Med. ann. Rev., 106

Keay, A. J. and Fleming, J. G. (1970) Further studies on the use of cephaloridine in the control of infections in the newborn. Postgrad. med. J. Suppl., **46**, 81

Klein, J. O. (1969) Consideration of gentamicin for therapy of neonatal sepsis. J. infect. Dis., **119**, 457

Leedom, J. M., Wehrle, P. F., Mathies, A. W. Jr., Ivler, D. and Warren, W. S. (1969) Gentamicin in the treatment of meningitis in neonates. J. infect. Dis., **119**, 476

Michael, A. F. and Sutherland, J. M. (1960) Comparison of the acute lethal toxicity of antibiotics in newborn and adult rats. Amer. J. Dis. Child., **100**, 615

Newman, R. L. and Holt, R. J. (1969) Gentamicin in infections of the central nervous system. J. infect. Dis., **119**, 417

Ross, S., Kraybill, E. N. and Kahn, W. (1970) Treatment of proteus meningitis with carbenicillin: a report of four cases. J. infect. Dis., **122**, suppl., 562

Schulkind, M. L. and Adler, W. H. III (1970) The treatment of Pseudomonas aeruginosa infections in children with carbenicillin. Advances in the management of Pseudomonas and Proteus infections. Excerpta med. (Amst.) 36

Sheng, K. T., Huang, N. H. and Promadhattavedi, V. (1964) Serum concentrations of cephalothin in infants and children and placental transmission of the antibiotic. Antimicrob. Agents Chemother., 200

Yaffe, S. J. (1965) Antibiotic dosage in newborn and premature infants. J. Amer. med. Ass., **193**, 162

Yaffe, S. J. and Simon, H. J. (1970) Clinical pharmacology of antibiotics in the neonate. The control of chemotherapy. (Ed) Watt. Page 37. E. & S. Livingstone, Edinburgh

21 Chemotherapy of Respiratory Infections

INTRODUCTION

Infections of the respiratory tract are responsible for a vast amount of morbidity and considerable mortality. Colds, coughs, bronchitis and pneumonia, demand a high proportion of doctors and particularly general practitioners time. Climate, occupation, smoking habits, atmospheric pollution, influence greatly the incidence of these disorders; in the United Kingdom the problem is formidable.

In this chapter the common respiratory infections are discussed; tuberculosis is dealt with in Chapter 18.

UPPER RESPIRATORY INFECTION

Infection of the upper respiratory tract is usually viral in origin but bacteria or fungi are sometimes responsible for primary infection. A more common sequence of events is for primary upper respiratory viral infection to be followed by bacterial infection which may involve not only the upper but also the lower respiratory tract. The first major problem confronting the clinician is in distinguishing between viral infection, which is almost without exception unresponsive to chemotherapy and infection due to other micro-organisms, particularly bacterial pathogens, which may well respond to available antibacterial agents. With the aid of bacteriological and virological measures it is often possible to confirm retrospectively the agent responsible for a particular illness; clinical diagnosis is difficult and frequently erroneous but the decision to treat will in most acute cases rest entirely on clinical judgement. A degree of failure and some confusion is therefore inevitable.

TREATMENT

When the clinical evidence points to acute bacterial infection such as tonsillitis or pharyngitis due to group A streptococci the course is clear; penicillin G should be administered. Similarly, results of culture may indicate the presence of pneumococci or in children Haemophilus influenzae; in the presence of symptoms these are probably best treated by penicillin G or ampicillin, respectively. If virus infection is suspected appropriate virological investigations may be carried out and symptomatic treatment prescribed. A viral infection due to Herpes simplex will often cause sufficiently characteristic lesions of gums and mucous membranes, particularly in children, for clinical recognition. Idoxuridine (see page 157) in dimethyl sulphoxide may relieve symptoms. The coxsackie group of viruses cause faucial eananthemata which when recognised clinically provide a contraindication to administration of chemotherapy. One of the commonest viral illnesses today is infectious mononucleosis which can be diagnosed clinically in the majority of cases and confirmed rapidly by finding atypical cells in the peripheral blood or a positive test for heterophile antibody (Paul-Bunnell). When this diagnosis is made antibiotics should be withheld.

Antibiotic prophylaxis of secondary bacterial infection, of colds and upper respiratory viral infections is of dubious value and as a routine measure should be avoided. There is a small group of patients subject to recurrent purulent sinusitis, and a much larger group who develop repeated lower respiratory infections in whom routine prophylaxis may be warranted. Ampicillin, tetracyclines and trimethoprim/sulphonamide are the drugs most likely to be effective.

LOWER RESPIRATORY TRACT INFECTIONS

CROUP

Croup is a descriptive term applied to a condition which occurs in infants and young children associated with a characteristic 'barking' cough which gives the condition its name. Croup includes both acute laryngo-tracheitis and acute epiglottis, the former is most frequently caused by influenza, para influenza and measles viruses; Corynebacterium diphtheriae is occasionally responsible. Acute epiglottitis usually results from infection with Haemophilus influenzae. The onset is sudden, with fever and stridor and sometimes the epiglottis may be seen to be swollen, and tracheotomy may be required. Both these acute and sometimes frightening conditions should be treated with ampicillin. Nursing the patient in a moist atmosphere and the administration of corticosteroids are useful adjuncts to treatment. When diphtheria is suspected antitoxin must be given in conjunction with penicillin G.

BRONCHITIS

Acute bronchitis may complicate an upper respiratory infection and present as a single acute episode; frequently it is an exacerbation, that is reinfection or possibly a recrudescence of a chronic bronchial infection. Ampicillin, trimethorprim/sulphonamide or tetracycline may be given 'blindly' before the result of sputum cultures are available. Penicillin combined with streptomycin may be given to seriously ill patients.

BRONCHIOLITIS

Bronchiolitis is an acute respiratory infection occurring in young children. This acute illness is due primarily to virus infection but staphylococci are also responsible and in most cases antistaphylococcal therapy is indicated. There is cough, fever, rapid respiration and widespread fine crepitations may be heard on auscultation. Pulmonary distension occurs and sometimes can be demonstrated radiologically. As there is always doubt about the precise cause, and as these infants are seriously ill it is justified to use an agent such as one of the cephalosporin derivatives which should be effective against staphylococci, *H. influenzae* as well as other bacterial pathogens. Cardiac failure develops quickly in these infants and must be treated appropriately. Corticosteroids have proved most helpful in the management of bronchiolitis.

PERTUSSIS

Although whooping cough is probably due in most cases to infection with *Haemophilus pertussis* and this organism is sensitive to a number of antibiotics there is no convincing evidence that administration of such drugs is helpful. At the moment the only place for chemotherapy is in the management of secondary bacterial infection.

Bacterial

- i *Strept. pneumoniae*
- ii *H. influenzae*
- iii *Staphylococci*
- iv Streptococci
- v Gram-negative
  - *Kl. pneumoniae*
  - *E. coli*
  - Pseudomonas
- vi *H. pertussis*
- vii *M. tuberculosis*

Non Bacterial

Viral
- i Influenza
- ii Adenovirus
- iii Respiratory syncytial
- iv Measles
- v Chicken pox

M. pneumoniae

R. burneti

Psittacosis agent

Protozoal
- i *Toxoplasma gondii*
- ii *Pneumocystis carinii*
- iii *E. histolitica*

Fungi

Physical Agents, eg toxic gases

Allergy: Eosinophilia. Collagen Disease.

Figure 9. Classification of pneumonia

PNEUMONIA

Figure 9 is a scheme indicating the aetiological agents responsible for pneumonia. Because of the requirement for a comprehensive list this scheme does not give sufficient emphasis to the **common** problem encountered by the clinician faced with a patient with an acute respiratory infection. The most practical approach is to consider the pathogens in two separate groups, bacterial and non-bacterial.

Bacterial Pneumonia

Typical lobar pneumonia in adults caused by Strep. pneumoniae accompanied by high fever, rigors, and physical signs of consolidation of lobar distribution can usually be recognised. Leucocytosis and radiological confirmation complete the indications for the administration of penicillin G. Blood cultures should be carried out. Bronchopneumonia, particularly in the older age groups has a less conspicuous onset, is usually bilateral and the bacterial pathogens are less certain and often multiple. A wide-spectrum antibiotic such as ampicillin is indicated. Staphylococci and Kl. pneumoniae are rather rarer causes of pneumonia and can often be suspected when the clinical features, bacteriological and radiological measures are assessed. In both conditions cavitation is common. Staphylococcal pneumonia demands treatment with penicillin and cloxacillin administered parenterally, at least in the initial phase, cephalosporin derivatives and fucidic acid may also be helpful. Pneumonia due to Kl. pneumoniae is often encountered in patients with serious underlying disease. This is a severe infection with marked toxicity and tenacious blood-stained sputum. Chloramphenicol combined with either streptomycin or gentamicin are probably the drugs of choice.

Non-bacterial Pneumonia

Non-bacterial infection results most often from infection with Mycoplasma pneumoniae — the Eaton agent of primary atypical pneumonia; less frequent causes are R. burneti and the agent responsible for psittacosis. In the whole group symptoms of non pulmonary origin are often conspicuous and it may well be only when radiological and laboratory investigations have been carried out that the true pulmonary nature of the infection becomes clear. Thus in non-bacterial pneumonia headache, generalised muscle pain, diarrhoea, arthralgia may be the patient's chief complaint rather than cough or haemophysis. In perhaps half of the cases due to M. pneumoniae there is a degree of haemolytic jaundice which may be appreciated clinically and which is accompanied by a positive Coombs test and often cold agglutinins showing (Anti I) specificity. In many cases of non-bacterial pneumonia the whole illness is rather less acute than pneumococcal pneumonia, the leucocyte count will probably show little variation from normal but the erythrocyte sedimentation rate may be markedly raised.

In treating mycoplasma pneumonia tetracycline is probably the drug of choice. Demethylchlortetracycline has been usually advocated but there is little to choose between any of the tetracyclines. In many cases the response is disappointing and it may be difficult to be certain that the drug has been of genuine value. Chloramphenicol and erythromycin can also be used but they seem to have no advantages over tetracyclines.

Patients with infection due to R. burneti or the psittacosis agent will often present with pyrexia of uncertain origin. Diarrhoea is sometimes a marked feature of psittacosis. Diagnosis in these conditions is confirmed serologically. In treating these infections tetracyclines or possibly chloramphenicol may be administered.

Viral Pneumonia

Pneumonia occurring during acute illness due to influenza, adeno, measles and chicken pox viruses is frequently of secondary bacterial origin and must be treated as such. Staphylococcal pneumonia complicating these viral infections has a high mortality, therefore in practice antistaphylococcal agents are administered. True virus pneumonia may occasionally occur but is unresponsive to chemotherapy.

PNEUMONIA OF UNKNOWN AETIOLOGY

Many pneumonic infections defy classification; even in retrospect when the results of all laboratory and radiological investigations are available it may be impossible to define the precise aetiology in some patients. Many of these are probably viral in origin, some have a bacterial origin representing superinfection with staphylococci, H. influenzae or Gram-negative pathogens. Others are a result of bronchial embolism — that is aspiration of upper respiratory mucous plugs causing local stasis and atelectasis rather than primary alveolar invasion by micro-organisms.

A Caused by specific organism
- i Staph. aureus
- ii Actinomyces israeli
- iii Kl. pneumoniae
- iv Entamoeba histolitica

B Due to bronchial occlusion
eg Carcinoma or foreign body

C Due to vascular embolism
- i Infarct
- ii Pyaemic

D Traumatic
Infected haematoma

E Non specific suppuration —
aspiration pneumonia

Figure 10. Classification of lung abscess

LUNG ABSCESS

The formation of a lung abscess represents an important development in a pulmonary infection in which suppuration and necrosis of varying degrees are present. No completely satisfactory classification is available, but Figure 10 (after Cleland, 1963) is practical.

When dealing with lung abscess it is important to keep in mind two major diseases which may be closely related to cavity formation – namely carcinoma and tuberculosis. The majority of lung abscesses are probably caused by Staph. aureus, Friedlander's bacillus, and mixed anaerobic organisms. Primary lung abscess is a misnomer. Even though in some cases aetiological factors cannot be identified they must be sought diligently, particularly important is a history of foreign body inhalation, evidence of recent dental manipulations or a history of episodes of unconsciousness, stupor or anaesthesia. Body posture during unconsciousness may explain the site of abscess formation. In some cases staphylococcal lung abscess are merely pulmonary manifestations of staphylococcal septicaemia and are usually accompanied by abscesses in other tissues.

TREATMENT

Treatment of lung abscess depends on specific chemotherapy, adequate bronchial drainage, and in some cases resection.

It is vital to obtain blood and sputum cultures for the bacteriological results may dictate therapy. In many instances it is possible to suspect on clinical grounds the correct aetiology and to institute appropriate therapy. Many staphylococcal cases will come in this category. Antistaphylococcal agents – penicillin G and one of the isoxaxole penicillins should be administered in large doses. Fucidic acid may be most helpful due to its ability to penetrate tissues. The antibiotic management of such acute staphylococcal infections has been outlined in the chapter on septicaemia (page 193). For abscesses caused by Kl. pneumoniae combined therapy with streptomycin and chloramphenicol is likely to be most effective; as this condition is often complicated by superinfection with mixed organisms tetracyclines, ampicillin, gentamicin and cephalosporin derivatives may also be used.

Thoracic actinomycosis should be treated with penicillin. Large doses for prolonged periods are necessary – most cases requiring therapy for at least two months. Nocardia asteroides is rarely encountered and treatment involves prolonged courses of sulphonamides possibly combined with erythromycin. Entamoeba histolitica occasionally causes lung abscess; where this diagnosis is suspected emetine hydrochloride (60 mg/day) may be given diagnostic trial. In chronic lung diseases, particularly tuberculosis, in which cavitation occurs the devitalised lung may be colonised by a variety of fungi. The most common offender is Aspergillus fumigatus and the ball-like mass of mycelia is given the generic term mycetoma. Treatment of this complication is by surgical resection; amphotericin B may be given in the operative period to prevent dissemination of fungus and fistula formation.

Non-specific lung abscess probably represents one of the extremes of a spectrum of pulmonary infections caused by aspiration in which anaerobic conditions predominate. The nature of the aspirated material and the severity of anaerobic conditions seem to determine the amount of cavitation and the bacteriological flora. Sputum cultures should give a guide to therapy.

CHRONIC PULMONARY INFECTIONS

CHRONIC BRONCHITIS

This condition is important medically, socially and industrially particularly in the United Kingdom, where each year over 30,000 men and women die because of this condition. Cigarette smoking is a major identifiable factor in its causation and in its persistence; atmospheric pollution and hereditary factors are also operative (Report RCP, 1971). In the expectorated sputum of bronchitic patients bacteria are frequently cultured, particularly Haemophilus influenzae and pneumococci, and less frequently staphylococci. It is natural that chemotherapy directed against these pathogens should be explored. The subject is considered in detail in Chapter 23. A summary of the main points is as follows:

Prophylactic Therapy

This is useful in some patients; intermittent rather than continuous therapy should be tried initially, ampicillin (1 G/day), trimethoprim/sulphonamide (tablets 2/day) or possibly tetracyclines (1 G/day) are most useful.

Acute Episode

This must be presumed to result from acute bacterial infection and treated as such even though bacteriological proof may be lacking, or an initiating viral infection suspected.

Ampicillin, combined penicillin and streptomycin, trimethoprim/sulphonamide are the most commonly effective agents. Chloramphenicol may well be effective but should be avoided except in desperate circumstances, in a condition notorious for recurrence.

BRONCHIECTASIS

The chemotherapy of bronchiectasis is similar to that of chronic bronchitis. Superinfection with staphylococci, Pseudomonas aeruginosa and other Gram-negative species may be very troublesome. In both these conditions it must be remembered that a patient admitted to a large ward with an exacerbation of infection due to H. influenzae may die from superinfection due to the prevalent (usually multiply resistant) strain of Staph. aureus.

MUCOVICIDOSIS

In cystic fibrosis it seems probable that the initial pathogen is Staph. aureus and after prolonged therapy the flora may be predominantly Gram-negative. Pseudomonas aeruginosa is the usual offender but the role of H. influenzae is not fully understood. Clearly in this situation the emphasis will be, initially, on antistaphylococcal agents and subsequent therapy will depend on the assessment of sputum cultures. Antibodies against particular organisms may be of help in deciding if these should be regarded as true pathogens and therefore deserving of specific chemotherapy.

REFERENCES

Cleland, W. P. (1963) 'Lung Abscess in Chest Diseases'. (Ed) Perry, Holmes Sellors. Volume 2, page 127. Butterworth, London

Report of the Royal College of Physicians (1971) 'Smoking and Health Now'. Page 69. Pitman Medical & Scientific Publishing Co. Ltd., London

22 Chemotherapy of Urinary Tract Infections

INTRODUCTION

Infection of the urinary tract is something of a paradox. It may be present without clinical features and occurs in the absence of urinary abnormalities; the presence of protein and cells in the urine while indicating inflammation in the urinary tract does not necessarily imply infection. Further, many, perhaps the majority of acute infections clear spontaneously or with therapy that may be considered appropriate while others progress to chronic infection and sometimes renal failure for no definable reason. Understanding of these paradoxical features is limited and therapy largely empirical.

In this chapter infections of the urinary tract other than tuberculosis and those due to venereal disease are discussed.

DEFINITIONS

A urinary tract infection is defined as a condition characterized by the persistence of actively multiplying bacteria in bladder urine. This occurs when 100,000 or more organisms are present in 1 ml of urine on two separate occasions. These must be clean voided samples or alternatively may be obtained by suprapubic aspiration. When infection is present white blood cells usually accompany bacteria. Mixed cultures, especially when unaccompanied by pus cells, indicate contamination rather than infection. Symptoms often, but not always accompany these laboratory findings.

Acute pyelonephritis describes a clinical situation in which loin pain, fever, rigors and frequency of micturition occur. In this condition it is presumed that there is bacterial involvement of the renal parenchymatous tissue and not infrequently there is blood stream invasion.

Chronic pyelonephritis found frequently at autopsy in subjects who during life have not complained of urinary symptoms brought attention to an histological abnormality that in subsequent studies was shown to be associated with asymptomatic bacteriuria. Chronic pyelonephritis has special significance in childhood, particularly those under five years, for the growing kidney may be more susceptible than the adult kidney to the damaging effects of infection (Asscher, 1970).

Asymptomatic bacteriuria is a laboratory finding and not a clinical condition; it is said to be significant when 100,000 or more organisms are present in 1 ml of clean voided urine. Most of the available data on asymptomatic bacteriuria has been obtained from pregnant women, chiefly by Kass and colleagues (see page 325). In non-pregnant women and in men the natural history of this laboratory finding is unknown so that the assessment of any therapeutic measures must be guarded and reconsidered frequently.

Cystitis is a condition in which frequency of micturition occurs, sometimes accompanied by fever and pain or tenderness confined to the suprapubic region. Urine cultures indicate infection. It is not clear if one is ever justified in assuming that simply because symptoms are confined to the bladder region, renal involvement can be excluded.

COLLECTING SAMPLES

Mid-stream samples are collected in adults and in older children who co-operate. The object is to use the initial phase of micturition to wash out contaminating organisms present in the anterior urethra. In women, the vulva need not necessarily be cleansed before obtaining a mid-stream sample (Murdoch et al, 1966).

In children and infants small sterile bags may be applied to the skin close to the external genitalia; if the skin has previously been thoroughly cleansed a clean sample can be obtained, but often the results are confusing. In selected cases suprapubic aspiration may be carried out; obtained in this way urine should be sterile.

Urine for bacteriological examination should reach the laboratory within an hour of being collected. If this is not possible it should be stored in a refrigerator at $4^{o}C$. In some situations the best solution is to use one of the dip-inoculum techniques. The culture medium comes on a plastic spoon or slide and is dipped into freshly voided urine which is then replaced in its sterile container for posting to the laboratory where examination is possible after overnight incubation.

BACTERIOLOGY

The majority of urinary tract infections are caused by Escherichia coli; in domiciliary practice a high proportion of these isolates are sensitive to sulphonamides, but in hospital many strains of E. coli are resistant not only to sulphonamides but also to antibiotics. It can be demonstrated by serotyping these bacteria that the strains present in the urinary tract are the same as those in the patient's bowel. Other bowel-derived organisms which cause urinary infections are Strep. faecalis, Proteus mirabilis, and Klebsiella aerogenes. In chronic infection, particularly when there has been instrumentation of the uretra, or when there is neurological abnormality Pseudomonas aeruginosa and occasionally Staph. aureus are encountered. In this group mixed infections are common.

INVESTIGATIONS

Assessment of infections of the urinary tract may require not only bacteriological confirmation of infection, but biochemical estimation of renal function and radiological procedures to define any anatomical abnormality. In selected cases renal biopsy may be undertaken.

RENAL FUNCTION

Glomerular function may be assessed by creatinine and urea clearances or estimations of plasma concentrations of urea and creatinine while tubule function can be estimated by water excretion tests (concentration and dilution) hydrogen ion excretion, and various electrolyte balances. At initial assessment at least one test of glomerular function and one of tubule function should be carried out. Repeated assessment may indicate alterations in function.

RADIOLOGICAL PROCEDURES

A plain X-ray of the abdomen is a simple procedure which can reveal renal calcification, calculi, or give some information about the size, shape and position of the kidneys.

Intravenous pyelography is probably the most helpful radiological investigation. Abnormalities not only in size and position of the kidneys but also any distortion of the calyces and ureteres can be distinguished. Retrograde pyelography is sometimes helpful, but it should be remembered that this technique can introduce infection. Cystography may define vesico-ureteric reflux and is an important investigation, especially in young children. Special techniques such as renal arteriography or cine radiography are sometimes helpful.

RENAL BIOPSY

Much has been learned about the natural history of renal disease from this investigation; however, in relation to the individual patient with a urinary tract infection renal biopsy is seldom indicated. Pyelonephritis can certainly be diagnosed histologically but in many cases the focal nature of lesion makes interpretation difficult.

DIAGNOSIS

ACUTE INFECTION

When urinary tract infection presents with fever, loin pain accompanied by tenderness and frequency of micturition the diagnosis is easily made. This clinical diagnosis is confirmed by finding proteinuria, together with high bacterial counts in the urine and often increased white cell excretion. The presence of a known predisposing factor such as pregnancy, sexual intercourse or instrumentation of the bladder completes the clinical picture.

RECURRENT ACUTE INFECTION

Repeated, and apparently isolated episodes of urinary tract infection occur. Such repeated attacks may be relapses due to infection with the same organism or to reinfection with different organisms. This distinction can be accomplished by serotyping strains of E. coli. When the same serotype is held responsible for a number of episodes this is in favour of a local renal tract abnormality. Occasionally such repeated infections may be caused by protoplast formation in the renal medulla which is favoured by hyperosmolality. Protoplasts – cell wall deficient variants of bacteria – are not inhibited by antibiotics the main action of which is directed against synthesis of cell wall constituents.

CHRONIC URINARY TRACT INFECTION

Chronic pyelonephritis may produce no symptoms; occasionally there is vague abdominal pain and ill health and there may be episodes of acute pyelonephritis. In children failure to thrive is commonly due to chronic urinary tract infection which may also present with bouts of unexplained fever and vomiting. In some cases the late complication of anaemia, uraemia, or cardiovascular catastrophe may be the first manifestation of unsuspected chronic pyelonephritis. In patients with significant bacteriuria pyelonephritis must be presumed and it is this group which requires the full gamut of biochemical, radiological and bacteriological investigation. In children the demonstration of vesico-ureteric reflux is an important finding for the planning of therapy will to some extent be governed by its presence.

DRUGS

The metabolism of antibacterial drugs in relation to the kidney in general and with particular emphasis on renal failure is discussed in Chapter 20 (page 257). Here a summary of useful drugs and techniques of practical importance are discussed.

URINARY pH

The pH of urine fluctuates, rising after meals and falling at night. Infection with organisms which produce urea-splitting enzymes result in the production of an alkaline urine; Proteus species is most likely to produce this change. Deliberate alteration of urinary pH influences the action of some antibiotics and acidification is essential for certain agents. These are listed in Figure 11.

URINE

Acid		Alkaline	
Essential:	Hexamine Mandelic acid Mandelamine	Enhances:	Sulphonamides Aminoglucodies: streptomycin, kanamycin, gentamicin Penicillin G
Enhances:	Tetracyclines Nitrofurantoin		

Figure 11. The influence of urine pH on the action of some agents used in treating urinary infections

Urine may be made acid by the administration of ammonium chloride (6-12g/day orally), methionine (3-10g/day orally) or ascorbic acid (4g/day orally). When ammonia producing organisms or renal failure are present attempts to acidify the urine may result in dangerous acidosis. Alkalinization can be produced by sodium bicarbonate or acetazolamide.

URINARY ANTISEPTICS

Hexamine and mandelic acid are two synthetic compounds which exert antibacterial activity in acid urine. In the past they had considerable popularity when used together as the compound Mandelamine.

Nitrofurantoin (page 123) achieves high concentrations in the urine after oral administration. Plasma and tissue levels are not satisfactory for treating parenchymatous renal infection.

Nalidixic acid (page 121) is excreted predominantly in the urine and this has led to its use in urinary tract infections. However, resistance develops quickly, making the drug almost valueless.

Soluble sulphonamides (page 133) excreted predominantly in the urine are bacteriostatic agents frequently used in treating urinary tract infections as many strains of E. coli, particularly in domestic practice, are sensitive to their action. Trimethoprim, together with the sulphonamide sulphamethoxazole (page 138), exert a synergistic bactericidal action against a wide range of bacteria and provides a recent addition of considerable importance in the treatment of urinary tract infections. Given together as a single tablet (Septrin: Bactrim) this is a highly effective therapy in many urinary infections.

ANTIBIOTICS

Ampicillin (page 31) active against many urinary pathogens may be administered orally or parenterally. It is often effective but resistant strains of E. coli do emerge. If used repeatedly this drug tends to encourage infection with resistant strains of Klebsiellae.

Cephalosporins (page 41). Both cephaloridine and cephalothin administered parenterally have a place in renal tract infections, particularly if accompanied by septicaemia. Large doses of cephaloridine can produce renal failure. Cephalexin (page 45) is an orally absorbed cephalosporin derivative which has some place in treatment of urinary tract infections, but it is too early for full assessment of this drug.

Kanamycin (page 89) and gentamicin (page 110) are two aminoglucoside antibiotics that may be extremely useful in treating acute urinary infections, especially when accompanied by septicaemia. They are unlikely to be drugs of first choice unless there is repeated infection with resistant organisms.

Carbenicillin (page 33) achieves very high concentrations in the urine and can be used to treat infections due to Pseudomonas aeruginosa or Proteus species. As these are most difficult, if not impossible to cure, combined therapy with gentamicin may be warranted.

Cycloserine (page 239) best known for its antituberculous action has some advocates for its use in urinary tract infection. Murdoch (1968) and Syme (1961) and their colleagues used cycloserine for treating both acute infections (250 mg thrice daily) and long term management (250 mg alternate days). Full doses may produce toxic effects predominantly in the central nervous system. Blood levels should not exceed 20-25 μg/ml.

Chloramphenicol, while it is effective against many urinary pathogens, is at a disadvantage in that renal excretion is limited and chloramphenicol urinary metabolites have little antibacterial action.

Tetracyclines also are best avoided in urinary tract infections. These compounds can cause deterioration in renal function and induce azotaemia (see page 70).

THERAPEUTIC PLAN

The treatment of urinary tract infections can be considered under four separate heads: (i) predisposing causes — seeking and if possible correcting anatomical abnormalities (eg congenital, traumatic, disease induced); (ii) initial chemotherapy; (iii) long-term chemotherapy; (iv) prophylaxis.

(i) **Predisposing causes**

Some precipitating factors are easily recognized and in this category come: renal calculi, major anatomical abnormalities such as duplex ureters, diverticula or tumour of the bladder. Many of these causes can be diagnosed by intravenous pyelography. On physical examination of children certain congenital defects should be sought for there is a close association between some defects and renal tract anomalies. These defects include: single umbilical artery, low-set malformed ears, genital malformation and spina bifida. Children with vesico-ureteric reflux who either have urinary symptoms or bacteriuria or both should receive chemotherapy – probably for very long periods.

(ii) **Initial therapy**

The patients selected for initial therapy are:

Those with acute symptomatic pyelonephritis;
Those with asymptomatic bacteriuria of pregnancy;
Those with an anatomical anomaly while awaiting its correction;
Children with vesico-urteric reflux.

Chemotherapy will be dictated by the results of urine cultures. In practice most acute infections may be treated with one of the following:

	Adults	**Children**
Sulphadimidine	1g 4 times daily	0.25g - 1.0g 4 times daily
Ampicillin	500mg 4 times daily	100 mg/kg/day
Trimethoprim/ sulphamethoxazole	2 tablets twice daily	Paediatric suspension (40mg trimethoprim: 200mg sulphamethoxazole/5ml) 1 mth - 2 yrs: 2.5ml BD 2 - 6 yrs: 2.5 - 5ml BD 6 - 12 yrs: 5 - 10ml BD

For seriously ill patients with blood stream invasion, ampicillin kanamycin, gentamicin, or cephalosporins should be given parenterally. This treatment should continue for at least 10 days and in the absence of symptoms and with sterile urine this treatment can be considered successful. However, even in what may seem the simplest cases a further period of therapy is almost certainly warranted. Six weeks, on reduced doses may be sufficient but we do not have sufficient evidence to say categorically whether this period should be extended to six months or even longer.

(iii) **Long term therapy**

This implies that initial therapy and such surgical measures as have been carried out have not been curative and that long term treatment with drugs may offer relief of symptoms, or possibly reversal of some abnormality such as reflux. The crucial question of whether such therapy will prevent progression of renal damage cannot be answered at present.

A choice may be made from:

	Adults
Sulphidimidine	1g/day
Ampicillin	500mg/day
Nitrofurantoin	100mg/day
Trimethoprim/sulphamethoxazole	tab. 1/twice daily
Cycloserine	250mg/day

Whether treatment initial or long term is successful or not it is axiomatic that there should be adequate follow up. This may sometimes require that patients are referred to special centres and this particularly applies to children.

(iv) Prophylaxis

The most important measure in the prevention of urinary tract infection is the avoidance of catheterisation and instrumentation of the renal tract but these measures are sometimes essential and subsequent bacteriuria common. Cultures should be made to determine the pathogen but prophylactic antibacterial agents should not be used routinely; if they are administered in this context they ensure that the resulting infection is due to resistant strains or to invasion with intractable pathogens such as Pseudomonas aeruginosa. This subject is considered in detail on page 324.

REFERENCES

Asscher, A. W. (1970) Screening for urinary tract infections. J. roy. Coll. Phycns. Lond., **4**, 224

Murdoch, J. McC, Geddes, A. M., Tulloch, W. S., Newsam, J. E., Thomson, W. N., Bidwell, D. and Wallace, E. T. (1966) The problem of pyelonephritis. Practitioner, **196**, 800

Syme, J., Sleigh, J. D., Richardson, J. E. and Murdoch, J. McC. (1961) Cycloserine in infections of the urinary tract. Brit. J. Urol., **33**, 261

23 Chemoprophylaxis

INTRODUCTION

In writing of chemoprophylaxis it should be made clear at the outset that it is a subject bristling with inconsistencies, unproved assumptions and entrenched prejudices. It includes topics in which there is a large measure of agreement on the indications and efficacy of prophylaxis as in the prevention of recurrent episodes of rheumatic fever, but also those subjects in which opposing views may appear equally convincing, as in the case of prophylactic antibiotic therapy in the preparation of the bowel for surgery, or the usefulness of drugs in the prevention of recurrence of chronic pulmonary infection.

Chemoprophylaxis is mainly used in four situations:

(i) To protect healthy individuals who are expected to be exposed to pathogenic micro-organisms.

(ii) To protect individuals from the effects of infection with organisms to which they have been shown to be hypersensitive.

(iii) To prevent, or render less severe, acute episodes in patients with chronic disease.

(iv) To reduce or prevent infection in those considered to be at increased risk, as in comatose patients or in those suffering from acute viral infections.

Taking a broad view one is impressed with the lack of success of chemoprophylaxis. Even allowing for the difficulty in obtaining adequate information on the results of prophylactic antibiotic therapy, the few situations where success is conspicuous represent a small proportion of the field. This disenchantment with prophylactic therapy has come about mainly because of three factors.

1. Difficult as it may be in the acute process to explain what factors are responsible for infection, it is usually impossible to know with any degree of certainty how to explain (and therefore prevent) infection which may occur in the future. For instance, in the situation where most information is available, that of the relation of group A streptococcal infection to recurrences of rheumatic fever, there are still

many inconsistencies; the presence of streptococci in the pharynx of susceptible individuals does not always result in an episode of rheumatic fever, and an acute attack may follow an illness when streptococci cannot be cultured from the throat. These are well substantiated facts.

2. The aims of prophylaxis are often confused. It is not always clear if one is trying to protect against one group of organisms or to prevent infection with all bacteria.

3. Occasionally side effects produced by the drugs overshadow the disease which they are expected to prevent. The most dramatic instance is probably staphylococcal entero-colitis occurring in those receiving oral wide-spectrum antibiotics.

With regard to the efficacy of chemoprophylaxis two generalizations apply; these have been well summarized by Weinstein (1955), and I quote verbatim:

> " (a) When a single potent drug is used to avoid implantation of a specific organism or to eradicate it immediately or shortly after it has become established, chemoprophylaxis is with uncommon exception highly successful.
>
> " (b) If the aim of prophylaxis is to prevent colonization and/or infection by any and all organisms that may be present in the internal or external environment of a patient, failure is the rule."

CHEMOPROPHYLAXIS OF GROUP A STREPTOCOCCAL INFECTIONS

(i) **Tonsillitis, Pharyngitis**

Epidemics of streptococcal throat infections are not uncommon in semi-closed communities such as boarding schools, hostels and military camps. In this situation all those suffering from tonsillitis and those from whom Group A streptococci are isolated, should be treated with bactericidal doses of penicillin G for ten days. Rheumatic fever, which can occur in up to 10% of those exposed, may be prevented by this measure.

Sulphonamides which may be satisfactory in the prevention of recurrences of rheumatic fever should not be used for the treatment of existing streptococcal infection as they are not effective in the prevention of initial attacks of rheumatic fever.

(ii) **Rheumatic fever**

INITIAL ATTACKS

There is some evidence that effective chemotherapy of streptococcal infections prevents the initial manifestation of acute rheumatic fever. One study suggested that treatment with penicillin prevented acute rheumatic fever if the antibiotic were administered up to 9 days after the onset of the streptococcal infection (Catanzaro et al, 1954). Even if this is accepted it has never

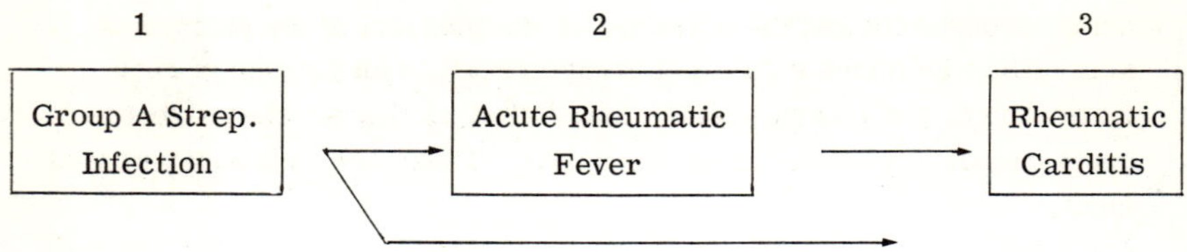

Figure 12. Penicillin given early in 1 may prevent 2 but does not necessarily reduce incidence of 3. Penicillin given in 2 does not prevent 3

been substantiated that effective antibiotic therapy prevents the development of rheumatic carditis, and the incidence of valvular heart disease is not reduced by penicillin therapy of acute rheumatic fever (Rammelkamp, 1965). The sequence of events, so far elucidated, is presented schematically in Figure 12, in an attempt to clarify this complex relationship. The implications for therapy are clear, streptococcal infections should be treated early and energetically with bactericidal doses of penicillin. Because there is often doubt about the precise time relation between streptococcal infection and rheumatic fever penicillin therapy should be administered in the initial stages of this condition.

RECURRENCES

Although acute rheumatic fever is less common in the United Kingdom than it has ever been, approximately one thousand children suffer first attacks each year. In the absence of preventive measures the likelihood of recurrences will depend on the frequency and degree of exposure of the upper respiratory tract to group A β haemolytic streptococci (Report Standing Medical Advisory Committee. MOH, 1965). Within five years of the initial attack, when chemoprophylaxis is not used, one quarter to one half of these children suffer recurrences. The rationale of chemoprophylaxis is to prevent or reduce streptococcal throat infection and therefore subsequent attacks of rheumatic fever. Recurrences do not occur in more than 5% of children receiving continuous chemoprophylaxis with penicillin or a suitable sulphonamide for a period of five years or until leaving school, whichever is the longer (Reports WHO, 1957; Royal College Physicians, London, 1957). Extensive trials in the United States are in agreement with these findings.

CATEGORIES IN WHOM PROPHYLAXIS SHOULD BE USED

Continuous chemoprophylaxis should be offered to patients who have had an attack of acute rheumatic fever. This is particularly important in school children; there is some evidence that boys in large schools are most vulnerable (Bates, 1967). Prophylaxis should be continued to the age of 35 and probably much longer.

SPECIAL CIRCUMSTANCES

1. When individuals, known to be receiving prophylactic therapy, enter an environment where excessive exposure to group A streptococci may occur as in a general hospital ward, the dose of prophylactic drug should be doubled.

2. When patients who have had rheumatic fever develop streptococcal infection they should be given ten days' penicillin therapy in bactericidal doses even though they are having continuous prophylactic therapy.

3. Surgical and dental procedures require extra antibiotic cover. One hour previously penicillin G 1 M.u. and 300,000 u procaine penicillin are given intramuscularly. As some patients harbour resistant mouth organisms, it is probably better to use another drug (eg cephaloridine 1g). The object of these measures is to prevent bacterial endocarditis.

DRUGS AND DOSES

Sulphonamide

A suitable drug is sulphadimidine in daily doses of 0.5 to 1.0g by mouth. This is effective in preventing recurrences, but reactions are more likely to occur than when penicillin is used, and therefore it is not recommended as first choice.

Penicillin

Two schedules are available for continuous prophylaxis, oral and intramuscular. Both routes have advantages and disadvantages; the intramuscular route is probably more effective.

Oral

Phenoxymethyl penicillin tablets (Penicillin V tablets) 125mg twice daily or Benzyl penicillin tablets BP 200,000 u twice daily is given.

Intramuscular

Monthly intramuscular injections of 1.5 mega units (5 ml) of benzathine penicillin may be used. This injection often causes considerable pain which may persist for several days.

Patients allergic to penicillin

Sulphonamides may be used, but erythromycin is to be preferred; Tidewell and Lewis (1959) showed that in children, either 100 mg (tablet) or 125 mg (syrup) erythromycin daily was effective. Side effects were few and bacterial resistance was not encountered. Another drug which may prove useful in this context is lincomycin or its derivative clindamycin.

(iii) **Glomerulonephritis**

There is a similar complex relationship between streptococcal infection and acute glomerulonephritis as exists between rheumatic fever and streptococcal infection. Certain types of group A streptococci have been shown to be nephritogenic. The majority of cases of glomerulonephritis recover completely and do not show increased susceptibility to recurrence. This is most plausibly explained by postulating type specific immunity to the nephritogenic strain of streptococci. As exposure to further infection with a similar nephritogenic strain is thought to be unlikely these patients are not usually offered continuous prophylaxis.

Penicillin therapy (10 days bactericidal) should be offered to those (i) who develop acute glomerulonephritis; (ii) contacts of (i) who have symptoms of streptococcal infection or are found to have group A streptococci on culture. The object is to eradicate the nephritogenic strain of streptococci in semi-closed communities. There is insufficient data to be certain if these measures reduce the incidence of glomerulonephritis. Patients with chronic nephritis of whatever aetiology may have an exacerbation when infected with group A streptococci of any type (Rammelkamp, 1965) and in those in whom renal function deteriorates continuous penicillin prophylaxis may be warranted. Adequate studies on the efficacy of this procedure are not available.

CHRONIC PULMONARY INFECTION

(i) **Chronic Bronchitis**

Chronic bronchitis is a condition in which changes in bronchopulmonary anatomy are associated with infection; the presence of cough and increased quantities of sputum are marked features of the disease. The sputum is frequently purulent, especially during exacerbations which characterize the condition, and culture produces in the majority of cases either Str. pneumoniae or H. influenzae. As there are antibiotics which are capable of inhibiting the growth of these organisms it is logical that they should be used in an attempt to suppress or even cure bronchial infection; for the most part antibiotics given prophylactically have been disappointing in this context. This arises because the aetiology of chronic bronchitis cannot be ascribed to a single factor; infection is in a sense secondary, being only one cause of bronchial mucous gland hypertrophy, smoking, air pollution and heredity, all having some part to play. Further, there is great individual variation from patient to patient, some, for instance, are never free from purulent sputum, others seem to have a chronic disease with episodes of acute infection and partial bronchial obstruction initiated perhaps by respiratory viral infection or alteration in climatic conditions. Many of the antibiotics administered probably never reach the bronchial secretions in effective concentrations; dosage and toxicity become crucial.

TABLE XXXI

Authors	Year	No. of patients	Therapy	Duration	Comments
Elmes et al	1957	88	1g/day Oxytetracycline	7 days (exacerbation)	Treated group lost less time from work. Difference could have occurred by chance 1:10
Pridie et al	1960	151	1. Oxytetracycline 0.5g/day, or 2. Penicillin and Sulph. (500mg + 2g)	24 weeks (continuous)	1. Small reduction in length of exacerbation 2. Both treatments reduced the number and incidence of Str. pneumoniae but not H. influenzae 3. "...neither therapeutic regime at the continuous daily level can be recommended..."
Francis et al	1964	470	1. Penicillin V 624mg/day, or 2. Tetracycline 1g/day, or 3. Erythromycin estolate, or 4. Sulphamethoxy-pyradazine 500mg/day	140 days (continuous)	1. Sulphonamide inferior to others in suppressing H. influenzae 2. Impossible to decide which of other regimes used is best 3. Drugs used should be capable of suppressing both H. influenzae and Str. pneumoniae
MRC Report	1966	373	1. Oxytetracycline (continuous) with 2. Chloramphenicol or Sulphamethoxy-pyradazine in exacerbations	Sept-April for 5 years	1. "Oxytetracycline...by itself appeared to have no effect on the number of illnesses." 2. Oxytetracycline with chloramphenicol reduced the number who had many illnesses. Neither prophylaxis nor therapy had any effect on the decline of FEV or on volume and purulence of sputum

The economic implications of this disease cannot be ignored; between June, 1952 and June, 1954, for instance, male insured workers in Great Britain lost nearly 15 million days work owing to sickness diagnosed as bronchitis. If sickness benefits and wages are considered together, this represents a loss to the community of about £30 million (Elmes et al, 1957).

There have been many trials using various drugs; the overall impression is that some patients may benefit, but there seems no easy way of selecting those who are most likely to respond satisfactorily. Measuring the days lost from work during a given period of time in a double blind trial is probably the most satisfactory design; both continuous prophylaxis and early treatment of exacerbations may be used. Table XXXI summarizes the results obtained in four trials during the past ten years, giving some of the authors' own comments. Some general conclusions can be drawn from these publications:

1. All the results are disappointing; there is great individual variation; tetracyclines have been most used.
2. Early treatment of exacerbations seems as effective as continuous prophylaxis.
3. Sulphonamides should not be used.
4. Any drug used should be effective against H. influenzae and Str. pneumoniae.

As ampicillin is effective against these organisms it would seem to be an obvious choice of therapy. One of the difficulties is in achieving a bactericidal concentration of the drug in the sputum and maintaining this high level until the majority of the organisms have been killed. Although serum levels increase as the dose is increased the levels in sputum reach a plateau even though the serum level continues to rise. The transfer of ampicillin from serum to sputum is therefore not by simple diffusion; there must be an active transport mechanism which becomes saturated at relatively low blood levels (May, 1966).

The majority of trials using ampicillin in chronic bronchitis have involved fairly small numbers of patients; Piane et al (1966) treated 18 patients with various antibiotics and considered ampicillin most effective in preventing relapses; a trial on a group of 58 patients, approximately half of them receiving ampicillin continuously from October to March showed the main value of the drug to be a clearing effect on the sputum and a lesser effect in reducing the incidence of exacerbations (Murray, 1964). Great individual variation from patient to patient makes statistical assessment in small groups almost valueless. Despite the absence of clear-cut results there is an overall impression that ampicillin in high doses may be more beneficial than any other available agent.

RECOMMENDATIONS

1. Sulphonamides should not be used; chloramphenicol may be effective but is not advised; the best choice is either tetracycline or ampicillin with a bias in favour of the latter.
2. Early treatment of exacerbations is as effective as continuous prophylaxis in the majority of patients.
3. In an acute attack, ampicillin 1g 6 hourly by mouth, perhaps combined with probenecid 0.5g twice daily, will usually clear purulent sputum. When these high doses have been successful, lower doses may be continued for days or even weeks in some patients.

(ii) **Cystic Fibrosis**

In cystic fibrosis the main problem is the susceptibility of children to pulmonary infection and death is attributable to this cause in some 90% of cases. The maxillary antra usually contain pus; in the bronchi the primary disorder is not infection but the presence of excessive quantities of viscid sputum. Infection in these circumstances is probably inevitable. Interestingly the bacteria usually isolated are not the Str. pneumoniae and H. influenzae of adult bronchitis, but staphylococci and Gram-negative species, especially Pseudomonas aeruginosa. This bacterial flora probably reflects the environment of the child and may well be related to antibiotic therapy.

Continuous prophylactic therapy is probably best avoided; the doubtful benefits of this form of treatment are offset by a high incidence of bacterial resistance and side effects. In acute exacerbations clearly the bacteriology will dictate the choice of drug and this is likely to include cloxacillin, ampicillin and possibly chloramphenicol.

Fucidic acid given for 12 to 36 months to a group of thirteen children kept four free from staphylococci for more than one year and four were free from 6 to 12 months. Five continued to have staphylococci in the sputum, and no instance of staphylococcal resistance to fucidic acid was encountered (Norman, 1967).

CHEMOPROPHYLAXIS IN SURGERY

(i) 'Clean' Surgery

This term is used to describe elective operations such as herniorrhaphy, hysterectomy and many orthopaedic operations. In the majority of published series dealing with these types of operations the infection rate in those patients receiving antibiotics has in general terms been higher in the treated group. The percentage difference in the two groups is often small, but the overall impression is that in patients underoing 'clean' surgical operations prophylactic antibiotics have no place. As would be expected, when infection occurs in patients receiving antibiotics the organisms are often resistant to the drug which has been used prophylactically.

(ii) Surgery of the colon

Whether or not one should prescribe antibiotics to patients about to have operations on the bowel and particularly the colon has aroused much debate; the subject is often used as a prototype argument for or against prophylactic therapy. This public argument continues (Ingelfinger et al, 1966).

While it may seem logical to consider operation on the large bowel in the same category as operation on grossly contaminated wounds and to use antibiotics prophylactically to good purpose in both situations, in practice it has not proved easy to demonstrate consistently superior results for those patients undergoing colonic surgery treated with chemotherapeutic agents. The intestinal flora lives in symbosis with its host, the major constituents for an individual being remarkably constant and there is some evidence that this stable flora is a defence mechanism against infection (Bohnhoff et al, 1962). Interference with the subtle mechanism of bacterial population control may result in increased numbers of organisms becoming opportunist pathogens. Despite these somewhat theoretical considerations a reduction in size of bowel flora before surgery is desirable. Mechanical methods can cause drastic reduction in the total intestinal population. Antibiotics effect a selective reduction which is temporary and may be followed by a total bacterial population greater than the original. There are many bacteriological studies indicating that for a short period of time the bowel flora (that is those constituents which are easily cultured) may be reduced by about 50% when various antibiotics are used. The assessment of the clinical outcome of these patients in relation to untreated patients is unfortunately much more difficult. The results have a certain unpredictability, for instance, patients receiving a one day kanamycin regime for pre-operative bowel preparation showed a curious divorce between morbidity and mortality (Hulbert & Blair, 1967). Side effects may not be common but superinfection, especially with resistant organisms, may occasionally prove fatal. A further factor may have to be taken into consideration, if the animal studies of Vink (1953) and Cohn and Atik (1960) showing higher incidence of tumour recurrence in antibiotic treated rabbits, prove to have any application to the human situation.

The only conclusions that can be drawn from the mass of contradictory evidence in the literature are:

1. Routine antibiotics are no substitute for good surgical technique.
2. Routine chemoprophylaxis is probably unwarranted.
3. Chemoprophylaxis in selected cases, when infection exists, is probably justified.

(iii) Cardiac Surgery

The advances made in cardiac surgery and in the related anaesthetic problems have enabled surgeons to correct cardiac defects, and to replace diseased or defective heart valves by a variety of prostheses. A small proportion of these patients have developed endocarditis, which in these circumstances has a high mortality. Of 1,263 patients reviewed by Denton (1957) 20 developed bacterial endocarditis; one of these occurred among 374 cases of congenital heart disease and 19 among 1,889 cases of acquired valvular heart disease. More recently, Armoury et al (1966) reviewed 568 open-heart operations performed from September, 1956 to January, 1965; 357 patients required intracardiac prostheses, 223 intercardiac patches were used for closure of septal defects and 154 valve replacements were performed on 134 patients. Thirteen patients developed endocarditis in this series, only one of which had congenital heart disease.

The recognition of endocarditis in this context presents some difficulties, for classical features such as emboli may be lacking. Mild fever, anaemia, tachycardia and sometimes splenomegaly are the usual findings. The commonest infecting organism in the majority of reported series is the staphylococcus, the coagulase negative variety predominating. Lord and associates (1961) collected 18 cases, staphylococci being responsible for half, Candida, Achromobacter and Pseudomonas were the other species identified in this group. Diphtheroid organisms were reported in three patients (Davis et al, 1963).

The treatment of this form of endocarditis is often extremely difficult, infection in some cases persists due to the formation of foreign body granuloma; removal of catgut sutures or replacement of valves may occasionally effect cure. Also, the organisms recovered on blood culture in these patients may be markedly resistant to antibiotics; the relationship of degree of resistance and the frequency of resistant strains to prophylactic antibiotic therapy is not clear.

In planning prophylactic antibiotic regimes no precise recommendations can be made; in the absence of sufficient data the following general measures are suggested:

1. Frequent blood cultures should be carried out post-operatively; when infection is discovered therapeutic doses of the appropriate drugs should be administered — probably for a period of six weeks. This is the most rational approach in the present stage of knowledge.
2. If prophylactic antibiotics are administered, they should be given for a short period (eg 5 days) using high doses starting just prior to surgery. The drug or drugs used should have adequate activity against staphylococci and should include a hindered penicillin compound. With this type of regime the incidence of staphylococcal endocarditis may be reduced, but it is possible that infection with Gram-negative species, yeasts and fungi may be increased.
3. There is good evidence that prophylactic antibiotics reduce the incidence of bacteraemia in patients undergoing cardiac catheterization.

(iv) **Neurosurgery**

Infections after neurosurgery are now unusual and treatment of the rare case of established meningitis differs in no major respect from treatment of primary meningitis. One problem which sometimes arises is that a pleocytosis in the cerebrospinal fluid, perhaps accompanied by meningeal irritation, may result from blood in the subarachnoid space. Interpretation of these findings and differentiation from bacterial meningitis may be difficult. It is usual to obtain cerebrospinal fluid daily or twice daily either by lumbar or ventricular puncture and to administer a sulphonamide if the changes in the fluid are suggestive of infection (Pennybacker, 1966). Some surgeons leave antibiotics (eg penicillin) in the cavity from which a cerebral tumour has been excised or in the subdural space before closing the dura. The closed dura is dusted with an antibiotic powder such as polybacterin. It is impossible to know what effects these measures have on the prevention of infection.

A special situation probably justifying prophylactic therapy is the insertion of various types of implants into the region of the pituitary gland when the skull is entered by way of the nasal cavity. Preparation of the area with antiseptic solutions may reduce bacterial counts and prevent grossly contaminated material entering the skull. Meningitis following this procedure is often due to pneumococci and prophylactic measures directed against this organism would seem most logical until there is more information on the incidence, bacteriology and prevention of this form of meningitis.

(v) Urology

In urology there are three aspects to the use of prophylactic antibiotics as reviewed by Walker (1966). The first of these is when a patient requires an indwelling catheter, the second before instrumentation of the urethra, and the third in association with major surgical procedures.

CATHETERIZATION AND INSTRUMENTATION

Symptomatic cystitis follows single catheterization in from 2% to 5% of patients and asymptomatic bacteriuria may be much more common. When a catheter is left in the bladder urinary tract infection occurs in 98% of patients within 48 hours (Kass, 1955). It might be assumed that prophylactic antibiotic therapy would be logical in this context. Petersdorf and associates (1957) examined the efficacy of this practice; 38 patients receiving prophylactic penicillin and streptomycin, nitrofurantoin, or sulfasoxazole developed bacteriuria. In 17 of the 38 patients the urinary flora changed from *E. coli* to *Alk. aerogenes* Proteus, Pseudomonas or resistant *Staphylococcus aureus*. In 11 patients with indwelling catheters, not receiving antibiotics, bacteriuria was present in all, but infection with more resistant organisms supervened in only one case. The impressive finding that about half the patients given antibiotics changed their flora to resistant organisms has been found by others (eg Riley & Knight, 1958; Shubin & Weil, 1963) and points a clear contraindication to the use of prophylactic antibiotic therapy in this context. Very careful technique, closed drainage systems avoiding bubbles passing up the tube, proper use of acidifying agents and increased urine flow, are some of the measures which may produce better results than routine antibiotic 'cover'.

MAJOR UROLOGICAL SURGERY

From a study of several hundred cases Jonsson and Erlanson (1954) concluded that chemotherapy did little to prevent infection following surgery for prostatic disease or tumours of the bladder where an indwelling catheter or spurapubic drainage was necessary. In a controlled trial of 100 cases of transurethral resection of the prostate in which chloramphenicol was given either pre- or post-operatively Appleton and Waisbren (1956) concluded that the drug had no effect as judged by the occurrence of post-operative bacteraemia, pyuria, fever, period of stay in hospital, or mortality.

Patients presenting with acute urinary tract infection require appropriate antibiotic therapy; routine prophylactic therapy is clearly not warranted.

(vi) Infected Wounds: Burns

When infected wounds require surgery or grafting, it is wise to obtain cultures from the infected areas and institute appropriate antibiotic therapy. The mere presence of small numbers of organisms without evidence of infection is not an indication for specific therapy. In wounds involving a good deal of muscle damage and tissue necrosis high doses of penicillin G should be prescribed.

Chemoprophylaxis in burns seldom prevents colonization with bacteria and results frequently in the presence of resistant strains, especially staphylococci and Pseudomonas aeruginosa. In large burns requiring urgent grafting the local application of several antibiotic preparations in rotation as suggested by Lowbury (1958) may offer the best hope of satisfactory result. He has put forward the idea (Lowbury, 1966) that selected prophylaxis against the main pathogens (Str. pyogenes, Ps. pyocyanea, and Staph. aureus) should be attempted while permitting bacteria that appear to be less injurious to colonize burns. This is almost what happens when a cream containing neomycin, chlorhexidine and polymyxin is applied.

OBSTETRICS

(i) Ruptured membranes

In obstetric patients in whom the membranes have ruptured and labour is prolonged or delayed, there is suggestive evidence that antibiotics may reduce post-partum sepsis and morbidity. The evidence is far from conclusive and better studies are required, but a short period of administration of an antibiotic such as ampicillin is justified in these circumstances.

(ii) Asymptomatic bacteriuria in pregnancy

Urine is normally sterile; a proportion of people, especially diabetics may have asymptomatic bacteriuria. Significant asymptomatic bacteriuria is usually defined as the presence of 100,000 organisms per ml urine in a clean-voided sample. In asymptomatic patients the same organism should be present in at least two consecutive cultures before the diagnosis is established. The natural history of significant asymptomatic bacteriuria is unknown, but it seems likely on present evidence that it is a precursor of some cases of chronic pyelonephritis. Having made a diagnosis of significant asymptomatic bacteriuria (which is not a disease but a laboratory finding and a theoretical concept) we cannot estimate the risks of severe renal disease developing in an individual patient. In pregnant women the situation is somewhat different. Kass (1960) has shown that 6% to 7% of prospective mothers at the Boston City Hospital had significant bacteriuria. In the absence of treatment 40% developed symptomatic pyelonephritis in late pregnancy or shortly after delivery, while in the group treated with sulphonamides there were no clinical manifestations of pyelonephritis. Similar results have been produced in other studies by Kaitz and Hodder (1961) and Turner (1961). The implication for chemoprophylaxis of significant bacteriuria in pregnant women is that if we wish to prevent a fairly high proportion of symptomatic acute urinary tract infections we may do so by the use of continuous sulphonamide therapy throughout pregnancy. The relationship of the success or failure of this prophylactic therapy to the development of chronic pyelonephritis is uncertain.

Kass (1962) considered that bacteriuria in pregnancy may contribute to the occurrence of prematurity and neonatal death. Henderon et al (1962) confirmed these findings, but several others (Kaitz et al, 1961; Turck et al, 1962; Sanford et al, 1963) failed to substantiate this relation.

The dangers to the pregnant woman of continuous sulphonamide prophylaxis (providing long acting compounds are avoided) during the whole course of pregnancy are probably not very great; the dangers to her child are greater for sulphonamides taken in late pregnancy can cause dangerously high levels of unbound bilirubin which may result in kernicterus. Even though the principle of treating this category of patient may be accepted, the choice of drug has to be settled; nalidixic acid might perhaps be substituted for sulphonamide.

Available evidence permits the individual doctor to choose between:

(i) Continuous chemoprophylaxis throughout pregnancy in women with significant asymptomatic bacteriuria.

(ii) Treating symptomatic acute urinary tract infections when they arise.

CHEMOPROPHYLAXIS IN THE NEONATAL PERIOD

Although it is usually assumed that premature infants are more susceptible to infection than full term infants, and that those born to mothers who have had premature rupture of the membranes are particularly vulnerable, proof of these assumptions has been neither consistent nor convincing. When a premature infant dies the only abnormality demonstrable at autopsy may be a lung infection which may lead to the perhaps erroneous assumption that pneumonia was responsible for death. There are many studies indicating that premature infants have on the one hand either a reduced or alternatively an increased mortality when prophylactic antibiotics are administered. In a very full review of bacterial infection in cases of perinatal death Olding (1966) took post-mortem cultures from various sites and showed that in general cases treated with antibiotics gave a higher yield of positive cultures than those not treated. The exception to this was the blood, treated patients having a lower incidence of positive cultures. Petersdorf and associates (1961) reviewed the subject and concluded 'although better studies are needed, the results to date suggest but do not prove that antibiotics given to mothers and infants may favourably affect infant and maternal mortality in cases of prolonged, difficult labour .

In recent years there has been a tendency for pathogenic staphylococci to be replaced by Gram-negative organisms, especially Ps. aeruginosa, as a cause of severe and endemic infections in premature baby units. Once established these infections are particularly difficult to treat successfully. An approach which may well prove rewarding is passive immunisation with gamma globulin (provided the content of IgM is sufficiently high) of infants considered to be at special risk. If hyperimmune gamma globulin can be produced this would appear to be the technique of choice. Active immunisation against pseudomonas infection is not yet available.

CHEMOPROPHYLAXIS IN TUBERCULOSIS

In tuberculosis the use of chemoprophylaxis is as controversial as in most other aspects of this subject. A brief resume only relating to some of the problems will be given here.

PREVENTION OF TUBERCULOUS DISEASE

(i) Children under 4 years of age who are found to have a positive Mantoux reaction should be treated with antituberculous drugs for at least one year. Izoniazid alone (10-20mg/kg daily) or in conjunction with aminosalicylic acid has been administered. Using these drugs in this or a similar way reduces complications by 80% or more within a year of Mantoux conversion (Debre, 1956; Lambert, 1959). Vaccination with isoniazid-resistant BCG would be desirable in these children.

(ii) It may be occasionally necessary to offer chemoprophylaxis to some individuals at special risk such as Mantoux-negative nurses and medical students working in tuberculosis wards. These groups should not normally have access to the wards unless they are Mantoux positive.

(iii) Prophylactic treatment of adult Mantoux converters is unsettled; if there has been recent contact with a proved case prophylactic therapy is probably justified.

(iv) Young adults with pleural effusions of tuberculous origin should receive prophylactic therapy. This treatment usually has little effect on the effusion, but reduces the incidence of subsequent parenchymatous pulmonary lesions.

(v) On the basis of the study by Ferebee et al (1963) routine prophylactic therapy does not seem warranted in household contacts of known sufferers from tuberculosis.

CHEMOPROPHYLAXIS IN MISCELLANEOUS CONDITIONS

(i) **Upper respiratory tract infections**

The majority of these infections are not caused by bacterial pathogens and do not respond to antibiotic therapy. If the only presenting feature is 'sore throat' a proportion will be due to streptococci and may be expected to respond to antibiotics. The correct procedure is to obtain cultures and if pathogenic organisms are present then a therapeutic course of drug, usually penicillin, should be given. Routine chemoprophylaxis should be avoided.

(ii) **Measles**

Routine chemotherapy should not be used. Some authors, chiefly Karelitz et al (1954) have produced studies indicating that bacterial complications are reduced in measles when prophylactic antibiotics are administered. On the other hand Weinstein (1955) showed that prophylaxis may be not only ineffective but dangerous. A review of 4,728 cases of measles reported by members of the College of General Practitioners (1956) in Great Britain concluded that routine administration of antibiotics are largely unnecessary, that sulphonamide drugs increased rather than decreased complications, but that some severe cases may have benefited from antibiotic therapy.

(iii) **Unconscious patients**

These are patients in coma for various reasons, barbiturate intoxication, head injury, diabetic acidosis, cerebro-vascular accidents and the like. Some of these patients die and their lungs at post-mortem reveal evidence of bronchopneumonia. So variable are these conditions that a controlled trial is impossible. Petersdorf and co-workers (1957) attempted a trial which indicated the uselessness of antibiotics in this context.

(iv) **Patients receiving corticosteroids**

The evidence that antibiotics prevent severe infections in patients receiving long term therapy with corticosteroid drugs is unconvincing.

(v) **Meningococcal Infection**

Chemoprophylaxis with sulphonamides is capable of markedly reducing the carrier rate and the incidence of infections in semi-closed communities. Most of this evidence comes from military establishments in the United States. In recent years the presence of sulphonamide-resistant meningococci has markedly reduced the efficacy of sulphonamide prophylaxis. An effective alternative does not seem to have been found for providing prophylaxis in communities where sulphonamide-resistant meningococci are prevalent.

(vi) **Gonorrhoea**

A single tablet of 100,000 or 250,000 units of buffered penicillin G taken up to 4 hours after sexual contact will protect most individuals from gonorrhoea. There is no evidence that this treatment suppresses syphilis (Finland, 1960). Larger doses may be required in future as a proportion of gonococci have become relatively penicillin-resistant.

(v) **Syphilis**

Large doses of penicillin given for at least several days during a period of up to 3 months after sexual exposure reduced the incidence of syphilis from 25% among untreated controls to 4% in those receiving chemotherapy (Plotke et al, 1949).

Adequate penicillin therapy is indicated in the treatment of the pregnant syphilitic woman to prevent congenital syphilis in the newborn. This chemoprophylaxis is highly successful.

(vi) **During Peritoneal Dialysis**

The addition of antibiotics to the fluid used in peritoneal dialysis does not seem to reduce the incidence of peritonitis. Stewart and associates (1965) found that when a combination of penicillin and streptomycin or methicillin and polymyxin B was added to the fluid, there was a total of 14 infections out of 79 patients dialysed. There were six cases of peritonitis in 26 patients dialysed without the addition of antibiotics to the fluid. In three patients chloramphenicol was added to the fluid and there were no infections.

TABLE XXXII. Chemoprophylaxis

Prophylaxis likely to succeed	Prophylaxis of doubtful value; great variation	Chemoprophylaxis NOT indicated
1. Group A Streptococcal Infections Rheumatic fever Chronic glomerulonephritis (some cases) 2. Bacterial Endocarditis 3. Infected Wounds 4. Significant asymptomatic bacteriuria of pregnancy 5. Tuberculosis i. Mantoux positive children under 4 ii. Special risk group - eg nurses iii. TB pleural effusion 6. Meningococcal infection 7. Gonorrhoea 8. Syphilis	1. Chronic bronchitis 2. Cystic fibrosis 3. Surgery of the colon 4. Cardiac Surgery 5. Prevention of meningitis after pituitary implants 6. Prolonged labour with ruptured membranes 7. Neonates 8. Severe burns	1. 'Clean' Surgery 2. Cardiac catheterization 3. Instrumentation of the bladder 4. Major urological surgery 5. Neurosurgery 6. Virus Infections 7. Coma 8. Patients receiving corticosteroids 9. In peritoneal dialysis fluid

SUMMARY

In this chapter on the prophylactic use of antibiotic drugs I have tried to provide a guide to those seeking advice in a number of clinical situations. Where conclusions have seemed possible I have made them; frequently no firm conclusion can be made and I have attempted to provide a short discussion of the most relevant evidence, leaving the individual doctor to decide his own course of action. By way of summary the various conditions discussed in the chapter are divided into three groups, those in which prophylactic therapy has a high chance of success, conditions in which prophylactic antibiotics may sometimes be successful, but in which the drugs are usually contraindicated, and a third group in which antibiotics should not be used. The barriers between these groups must not be regarded as being rigid, and they reflect to a considerable extent personal bias.

REFERENCES

Appleton, D. M. and Waisbren, B. A. (1956) Prophylactic use of chloramphenicol in transurethral resection of the prostate gland. J. Urol. (Baltimore), **75**, 304

Armoury, R. A., Bowman, F. O. and Malm, J. R. (1966) Endocarditis associated with intracardiac prostheses. J. thorac. cardiovasc. Surg., **51**, 36

Bates, M. M. (1967) Acute rheumatism in approved schools in England and Wales 1960-65. Mon. Bull. Min. Hlth. & PHLS, **26**, 132

Bohnhoff, M. and Miller, C. P. (1962) Enhanced susceptibility to Salmonella infection in streptomycin treated mice. J. infect. Dis., **111**, 117

Catanzaro, F. J., Stetson, C. A., Morris, A. J., Chamovitz, R., Rammelkamp, C. H . Jr., Stolzer, B. L. and Perry, W. D. (1954) The role of the streptococcus in the pathogenesis of rheumatic fever. Amer. J. Med., **17**, 749

Cohn, I. and Atik, M. (1960) The influence of antibiotics on the spread of tumors of the colon. Ann. Surg., **151**, 917

College of General Practitioners: The Complications of Measles (London, 1956); quoted in an editorial: Treatment of Measles. Brit. med. J., **2**, 90

Davis, A., Binder, M. J., Burroughs, J. T., Miller, A .B. and Finegold, S. M. (1963) Diphtheroid Endocarditis after cardio pulmonary bypass surgery for the repair of cardiac valvular defects. In Antimicrob. Agents Chemother. American Soc. for Microbiology. Pages 643-656

Debre, R. (1956) Systemic treatment of primary tuberculosis. New Engl. J. Med., **255**, 794

Denton, C., Pappas, E. G., Uricchio, J. F., Goldberg, H. and Likoff, W. (1957) Bacterial Endocarditis following cardiac surgery. Circulation, **15**, 525

Elmes, P. C., Fletcher, C. M. and Dutton, A. A .C. (1957) Prophylactic use of oxytetracycline for exacerbations of chronic bronchitis. Brit. med. J., **2**, 1272

Ferebee, S. H., Mount, F. W. and Comstock, G. W . (1963) The use of chemotherapy as a prophylactic measure in tuberculosis. Ann. NY Acad. Sci., **106**, 151

Finland, M. (1960-July) Chemoprophylaxis of Infectious Diseases (part II). Disease-a-Month, Chicago. Page 5

Francis, R. S., May, J. R. and Spicer, C . C. (1964) Influence of daily penicillin, tetracycline, erythromycin, and sulphamethoxy pyridazine on exacerbations of chronic bronchitis. Brit. med. J., **1**, 728

Henderson, M., Entwistle, G. and Tayback, M. (1962) Bacteriuria and pregnancy outcome; preliminary findings. Amer. J. publ. Hlth., **52**, 1887

Hulbert, J. and Blair, D. W. (1967) One day kanamycin regime for preoperative bowel preparation. Post. Med. Jnl. Suppl., May 1967. Pages 27-32

Ingelfinger, F. J., Relman, A . S . and Finland, M. (1966) Controversy in internal medicine. W. B. Saunders, Philadelphia. Pages 605-614

Jonsson, G. and Erlanson, P. (1954) Effect of chemotherapy and evaluation of sensitivity tests in vitro in surgical urinary infections. Acta chir. scand., **107**, 1

Kaitz, A. L. and Hodder, E. W. (1960) Bacteriuria and pyelonephritis of pregnancy. A prospective study of 616 pregnant women. New Eng. J. Med., **265**, 667

Karelitz, S. and Isenberg, H. D. (1959) The antibiotic prophylaxis of bacterial complications of measles. J. Pediat., **54**, 1

Kass, E. H. (1955) Chemotherapeutic and Antibiotic Drugs in management of infections of urinary tract. Amer. J. Med., **18**, 764

Kass, E. H. (1960) Hormones and Host Resistance to Infections. Bact. Rev., **24**, 177

Kass, E. H. (1962) Prevention of apparently non-infectious disease by detection and treatment of infections in the urinary tract. J. chron. Dis., **15**, 665

Lambert, H. P. (1959) Chemoprophylaxis of tuberculosis. Amer. Rev. resp. Dis., **80**, 648

Lord, W. J. Jr., Imparato, A. M., Hackel, A. and Doyle, E. F. (1961) Endocarditis complicating open-heart surgery. Circulation, **23**, 489

Lowbury, E. J. L. (1958) Hospital Infection. Proc. roy. soc. Med., **51**, 807

Lowbury, E. J. L. (1966) in 'The Therapeutic Use of Antibiotics in Hospital Practice'. (Ed) Ridley and Phillips. E. & S. Livingstone Ltd., Edinburgh. Pages 203-220

May, J. R. (1966) Ampicillin in chronic bronchitis. Ampicillin Therapy Symposium, Brussels. Pages 67-72. Excerpta Medica Foundation. June, 1966

Murray, E. A. (1964) A trial of ampicillin in chronic bronchitis. J. Coll. gen. Practit., **7**, 244

Norman, A. P. (1967) Fucidic acid in cystic fibrosis (c). Lancet, **ii**, 516

Olding, L. (1966) Bacterial infection in cases of perinatal death. Acta paediat. scand. Suppl. 171

Pennybacker, J. (1966) Personal communication

Petersdorf, R. G., Browder, A. A. and Feinstein, A. R. (1961) Protection against infection in susceptible individuals. J. Pediat., **58**, 174

Petersdorf, R. G., Curtin, J. A., Hoeprich, P. D., Peeler, R. N. and Bennett, I. L. Jr. (1957) A study of antibiotic prophylaxis in unconscious patients. New Engl. J. Med., **257**, 1001

Piane, C., Castelluccio, A and Morbelli, E. (1966) Il trattamento antibiotico profilattico della riacutizzacioni della bronchite cronica. Rif. med., **80**, 201

Plotke, F., Eisenberg, H., Baker, A. H. and Laughlin, M. E. (1949) Penicillin in the abortive treatment of syphilis. J. Ven. Dis. Inform., **30**, 252

Pridie, R. B., Datta, N., Massey, D. G., Poole, G. W., Schneeweiss, J. and Stradling, P. (1960) A trial of continuous winter chemotherapy in chronic bronchitis. Lancet, **ii**, 723

Rammelkamp, C. H .Jr. (1965) Prophylaxis of bacterial disease with antimicrobiol. drugs. Amer. J. Med., **39**, 804

Report to Medical Research Council (1966) Value of chemoprophylaxis and chemotherapy in early chronic bronchitis. Brit. med. J., **1**, 1317

Report: Royal College of Physicians of London (1957) (Rheumatic Fever Committee)

Report: Prevention of initial attacks and recurrences of rheumatic fever (1965) Standing Medical Advisory Committee, Central Health Services Council, MOH. HMSO, London

Report: World Health Organization (1957) Wld. Hlth. Org. tech. Rep. Ser. No.126

Riley, H. D. Jr. and Knight, V. (1958) Urinary tract infections in paralytic poliomyelitis. Medicine, **37**, 281

Sanford, J. P., Bryant, R. E., Windom, R. E. and Vineyard, J. P. Jr. (1963) Asymptomatic bacteriuria in pregnancy and its association with prematurity. Clin. Res. (Proceedings), **2**, 212

Shubin, H. and Weil, M. H. (1963) Bacterial Shock. A serious complication of urological practice. J. Amer. med. Ass., **185**, 850

Stewart, J. K., Tuckwell, L. A., Sinnett, P. F., Edwards, K. D. G. and

Whyte, H. M. (1965) Peritoneal and haemodialysis: a comparison of their morbidity, and of the mortality suffered by dialysed patients. Quart. J. Med., **35**, 407

Tidwell, R. A. and Lewis, D. (1959) Erythromycin prophylaxis:a four year study. Antibiotic Med. clin. Ther., **6**, 395

Turck, M., Goffe, B. S. and Petersdorf, R. G. (1962) Bacteriuria of pregnancy, relation to socio-economic factors. New Engl. J. Med., **266**, 857

Turner, G. (1961) Bacilluria in pregnancy. Lancet, **ii**, 1062

Vink, M. (1953) Local recurrence of cancer in the large bowel: the role of implantation metastases and bowel disinfection. Brit. J. Surg., **41**, 431

Walker, R. M. (1966) In 'The Therapeutic Use of Antibiotics in Hospital Practice'. (Ed) Ridley and Phillips. E. & S. Livingstone, Edinburgh. Page 165

Weinstein, L. (1955) The complications of antibiotic therapy. Bull. NY Acad. Med., **31**, 500

Weinstein, L. (1955) Failure of chemotherapy to prevent the bacterial complications of measles. New Engl. J. Med., **253**, 679

Index